Implantable Cardioverter-Defibrillators
Step by Step
AN ILLUSTRATED GUIDE

Companion Website

With this book you are given free access to a companion resources site.

www.wiley.com/go/icdstepbystep

- The website includes over 150 images taken from this book
- You are free to download these images and use them in your own presentations to students*

How to access the website:

- Look under the label on the front inside cover of the book to see your unique access code.
- Enter this code when prompted when you access the site.

*Please note that these images are for your own use for study and instruction. If you are using these images in a presentation, the reference to the book should always be displayed along with the image. See website for full copyright information.

Implantable Cardioverter-Defibrillators Step by Step

AN ILLUSTRATED GUIDE

Roland X. Stroobandt
MD, PhD
Professor of Medicine
Heart Center, University Hospital Ghent, Belgium
Department of Cardiology, A.Z. Damiaan Hospital, Ostend, Belgium

S. Serge Barold
MD, FRACP, FACP, FACC, FESC, FHRS
Clinical Professor of Medicine,
University of South Florida Cardiology Division,
Tampa General Hospital, Tampa, Florida, USA

Alfons F. Sinnaeve
Ing, MSc
Professor Emeritus of Electronic Engineering
Technical University KHBO, Department of Electronics,
Ostend, Belgium

WILEY-BLACKWELL
A John Wiley & Sons, Ltd., Publication

Blackwell Publishing was acquired by John Wiley & Sons in February 2007. Blackwell's publishing program has been merged with Wiley's global Scientific, Technical and Medical business to form Wiley-Blackwell.

Registered office: John Wiley & Sons Ltd, The Atrium, Southern Gate, Chichester, West Sussex, PO19 8SQ, UK

Editorial offices: 9600 Garsington Road, Oxford, OX4 2DQ, UK
The Atrium, Southern Gate, Chichester, West Sussex, PO19 8SQ, UK
111 River Street, Hoboken, NJ 07030-5774, USA

For details of our global editorial offices, for customer services and for information about how to apply for permission to reuse the copyright material in this book please see our website at www.wiley.com/wiley-blackwell

Library of Congress Cataloging-in-Publication Data
Stroobandt, R. (Roland)
    Implantable cardioverter-defibrillators step by step : an illustrated guide / Roland X. Stroobandt, S. Serge Barold, Alfons F. Sinnaeve.
        p. ; cm.
    Sequel to: Cardiac pacemakers step by step / S. Serge Barold, Roland X. Stroobandt, Alfons F. Sinnaeve. c2004.
    ISBN 978-1-4051-8638-4
    1. Implantable cardioverter-defibrillators—Handbooks, manuals, etc.   I. Barold, S. Serge.   II. Sinnaeve, Alfons F.   III. Barold, S. Serge. Cardiac pacemakers step by step.   IV. Title.
    [DNLM: 1. Defibrillators, Implantable—Handbooks.   2. Tachycardia, Ventricular—therapy—Handbooks.
3. Death, Sudden, Cardiac—prevention & control—Handbooks.   4. Ventricular Fibrillation—therapy—Handbooks.
WG 39 S924i 2009]
    RC684.E4S74 2009
    617.4'120645—dc22

                                                                                                  2008033369

ISBN: 9781405186384
A catalogue record for this book is available from the British Library.

Set in 9.5/12pt palatino by Graphicraft Limited, Hong Kong
Printed in Singapore by Markono Print Media Pte Ltd
1   2009

Contents

Preface

Implantable Cardioverter-Defibrillators Step By Step is the logical sequel to our first book, *Cardiac Pacemakers Step by Step*, published in 2004. The pacemaker book should obviously be studied before starting this book because pacing constitutes an integral part of the function of an implantable cardioverter-defibrillator (ICD). The original pacemaker book was so well received that we decided to keep the same format. In addition, 65 carefully selected ICD recordings have been included.

As one picture is worth a thousand words, we have tried to avoid unnecessary text and focused on visual learning. Many of the figures are self-explanatory and the text in the appendix provides a summary of the field. The relevant figures are cited in the appended text. This arrangement promotes learning as an enjoyable and fun experience.

We have discussed the electrophysiologic aspects of ICD implantation but omitted a description of the standard surgical implantation procedures, which are well described elsewhere. Furthermore, the major ICD trials are mentioned only briefly to avoid reduplication of the abundant literature on the subject. Barring these two issues, which might have rendered the work unwieldy, the book provides a comprehensive review of the basic and clinical aspects of ICD therapy. A section on cardiac resynchronization was added because most patients with such devices also receive an ICD. The rapid evolution of technology made our task a moving target, with the continual need to upgrade some of the material. Despite our efforts, it is possible that some dated material might have escaped our attention, and we apologize for this.

We have discussed only the devices from the three US manufacturers as models, merely for the sake of convenience. We are well aware that manufacturers outside of the United States produce excellent devices. Although a full description of non-US ICDs is beyond the scope of the book, such ICDs share many characteristics with US devices so that the book will be universally applicable to the clinical evaluation of all devices regardless of their origin. We are particularly indebted to representatives of Medtronic Inc., St. Jude Medical and Boston Scientific for helping and guiding us with this project. However, we remain responsible for any mistakes related to ICD technology.

Roland X. Stroobandt
S. Serge Barold
Alfons F. Sinnaeve

Carsten Israel MD (Frankfurt, Germany), Michael O. Sweeney MD (Boston, MA), Bengt Herweg MD (Tampa, FL), and representatives from Medtronic Inc., Boston Scientific and St. Jude Medical kindly provided a number of tracings.

Figure 13.381 was reproduced with permission from Mehdirad A, Fredman C, Bierman K, Barold SS. AV interval-dependent crosstalk. Pacing Clin Electrophysiol 2008;31:232–4.

Figure 13.36 was reproduced with permission from Stroobandt R, Hagers Y, Provenier F, Van Belle Y, Hamerlijnck R, Barold SS. Silent lead malfunction detected only during defibrillator replacement. Pacing Clin Electrophysiol 2006;29:67–9.

Figure 13.44 was reproduced with permission from Sung RJ, Lauer MR (eds) Implantable cardioverter-defibrillator therapy. In: Fundamental Approaches to the Management of Cardiac Arrhythmias. Dordrecht, The Netherlands: Kluwer Academic Publishers, 2000:287–416.

Parts of the following guideline were reproduced by permission of the American Heart Association.

Zipes DP, Camm AJ, Borggrefe M, Buxton AE, Chaitman B, Fromer M, Gregoratos G, Klein G, Moss AJ, Myerburg RJ, Priori SG, Quinones MA, Roden DM, Silka MJ, Tracy C, Smith SC Jr, Jacobs AK, Adams CD, Antman EM, Anderson JL, Hunt SA, Halperin JL, Nishimura R, Ornato JP, Page RL, Riegel B, Priori SG, Blanc JJ, Budaj A, Camm AJ, Dean V, Deckers JW, Despres C, Dickstein K, Lekakis J, McGregor K, Metra M, Morais J, Osterspey A, Tamargo JL, Zamorano JL. ACC/AHA/ESC 2006 Guidelines for Management of Patients With Ventricular Arrhythmias and the Prevention of Sudden Death—Executive Summary: A Report of the American College of Cardiology/American Heart Association Task Force and the European Society of Cardiology Committee for Practice Guidelines (Writing Committee to Develop Guidelines for Management of Patients With Ventricular Arrhythmias and the Prevention of Sudden Cardiac Death). Developed in collaboration With the European Heart Rhythm Association and the Heart Rhythm Society. J Am Coll Cardiol. 2006;48:e247-346.

Epstein AE, DiMarco JP, Ellenbogen KA, Estes NA 3rd, Freedman RA, Gettes LS, Gillinov AM, Gregoratos G, Hammill SC, Hayes DL, Hlatky MA, Newby LK, Page RL, Schoenfeld MH, Silka MJ, Stevenson LW, Sweeney MO, Smith SC Jr, Jacobs AK, Adams CD, Anderson JL, Buller CE, Creager MA, Ettinger SM, Faxon DP, Halperin JL, Hiratzka LF, Hunt SA, Krumholz HM, Kushner FG, Lytle BW, Nishimura RA, Ornato JP, Page RL, Riegel B, Tarkington LG, Yancy CW; American College of Cardiology/American Heart Association Task Force on Practice Guidelines (Writing Committee to Revise the ACC/AHA/NASPE 2002 Guideline Update for Implantation of Cardiac Pacemakers and Antiarrhythmia Devices); American Association for Thoracic Surgery; Society of Thoracic Surgeons. ACC/AHA/HRS 2008 Guidelines for Device-Based Therapy of Cardiac Rhythm Abnormalities: a report of the American College of Cardiology/American Heart Association Task Force on Practice Guidelines (Writing Committee to Revise the ACC/AHA/NASPE 2002 Guideline Update for Implantation of Cardiac Pacemakers and Antiarrhythmia Devices) developed in collaboration with the American Association for Thoracic Surgery and Society of Thoracic Surgeons. J Am Coll Cardiol. 2008;51:e1-62.

The authors would also like to thank the nurses and technicians: Veerle De Meyer, Myriam Peleman, Rudy Colpaert, Guy De Cocker of the University Hospital, Ghent, Belgium, and Filiep Vandenbulcke of the A.Z. Damiaan Hospital, Ostend, Belgium, for their dedicated care of ICD patients and ability to recognize the teaching value of a number of recordings included in this book.

Introduction

Sudden cardiac death remains a major public health problem and accounts for 450 000 deaths annually in the United States and 400 000 in Europe. Michel Mirowski began developing an implantable defibrillator in the mid-1960s. The first automatic defibrillator was finally implanted in a human patient in 1980. The device presently known as an implantable cardioverter-defibrillator (ICD) has proven effective in preventing sudden cardiac death. Since 1980, technologic advances in device therapy including miniaturization, improved leads, optimal waveforms and transvenous implantation have revolutionized the treatment of malignant ventricular tachyarrhythmias and sudden cardiac death. These advances have made ICDs easier and safer to implant and better accepted by patients and physicians. Thus, ICDs have evolved from a treatment of last resort to the gold standard for patients at high risk for life-threatening ventricular arrhythmias. Recent advances include dual-chamber ICDs, additional therapy for atrial arrhythmias, and ICDs combined with biventricular pacing for selected heart failure patients. Device-based monitoring of contemporary ICDs can also record data unrelated to arrhythmias such as activity and the status of lung fluid in patients with congestive heart failure. Finally, ICDs provide health benefits with efficiency comparable to other well-accepted forms of health care such as renal dialysis.

The ICD does not prevent arrhythmias from occurring, and it is sometimes likened to having a miniature ambulance crew inside the chest. Shock delivery is the final step in a cascade of events beginning with arrhythmia detection. The device can detect ventricular tachyarrhythmias, determine whether they should be converted to a normal rhythm with a shock or rapid ventricular pacing, and then administer therapy. After successful treatment, the device must recognize the nontachycardic rhythm and reset the therapy sequences for the next event. Afterwards, the device keeps a complete record of what it has done. An ICD also gives bradycardia and post-shock bradycardia support like a conventional pacemaker.

Cardioversion and defibrillation are both forms of high-energy therapy or shocks. If the patient is conscious at the time of a shock, it is painful and usually described as feeling like a kick in the chest. Patients should be advised of this in advance. Their families should be advised that someone touching them is not harmed if the ICD discharges.

ICDs are multiprogrammable devices capable of delivering therapy for ventricular tachyarrhythmias in the form of high-energy defibrillation shocks, low-energy (cardioversion) shocks or antitachycardia pacing, and conventional pacing therapy for bradyarrhythmias (Fig. 0.01). Today's devices have a longevity of about 5–7 years, depending on shock and pacing frequency.

WHAT IS AN ICD ?

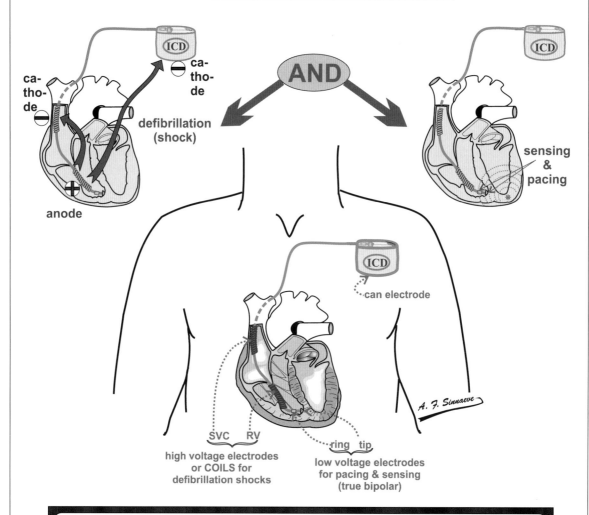

cathode

cathode

defibrillation
(shock)

anode

AND

sensing
&
pacing

can electrode

SVC   RV

high voltage electrodes
or COILS for
defibrillation shocks

ring tip

low voltage electrodes
for pacing & sensing
(true bipolar)

A. F. Sinnaeve

An ICD or implantable cardioverter-defibrillator is an electronic device implanted
in the body to protect against dangerous high ventricular rates. It is designed
to defibrillate the heart by delivering high voltage shocks or to stop malignant
tachycardias by antitachycardia pacing (short burst of rapid pacing sequence).
Contemporary ICDs also contain a classic pacemaker for bradycardia pacing.

Let's get this straight and avoid all confusion !

Pacing and shocking are done by electric impulses, therefore the electric current is
often depicted on the heart and the thorax. By international convention the electric
current flows from the positive connection (anode) to the negative connection
(cathode). This convention is used throughout the book !
Note that electrons (as in the metal wires) are flowing in the opposite direction. In
the body tissue, however, the electric current is due to the movement of ions.

ABBREVIATIONS : ICD = implantable cardioverter-defibrillator; SVC = superior vena cava ; RV = right ventricle ;
VT = ventricular tachycardia .

Figure 0.01

① CARDIAC TACHYARRHYTMIAS

* Cardiac Tachyarrhythmias - a summary
* Genesis of reentrant tachycardias
* Mechanisms of supraventricular tachycardias (SVT) - part 1
* Mechanisms of supraventricular tachycardias (SVT) - part 2
* Mechanisms of supraventricular tachycardias (SVT) - part 3
* Mechanisms of supraventricular tachycardias (SVT) - part 4
* Mechanisms of supraventricular tachycardias (SVT) - part 5
* Mechanisms of supraventricular tachycardias (SVT) - part 6
* Analysis of dual chamber EGMs - 1
    Tachycardia with 1:1 AV relationship
* Analysis of dual chamber EGMs - 2
    Tachycardia with 1:1 AV relationship
* Wide QRS tachycardias - part 1 Causes
* Wide QRS tachycardias - part 2 Stepwise approach
* Wide QRS tachycardias - part 3 Stepwise approach cont'd
* Bundle branch reentry tachycardia (BBR)
* Diagnosis of supraventricular tachycardia from stored EGMs
* Ventricular ATP with atrial entrainment and AV response after
    ventricular ATP
* Ventricular ATP with atrial entrainment and AAV response after
    ventricular ATP
* Ventricular ATP without atrial entrainment
* Ventricular ATP terminates the tachycardia without depolarization
    of the atria

Figure 1.00

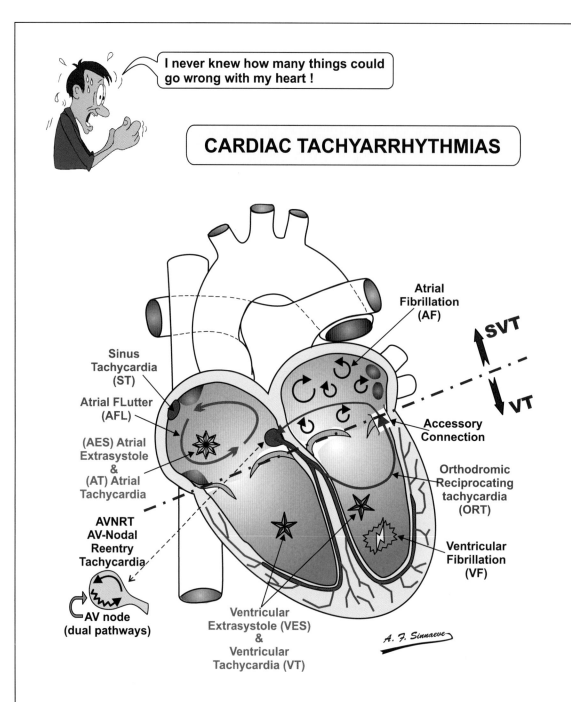

CARDIAC TACHYARRHYTHMIAS

Abbreviations : SVT = supraventricular tachycardia; VT = ventricular tachycardia;

Figure 1.01

GENESIS OF REENTRANT TACHYCARDIAS

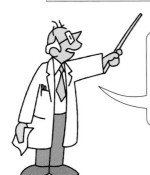

Reentry is considered the primary mechanism of ventricular tachycardias (VTs). Reentrant pathways may consist of bundle branches, Purkinje fibers with or without the surrounding muscle cells, as well as infarcted or fibrotic muscle cells. Most sustained monomorphic VTs are due to reentry involving a scar from an old myocardial infarction.

PREREQUISITES FOR A REENTRANT TACHYCARDIA TO OCCUR IN AN ANATOMIC CIRCUIT

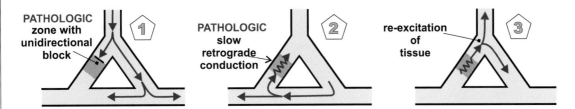

PATHOLOGIC zone with unidirectional block ①

PATHOLOGIC slow retrograde conduction ②

re-excitation of tissue ③

The tachycardia is sustained if the tissue proximal to the site of the (unidirectional) block is no longer refractory when it is excited by retrograde activation.

It follows that the total time to go around the circuit has to be shorter than the refractory period :

Refractory period $RP \leqq t_1 + t_2$

or :

$$RP \leqq \frac{L_1}{v_1} + \frac{L_2}{v_2}$$

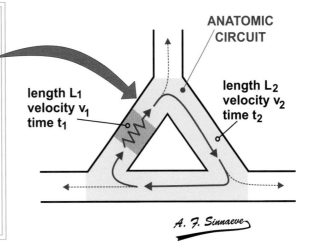

ANATOMIC CIRCUIT

length L_1 velocity v_1 time t_1

length L_2 velocity v_2 time t_2

A. F. Sinnaeve

A REENTRANT TACHYCARDIA CAN BE TERMINATED BY :
1. prolongation of the refractory period in the anatomical circuit (e.g. by drugs)
2. increase of the conduction velocity v_1 in the anatomical circuit
3. decrease of the length of the anatomical circuit ($L_1 + L_2$)
4. electrically-induced ventricular depolarization during the excitable gap which is the region in the circuit not yet activated by the circulating wavefront.

Figure 1.02

MECHANISMS of SUPRAVENTRICULAR TACHYCARDIAS (SVT) - part 1

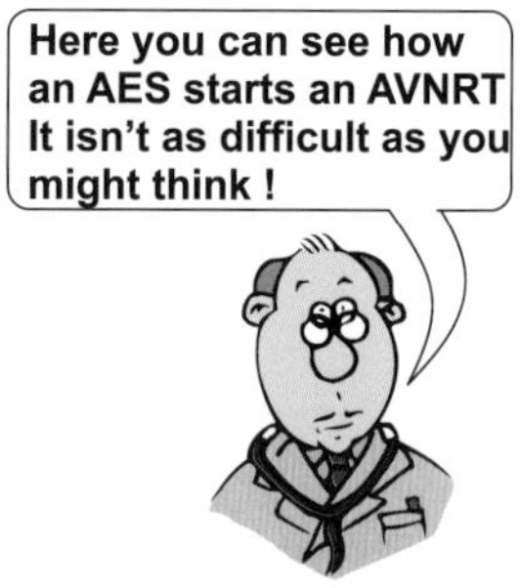

Here you can see how an AES starts an AVNRT
It isn't as difficult as you might think !

1 AV NODAL REENTRANT TACHYCARDIA (AVNRT)
common type : "Slow-Fast"

30% of the normal population has two pathways in their AV node (dual AVN physiology) but only a small fraction will develop AVNRT.
The fast pathway has a rather long refractory period and the slow pathway has a short refractory period.

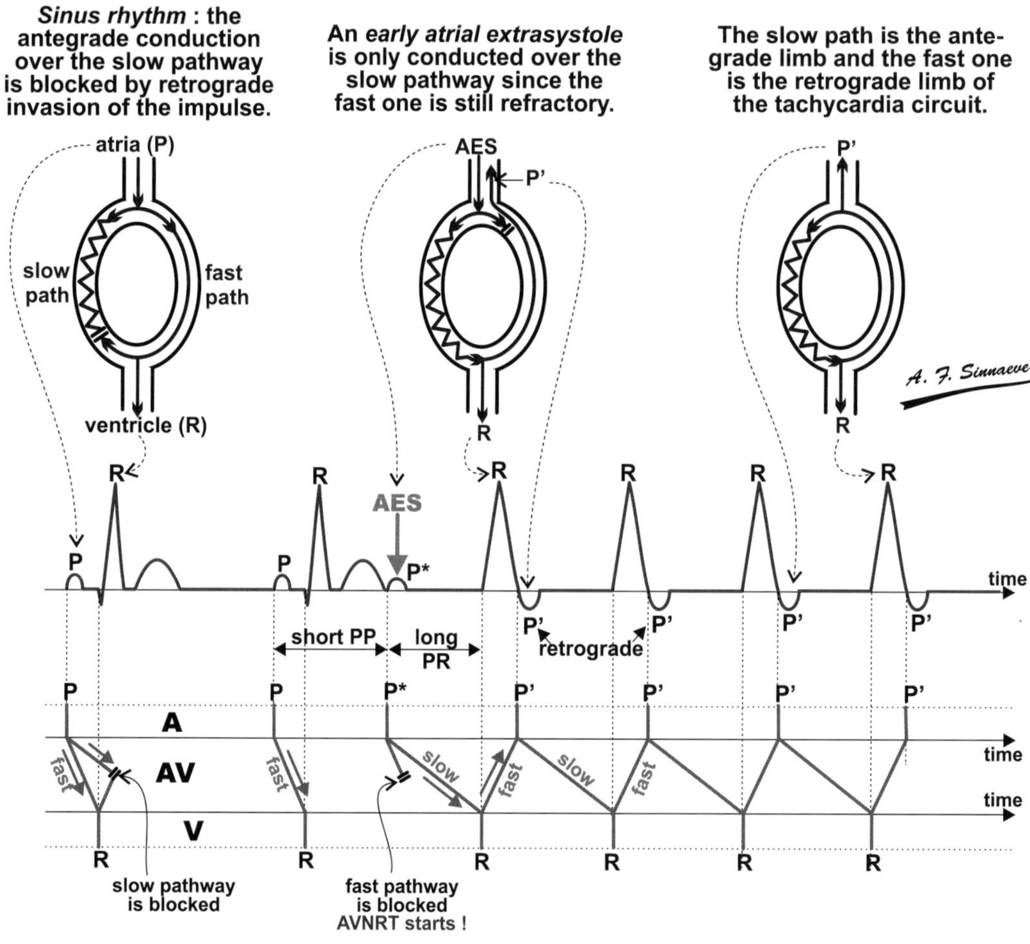

Sinus rhythm : the antegrade conduction over the slow pathway is blocked by retrograde invasion of the impulse.
An *early atrial extrasystole* is only conducted over the slow pathway since the fast one is still refractory.
The slow path is the antegrade limb and the fast one is the retrograde limb of the tachycardia circuit.
atria (P)
slow path
fast path
ventricle (R)
AES
P'
R
A. F. Sinnaeve
P
P*
time
short PP
long PR
retrograde
A
AV
V
fast
slow
slow pathway is blocked
fast pathway is blocked AVNRT starts !

Abbreviations : AES = atrial extrasystole ; AVNRT = AV nodal reentrant tachycardia .

Figure 1.03

MECHANISMS of SUPRAVENTRICULAR TACHYCARDIAS (SVT) - part 2

The mechanism of an ORT closely resembles that of an AVNRT. The difference is in the loop which is much larger for ORT !

2 ORTHODROMIC RECIPROCATING TACHYCARDIA (ORT)

* The accessory pathway conducts only in the retrograde direction during ORT.
* An ORT often starts with a ventricular premature complex (VPC).
* Since conduction over the AV node (AVN) is slower than the conduction over the accessory pathway (AccP), it follows that RP' < P'R (R = QRS complex and P' = retrograde P wave).
* The QRS complex is the same as during sinus rhythm unless there is rate related bundle branch aberrancy.

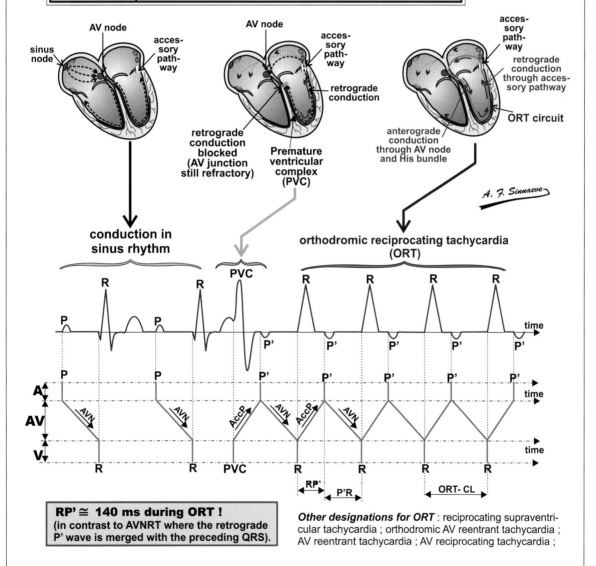

RP' ≅ 140 ms during ORT !
(in contrast to AVNRT where the retrograde P' wave is merged with the preceding QRS).

Other designations for ORT : reciprocating supraventricular tachycardia ; orthodromic AV reentrant tachycardia ; AV reentrant tachycardia ; AV reciprocating tachycardia ;

Abbreviations : AccP = accessory pathway ; AV = atrioventricular ; AVN = AV node ; AVNRT = AV nodal reentrant tachycardia ; PVC = premature ventricular complex ; ORT = orthodromic reciprocating tachycardia ; ORT-CL = ORT cycle length .

Figure 1.04

MECHANISMS of SUPRAVENTRICULAR TACHYCARDIAS (SVT) - part 3

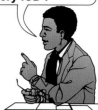

This is a tough task for the discriminators in every ICD !

3 **ATRIAL TACHYCARDIA (AT)**

* The morhpology of P waves during AT is different from those during sinus rhythm.
* P waves during AT are difficult to identify because they are often superimposed on T waves (e.g. when the AT gradually accelerates).
* The atrial rate is generally between 150 and 200 bpm (minimum 100 , maximum 250).
* On the ECG, there are isoelectric segments between the P waves.
* Since conduction to the ventricles occurs through the AV node, the QRS complex is the same as during sinus rhythm.

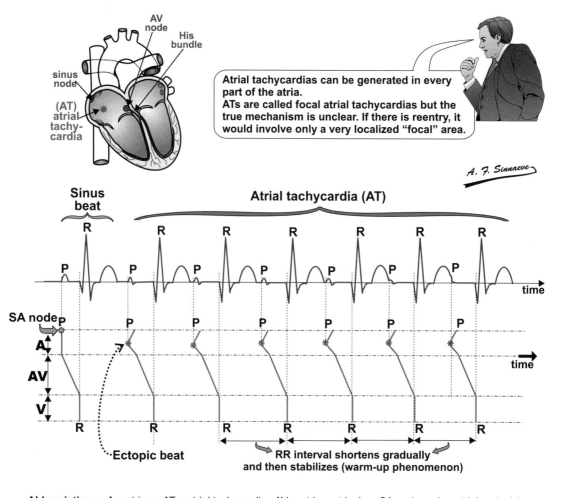

Atrial tachycardias can be generated in every part of the atria.
ATs are called focal atrial tachycardias but the true mechanism is unclear. If there is reentry, it would involve only a very localized "focal" area.

A. F. Sinnaeve

Abbreviations : A = atrium ; AT = atrial tachycardia ; AV = atrioventricular ; SA node = sino-atrial node (sinus node) ; V = ventricle ;

Figure 1.05

MECHANISMS of SUPRAVENTRICULAR TACHYCARDIAS (SVT) - part 4

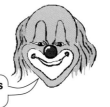

Did you know that my atrial flutter is caused by a circus movement ?!

4 **ATRIAL FLUTTER (AFL)**

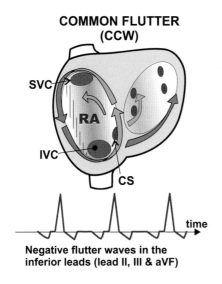

COMMON FLUTTER (CCW)

SVC
RA
IVC
CS

time

Negative flutter waves in the inferior leads (lead II, III & aVF)

COMMON "REVERSED" FLUTTER (CW)

SVC
RA
IVC
CS

time

Positive flutter waves in the inferior leads (lead II, III & aVF)

e.g. Atrial flutter with varying AV block 2:1, 4:1, etc.
(The atrial rate is 300 bpm and the ventricular rate varies from 150 bpm to 75 bpm)

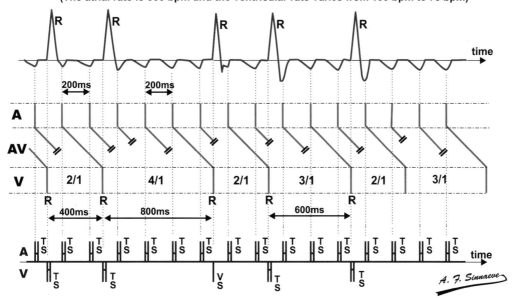

R   R   R   R   R

time

200ms   200ms

A

AV

V   2/1   4/1   2/1   3/1   2/1   3/1

R   R   R   R   R

400ms   800ms   600ms

A T T T T T T T T T T T T T T
    S S S S S S S S S S S S S S   time

V T T V T T
    S S S S S

A. F. Sinnaeve

Abbreviations : AFL = atrial flutter ; CCW = counterclockwise ; CW = clockwise ; CS = coronary sinus ; IVC = inferior vena cava ; SVC = superior vena cava ; TS = tachycardia sense ; VS = ventricular sense .

Figure 1.06

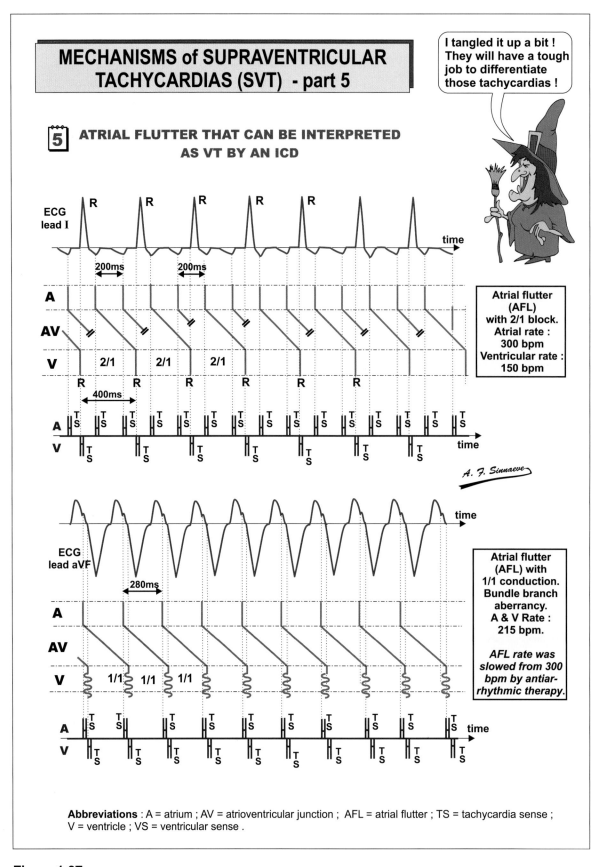

MECHANISMS of SUPRAVENTRICULAR TACHYCARDIAS (SVT) - part 5

5 ATRIAL FLUTTER THAT CAN BE INTERPRETED AS VT BY AN ICD

I tangled it up a bit ! They will have a tough job to differentiate those tachycardias !

ECG lead I — R R R R R

200ms   200ms

A

AV

V   2/1   2/1   2/1

R R R R R R
400ms

A TS TS TS TS TS TS TS TS TS TS TS TS TS TS

V TS TS TS TS TS TS TS

Atrial flutter (AFL) with 2/1 block. Atrial rate : 300 bpm Ventricular rate : 150 bpm

A. F. Sinnaeve

ECG lead aVF

280ms

A

AV

V   1/1   1/1   1/1

A TS TS TS TS TS TS TS TS TS TS TS TS

V TS TS TS TS TS TS TS TS TS TS TS

Atrial flutter (AFL) with 1/1 conduction. Bundle branch aberrancy. A & V Rate : 215 bpm.

AFL rate was slowed from 300 bpm by antiarrhythmic therapy.

Abbreviations : A = atrium ; AV = atrioventricular junction ; AFL = atrial flutter ; TS = tachycardia sense ; V = ventricle ; VS = ventricular sense .

Figure 1.07

MECHANISMS of SUPRAVENTRICULAR TACHYCARDIAS (SVT) - part 6

The electrophysiologic basis of atrial fibrillation remains unclear. Two major hypotheses prevail : (1) multiple wavelets of depolarization propagating within the atria, dividing, coalescing and extinguishing each other as they travel in an apparently random fashion seeking tissue that is excitable and (2) a single or a small number of high-frequency sources ("motors" or "drivers") of stable micro-reentry ("mother wave") primarily located at the left atrium/pulmonary vein junction with passive fibrillatory conduction giving rise to "daughter waves".
Both mechanisms may co-exist !

6 ATRIAL FIBRILLATION (AF)

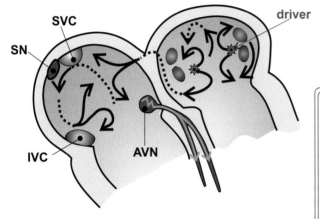
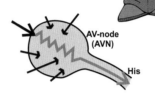

During AF the fibrillatory waves (f waves) have a rate of 350-500 per minute. Only some of the numerous atrial beats are transmitted at irregular intervals through the filter of the AV node to the ventricles. The single reliable diagnostic ECG feature therefore is the irregular ventricular response. Only in combination with complete AV block the ventricular rate is regular.

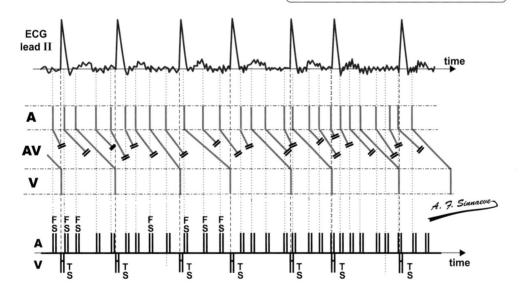

Abbreviations : A = atrium ; AV = atrioventricular junction ; AF = atrial fibrillation ; AVN = AV - node ; FS = fibrillation sense ; IVC = inferior vena cava ; SN = sinus node ; SVC = superior vena cava ; TS = tachycardia sense ; V = ventricle ;

Figure 1.08

ANALYSIS OF DUAL CHAMBER EGMs - 1
TACHYCARDIA with 1 : 1 AV RELATIONSHIP

If the atrial rate equals the ventricular rate (i.e. a 1:1 tachycardia), it is very hard for an ICD to differentiate between SVT and VT. Even a physician has to look very carefully !

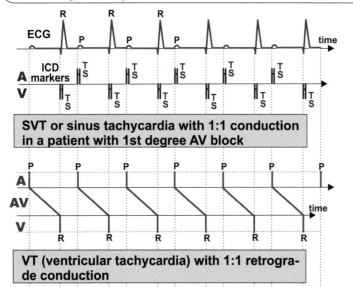

SVT or sinus tachycardia with 1:1 conduction in a patient with 1st degree AV block

The vast majority of tachycardias with 1:1 AV association are SVT mainly sinus tachycardia.
Normally an ST accelerates gradually with fairly stable PR interval.

VT (ventricular tachycardia) with 1:1 retrograde conduction

VT with 1:1 VA conduction constitutes 2-3% of VTs detected by ICDs.
Note : VT may exhibit a few beats of AV dissociation before stable 1:1 VA conduction becomes established.

NOTE : The chamber of onset may give an indication of the kind of tachycardia

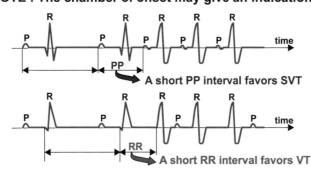

A short PP interval favors SVT

A short RR interval favors VT

Continuous registration and interpretation of the PP and the RR intervals may be used as an additional discriminator in ICDs !

A. F. Sinnaeve

VEGM morphology identical to that in sinus rhythm strongly suggests SVT. A VEGM morphology different from that of sinus rhythm indicates VT in about 90% of cases.

In tachycardias with 1:1 association :
* Transient AV block indicates SVT
* VA block during ATP is diagnostic of VT.

Abbreviations : *ATP = antitachycardia pacing; AV = atrioventricular; ST = sinus tachycardia; SVT = supraventricular tachycardia; TS (marker) = tachycardia sense; VA = ventriculoatrial; VEGM = ventricular electrogram; VT = ventricular tachycardia;*

Figure 1.09

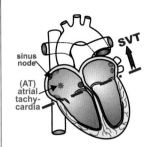

11

ANALYSIS OF DUAL CHAMBER EGMs - 2
TACHYCARDIA with 1 : 1 AV RELATIONSHIP

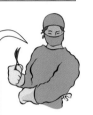

Important diagnostic information can be obtained about the mechanism of tachycardia by analyzing what happens with unsuccessful ventricular ATP.

If there is entrainment (i.e. the atrial rate accelerates during ventricular ATP and becomes equal to the stimulation rate), and the original tachycardia resumes with an AAV response at the end of the ATP sequence, the arrhythmia is AT.

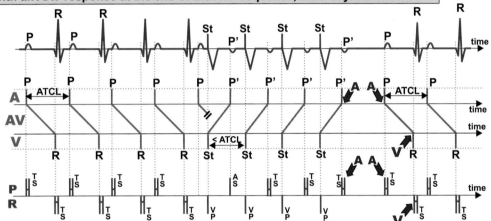

SVT is the most probable diagnosis if the atrial rate remains constant. Note : the ATP rate is faster than the AT rate !

A. F. Sinnaeve

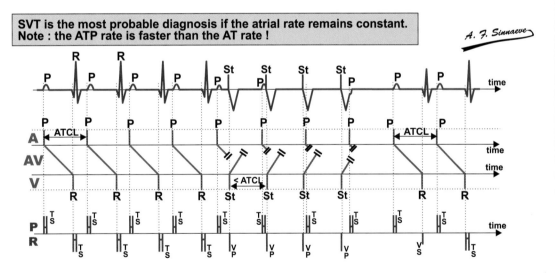

SUMMARY : Atrial response to ventricular ATP

VT vs SVT	No acceleration of atrial rate	Acceleration of atrial rate
No termination of tachycardia by ATP	Highly suggestive of AT *if* atrial rate remains constant	AT *if* AAV response
Termination of tachycardia by ATP	*Not* AT	*Not* decisive

Abbreviations : AT = atrial tachycardia; ATCL = atrial tachycardia cycle length; < ATCL = shorter than ATCL; ATP = antitachycardia pacing; P' = retrograde P wave; St = stimulus;
Markers : AS = atrial sense; TS = tachycardia sense; VP = ventricular pace

Figure 1.10

WIDE QRS TACHYCARDIAS

CAUSES

Wide or broad QRS complex is defined as being ≥ 120 ms !

1 **VT is the most common form of wide QRS complex tachycardia (90% of cases)**

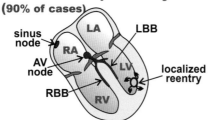

A regular wide QRS complex tachycardia should always be considered as being VT until proven otherwise.
VT is rare in structurally normal hearts.

2 **SVT (including ST, AT, AVNRT) with pre-existing or tachycardia-related BBB or functional aberrant conduction**

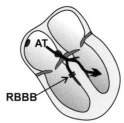

3 **Antidromic AVRT**

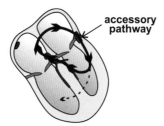

Pre-excitation (WPW); delta waves
Antidromic : anterograde over an accessory pathway and retrograde over the AV node

4 **Orthodromic AVRT with pre-existing or rate-related BBB or functional aberrant conduction)**

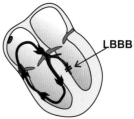

Orthodromic : anterograde over the AV node and retrograde over an accessory pathway

5 **SVT with conduction over an accessory pathway**

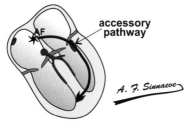

A. F. Sinnaeve

AF and conduction over an accessory pathway is always : *FBI* (fast, broad, irregular).
1:1 AV conduction of atrial flutter over the accessory pathway may result in very rapid ventricular rates

6 **Antidromic AVRT using Mahaim fiber**

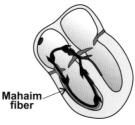

Mahaim fibers form an atriofasicular accessory pathway from the right atrium to the right bundle branch

Abbreviations : AF = atrial fibrillation ; AT = atrial tachycardia ; AVNRT = AV nodal reentry tachycardia ; AVRT = AV re-entrant tachycardia ; BBB = bundle branch block ; LBB = left bundle branch ; MI = myocardial infarction ; RBB = right bundle branch ; ST = sinus tachycardia ; SVT = supraventricular tachycardia ; VT = ventricular tachycardia ; WPW = Wolff-Parkinson-White .

Figure 1.11

WIDE QRS TACHYCARDIAS

STEPWISE APPROACH - part 1

We should know 3 things :
* What should be measured ?
* How should we measure correctly ?
* Which strategy do we have to follow ?

WHAT ?

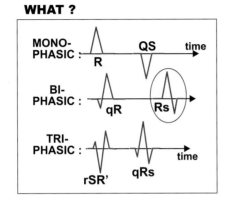

HOW ?

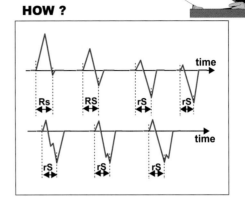

STRATEGY :

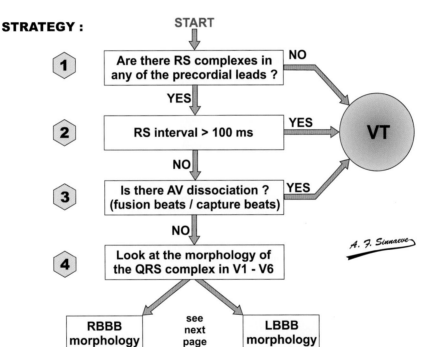

A. F. Sinnaeve

AV dissociation is present in approximately 50% of VTs but identified in the surface ECG in only half the patients with AV dissociation. Independent atrial and ventricular activity during wide QRS tachycardia is a hallmark of VT. In VT the ventricular rate is faster than the atrial rate in sinus rhythm. An ICD uses this information to make the diagnosis for VT.

Capture beats occur with complete ventricular activation over the AV conduction system.

Fusion beats are noted when activation of the ventricles occurs by both VT depolarization and activation over the AV conduction system.

Capture and fusion beats are uncommon and found mostly in relatively slower VTs

Abbreviations : AV = atrioventricular ; VT = ventricular tachycardia ; LBBB = left bundle branch block ; RBBB = right bundle branch block .

Figure 1.12

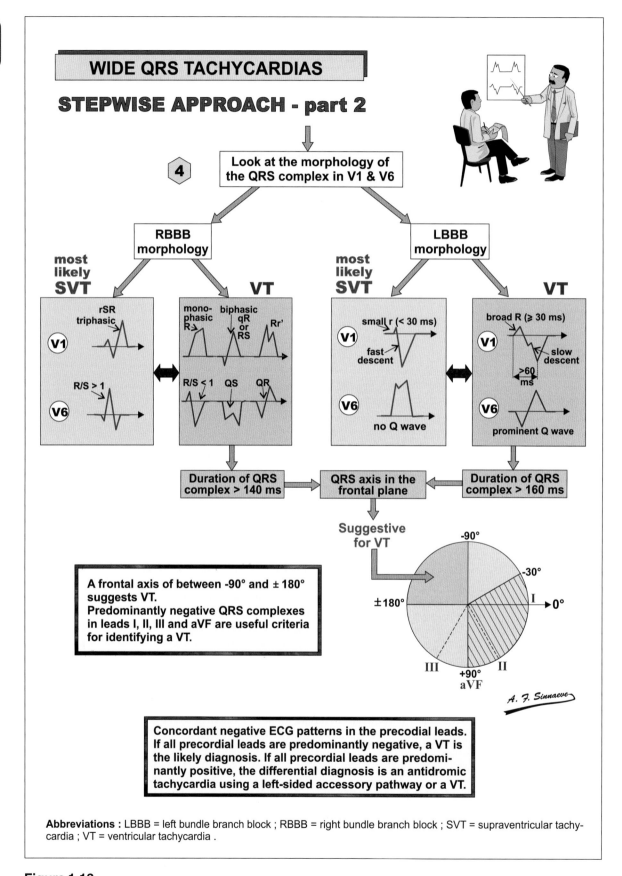

Figure 1.13

BUNDLE BRANCH REENTRY TACHYCARDIA (BBR)

① GENESIS

② CONTINUATION

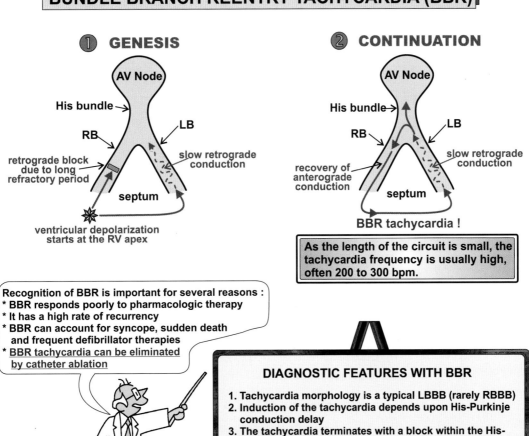

AV Node

His bundle →

RB

LB

retrograde block due to long refractory period

slow retrograde conduction

septum

ventricular depolarization starts at the RV apex

AV Node

His bundle →

RB

LB

recovery of anterograde conduction

slow retrograde conduction

septum

BBR tachycardia !

As the length of the circuit is small, the tachycardia frequency is usually high, often 200 to 300 bpm.

Recognition of BBR is important for several reasons :
* BBR responds poorly to pharmacologic therapy
* It has a high rate of recurrence
* BBR can account for syncope, sudden death and frequent defibrillator therapies
* BBR tachycardia can be eliminated by catheter ablation

DIAGNOSTIC FEATURES WITH BBR

1. Tachycardia morphology is a typical LBBB (rarely RBBB)
2. Induction of the tachycardia depends upon His-Purkinje conduction delay
3. The tachycardia terminates with a block within the His-Purkinje system
4. During BBR, a His potential precedes each QRS complex
5. Variations in the V-V intervals are preceded by similar changes in the H-H intervals

A. F. Sinnaeve

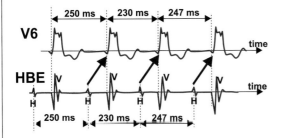

250 ms   230 ms   247 ms

V6

time

HBE

time

250 ms   230 ms   247 ms

Interfascicular tachycardia is also a possibility, usually proceeding in the anterograde direction over the LAF and retrograde through the LPF

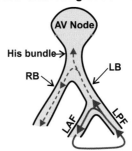

AV Node

His bundle →

RB

LB

LAF   LPF

Abbreviations : LAF = left anterior fasicle; LB = left bundle branch; LBBB = left bundle branch block; LPF = left posterior fasicle; RB = right bundle branch; RBBB = right bundle branch block; HBE = His bundle electrogram;

Figure 1.14

DIAGNOSIS OF SUPRAVENTRICULAR TACHYCARDIA FROM STORED ELECTROGRAMS

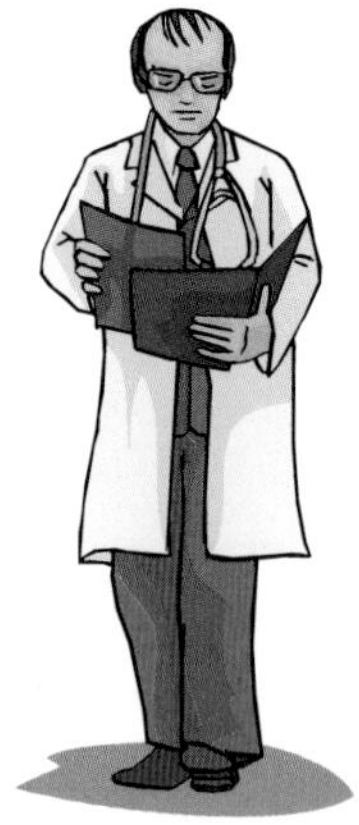

WHAT CAN BE REVEALED BY VENTRICULAR ATP (ANTITACHYCARDIA PACING) ?

 NO TERMINATION OF TACHYCARDIA BY ATP

1 **ACCELERATION** of the atrial rate to the ATP cycle length

    A After ATP, the tachycardia resumes with an **A-V RESPONSE** :

        A-V response is diagnostic for :
         * AV nodal reentrant tachycardia (AVNRT)
         * or Orthodromic reciprocating tachycardia (ORT)

        A-V response rules out atrial tachycardia (AT)

    B After ATP, the tachycardia resumes with an **A-A-V RESPONSE** :

        A-A-V response is diagnostic for :
         * Atrial tachycardia (AT)

        A-A-V response rules out AVNRT & ORT

2 **NO ACCELERATION** of the atrial rate to the ATP cycle length

    * Highly suggestive of AT if the atrial rate remains constant

    * Dissociation of A and V during ATP excludes ORT

 TERMINATION OF TACHYCARDIA BY ATP

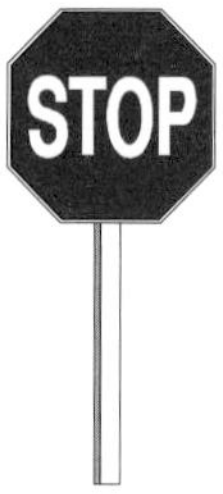

1 **ACCELERATION** of the atrial rate to the ATP cycle length

    * Not decisive if the atrial rate was entrained by RV pacing

2 **NO ACCELERATION** of the atrial rate to the ATP cycle length

    * Termination without atrial depolarization excludes AT

A. F. Sinnaeve

Figure 1.15

DIAGNOSIS OF SUPRAVENTRICULAR TACHYCARDIA FROM STORED ELECTROGRAMS - part 1

Ventricular ATP with atrial entrainment and AV reponse after ventricular ATP

1 **AV NODAL REENTRANT TACHYCARDIA (AVNRT)**

Antitachycardia pacing (ATP) at a slightly higher frequency than the tachycardia (i.e. overdrive pacing) may cause entrainment, i.e. the atrial cycle length (ACL) shortens to the ATP cycle length. All atrial electrograms are advanced.

If the AVNRT resumes after ATP, it will start at the last retrograde P' and an A-V sequence will be registrated by the stored atrial and ventricular electrograms.

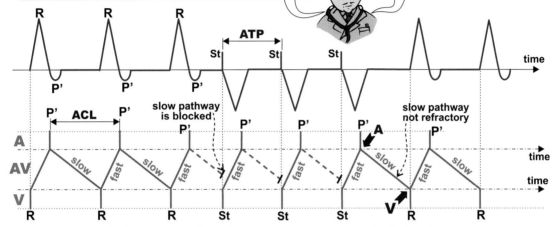

After the last ventricular paced beat in the ATP sequence, the antegrade limb of the tachycardia (slow pathway) is not refractory. The last retrograde atrial complex can therefore conduct to the ventricle producing a <u>DIAGNOSTIC AV RESPONSE</u>. This response RULES OUT AN ATRIAL TACHYCARDIA.

2 **ORTHODROMIC RECIPROCATING TACHYCARDIA (ORT)**

A. F. Sinnaeve

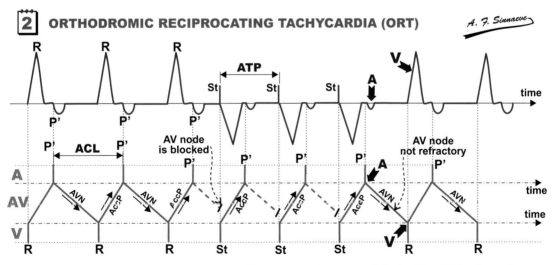

After the last ventricular paced beat in the ATP sequence, the antegrade limb of the ORT tachycardia (AV node) is not refractory. The last retrograde atrial complex can therefore conduct to the ventricle producing a <u>DIAGNOSTIC AV RESPONSE</u>. This response RULES OUT AN ATRIAL TACHYCARDIA.

Abbreviations : AccP = accessory pathway ; ACL = atrial cycle length ; ATP = antitachycardia pacing ; AVN = AV node = atrioventricular node ; St = stimulus .

Figure 1.16

DIAGNOSIS OF SUPRAVENTRICULAR TACHYCARDIA FROM STORED ELECTROGRAMS - part 2

Ventricular ATP with atrial entrainment and AAV reponse after ventricular ATP

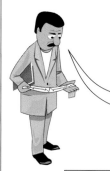
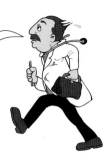

I have no time to lose. I have a diagnosis to make about the tachycardia of my ICD patient !

Take your time, John ! Haste makes waste ! Important diagnostic information can be obtained about the mechanism of a tachycardia by analyzing what happens after unsuccessful ventricular ATP.

If there is entrainment (i.e. the atrial rate accelerates during ventricular ATP and becomes equal to the stimulation rate), and the original tachycardia resumes with an *AAV RESPONSE* at the end of the ATP sequence, the *ARRHYTHMIA IS AT*. Retrograde VA conduction occurs through the AV node. Therefore the last retrograde atrial complex related to ventricular pacing (ATP) cannot conduct antegradely to the ventricle because the AV node is refractory for antegrade conduction, hence the AAV response.
AAV response *EXCLUDES AVNRT* and *ORT* as mechanism of the tachycardia.

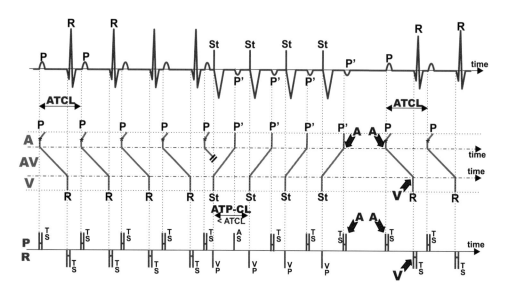

Abbreviations : AccP = accessory pathway ; ACL = atrial cycle length ; ATP = antitachycardia pacing ; AS = atrial sense ; AVN = AV node = atrioventricular node ; ATCL atrial tachycardia cycle length ; AVNRT = AV nodal reentrant tachycardia ; ORT = orthodromic reciprocating tachycardia ; St = stimulus ; TS = tachy sense ; VP = ventricular pace.

Figure 1.17

DIAGNOSIS OF SUPRAVENTRICULAR TACHYCARDIA FROM STORED ELECTROGRAMS - part 3

Ventricular ATP without atrial entrainment

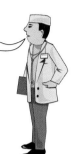

So, I have to pace in the ventricle at a pacing rate faster than the tachycardia rate and look if the atrial rate is changing. If I can note dissociation between ventricular and atrial rates, atrial tachycardia (AT) is very likely !?

Yes, make the cycle length of the ventricular pacing (ATP-CL) shorter than the cycle length of the tachycardia (ATCL).
AT IS THE MOST PROBABLE DIAGNOSIS if the atrial rate remains constant !
Note that dissociation between the tachycardia and the ventricular pacing, without termination of the tachycardia, **EXCLUDES** orthodromic reciprocating tachycardia (**ORT**).

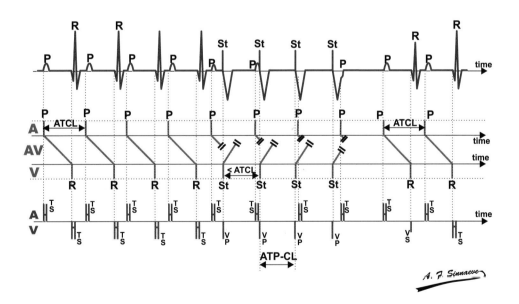

Abbreviations : ATCL = atrial cycle length ; AT = atrial tachycardia ; ATP = antitachycardia pacing ; ATP-CL = ATP cyle length ; AVN = AV node = atrioventricular node ; St = stimulus ; VP = ventricular pace ;

Figure 1.18

DIAGNOSIS OF SUPRAVENTRICULAR TACHYCARDIA
FROM STORED ELECTROGRAMS - part 4

Ventricular ATP terminates the tachycardia without depolarization of the atria

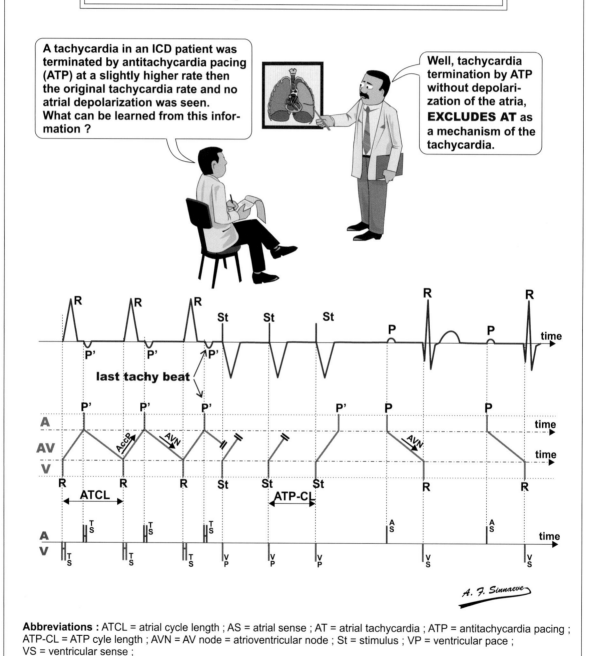

A tachycardia in an ICD patient was terminated by antitachycardia pacing (ATP) at a slightly higher rate then the original tachycardia rate and no atrial depolarization was seen. What can be learned from this information ?

Well, tachycardia termination by ATP without depolarization of the atria, **EXCLUDES AT** as a mechanism of the tachycardia.

Abbreviations : ATCL = atrial cycle length ; AS = atrial sense ; AT = atrial tachycardia ; ATP = antitachycardia pacing ; ATP-CL = ATP cyle length ; AVN = AV node = atrioventricular node ; St = stimulus ; VP = ventricular pace ; VS = ventricular sense ;

Figure 1.19

 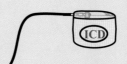

INDICATIONS

* Secondary vs primary prevention
* Classes and level of evidence
* Class I
* Class II
* Class III
* Action potential and action potential duration
* Action potential and ion channels
* The long QT syndrome (LQTS)
* LQTS as a source of arrhythmias
* LQTS : clinical symptoms & triggers of cardiac events
* The Brugada syndrome - characteristics
* The Brugada syndrome - classes
* The short QT syndrome (SQTS)
* Arrhythmogenic right ventricle dysplasia/cardiomyopathy (ARVD/C)
* Catecholaminergic polymorphic ventricular tachycardia (CPVT)
* Hypertrophic cardiomyopathy (HCM)
* Risk stratification in HCM

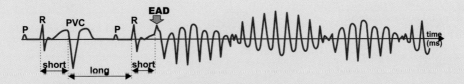

Figure 2.00

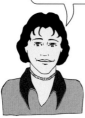

Can you tell me the difference between primary and secondary prevention ?

INDICATIONS FOR ICD THERAPY - 1

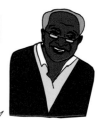

Well, that's easy !
* *SECONDARY PREVENTION* is the prevention after a prior life-threatening cardiac event. Since the probability for a second event is very high, secondary prevention is necessary !
* *PRIMARY PREVENTION* is to avoid any severe cardiac event from happening for the first time ! It is a preventive measure : prevention is better than cure.
Cardiomyopathy is a case in point :

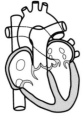

NORMAL

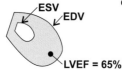

ESV
EDV
LVEF = 65%

NONISCHEMIC DILATED CARDIOMYOPATHY (DCM)

What is nonischemic CM ?
Nonischemic CM is a chronic heart muscle disease characterized by cavity enlargement and impaired systolic function of the left or both ventricles.
Most cases of nonischemic CM are idiopathic (i.e. no exact cause can be found)

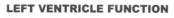

LEFT VENTRICLE FUNCTION

left ventricular ejection fraction
$$LVEF = \frac{EDV - ESV}{EDV} \times 100\%$$

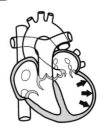

Nonischemic CM

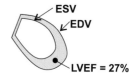

ESV
EDV
LVEF = 27%

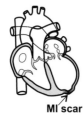

MI scar

ISCHEMIC CARDIOMYOPATHY

What is Ischemic CM ?
Ischemic cardiomyopathy (a lack of blood supply to the heart muscle) is the most common cause of dilated cardiomyopathy.
Ischemic CM is often associated with old MI.

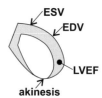

ESV
EDV
LVEF
akinesis

Factors associated with high risk

* Aborted sudden cardiac death (SCD)
* VT / VF
* unexplained syncope associated with poor LV function

Secondary prevention !

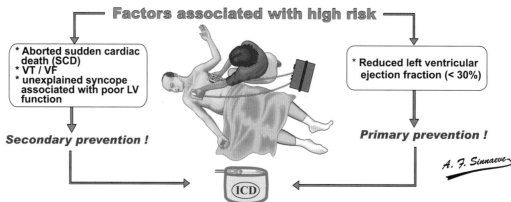

* Reduced left ventricular ejection fraction (< 30%)

Primary prevention !

A. F. Sinnaeve

ICD

Abbreviations : EDV : end diastolic volume ; ESV : end systolic volume ; LVEF : left ventricular ejection fraction ; MI : Myocardial infarction ; SCD : sudden cardiac death ; VF = ventricular fibrillation ; VT = ventricular tachycardia .

Figure 2.01

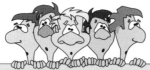

INDICATIONS FOR ICD THERAPY - 2

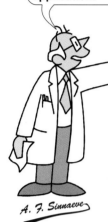

Learned societies in the USA (ACC, AHA, HRS or formerly NASPE) and in Europe (ESC,EHRA) have jointly published guidelines that are widely accepted and followed by physicians all over the world.
There are 3 classes ! The classification is based upon the level of evidence for each particular application.

Indications for ICD therapy

Class I : Clear evidence that procedure or treatment is effective
with 5 subdivisions

Class II : Conflicting evidence concerning usefulness or efficacy
Class IIa : Weight of evidence in favor of usefulness or efficacy
Class IIb : Usefulness or efficacy less well established
with 7 subdivisions

Class III : Evidence that procedure or treatment is not useful or effective and in some cases may be harmful
with 8 subdivisions

A. F. Sinnaeve

The weight of evidence is ranked :

Level A : highest level if data were derived from multiple *randomized* clinical trials that involved *large numbers* of patients.

Level B : intermediate if the data were derived from a limited number of rando-mized trials that involved comparatively *small numbers* of patients or from well-designed data analysis of *nonrandomized* studies or *observational* registries.

Level C : lower level when expert concensus is the primary basis for recommendation

TRIALS SUPPORTING PRIMARY PREVENTION

STUDY	Year	LVEF	Other inclusion criteria	Mortality reduction
MADIT	1996	≤ 35%	MI, asymptomatic nsVT, inducible VT at EPS not suppressed by a type I antiarrhythmic agent	54%
MUSTT	1999	≤ 40%	CAD, asymptomatic nsVT	51%
MADIT II	2002	≤ 30%	MI	31%
SCD HeFT	2005	≤ 35%	CHF	23%

MADIT = Multicenter Automatic Defibrillator Implantation Trial ; MUSTT = Multicenter Unsustained Tachycardia Trial ; SCD-HeFT = Sudden Cardiac Death in Heart Failure Trial ; CAD = coronary artery disease ; CHF = congestive heart failure ; LVEF = left ventricular ejection fraction ; MI = myocardial infarction ; nsVT = nonsustained ventricular tachycardia ; EPS = electrophysiologic study ; VT = ventricular tachycardia .
ACC = American College of Cardiology ; AHA = American Heart Association ; HRS = Heart Rhythm Society (NASPE = North American Society of Pacing and Electrophysiology) ; ESC = European society of Cardiology ; EHRA = European Heart Rhythm Association.

Figure 2.02

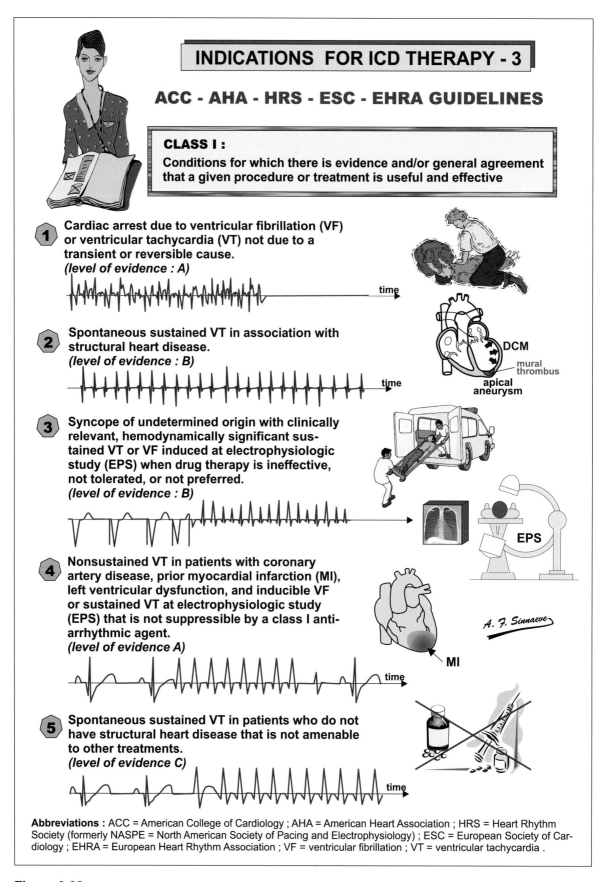

INDICATIONS FOR ICD THERAPY - 3

ACC - AHA - HRS - ESC - EHRA GUIDELINES

CLASS I :
Conditions for which there is evidence and/or general agreement that a given procedure or treatment is useful and effective

1 Cardiac arrest due to ventricular fibrillation (VF) or ventricular tachycardia (VT) not due to a transient or reversible cause.
(level of evidence : A)

time

2 Spontaneous sustained VT in association with structural heart disease.
(level of evidence : B)

time

DCM
mural thrombus
apical aneurysm

3 Syncope of undetermined origin with clinically relevant, hemodynamically significant sustained VT or VF induced at electrophysiologic study (EPS) when drug therapy is ineffective, not tolerated, or not preferred.
(level of evidence : B)

EPS

4 Nonsustained VT in patients with coronary artery disease, prior myocardial infarction (MI), left ventricular dysfunction, and inducible VF or sustained VT at electrophysiologic study (EPS) that is not suppressible by a class I anti-arrhythmic agent.
(level of evidence A)

time

A. F. Sinnaeve

MI

5 Spontaneous sustained VT in patients who do not have structural heart disease that is not amenable to other treatments.
(level of evidence C)

time

Abbreviations : ACC = American College of Cardiology ; AHA = American Heart Association ; HRS = Heart Rhythm Society (formerly NASPE = North American Society of Pacing and Electrophysiology) ; ESC = European Society of Cardiology ; EHRA = European Heart Rhythm Association ; VF = ventricular fibrillation ; VT = ventricular tachycardia .

Figure 2.03

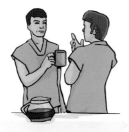

INDICATIONS FOR ICD THERAPY - 4

ACC - AHA - HRS - ESC - EHRA GUIDELINES

CLASS II :

Conditions for which there is conflicting evidence and/or a divergence of opinion about the usefulness/efficacy of a procedure or treatment

CLASS IIa :
Weight of evidence is in favor of usefulness/efficacy

1 Patients with LVEF of 30% or less, at least 1 month post-MI and 3 months post coronary artery revascularization surgery. *(level of evidence B)*

CLASS IIb :
Usefulness or efficacy is less well established

1 Cardiac arrest presumed to be due to VF when EPS is precluded by other medical conditions. *(level of evidence C)*

2 Severe symptoms (e.g. syncope) attributable to sustained ventricular arrhythmias in patients awaiting cardiac transplantation. *(level of evidence C)*

3 Familial or inherited conditions with a high risk for life-threatening ventricular tachyarrhythmias, such as LQTS or HCM. *(level of evidence B)*

4 Nonsustained VT with coronary artery disease, prior MI, LV dysfunction, and inducible sustained VT or VF at EPS. *(level of evidence B)*

5 Recurrent syncope of undetermined etiology in the presence of LV dysfunction and inducible ventricular arrhythmias at EPS when other causes of syncope have been excluded. *(level of evidence C)*

6 Syncope of unexplained etiology or family history of unexplained SCD in association with typical or atypical right bundle-branch block and ST-segment elevations (Brugada syndrome). *(level of evidence C)*

7 Syncope in patients with advanced structural heart disease in which thorough invasive and noninvasive investigation has failed to define a cause. *(level of evidence C)*

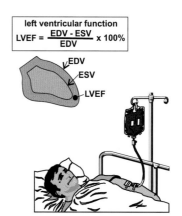

$$LVEF = \frac{EDV - ESV}{EDV} \times 100\%$$

left ventricular function

EDV
ESV
LVEF

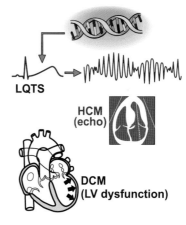

LQTS

HCM (echo)

DCM (LV dysfunction)

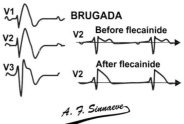

V1
V2
V3

BRUGADA
V2 Before flecainide
V2 After flecainide

A. F. Sinnaeve

Abbreviations : DCM = dilated cardiomyopathy ; EDV = end-diastolic volume ; EPS = electrophysiologic study ; ESV = end-systolic volume ; HCM = hypertrophic cardiomyopathy ; LQTS = long QT syndrome ; LV = left ventricle ; LVEF = left ventricular ejection fraction ; MI = myocardial infarction ; SCD = sudden cardiac death ; VF = ventricular fibrillation ; VT = ventricular tachycardia .

Figure 2.04

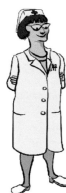

INDICATIONS FOR ICD THERAPY - 5

ACC - AHA - HRS - ESC - EHRA GUIDELINES

CLASS III :
Conditions for which there is evidence and/or a general agreement that the procedure or treatment is not useful/effective and in some cases may be harmful.

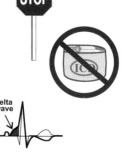

1. Syncope of undetermined cause in a patient without inducible ventricular tachyarrhythmias and without structural heart disease. *(level of evidence C)*

2. Incessant VT or VF. *(level of evidence C)*

3. VT or VF resulting from arrhythmias amenable to surgical or catheter ablation; e.g. atrial arrhythmias associated with the WPW syndrome, right ventricular outflow tract VT, idiopathic LV tachycardia, or fasicular VT. *(level of evidence C)*

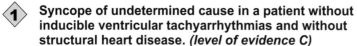

4. Ventricular tachyarrhythmias due to transient or reversible disorder (e.g. acute MI, electrolyte imbalance, drugs or trauma) when correction of the disorder is considered feasible and likely to substantially reduce the risk of recurrent arrhythmia. *(level of evidence B)*

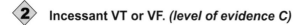

5. Significant psychiatric illnesses that may be aggravated by device implantation or may preclude systematic follow-up. *(level of evidence C)*

6. Terminal illnesses with projected life expectancy of 6 months or less. *(level of evidence C)*

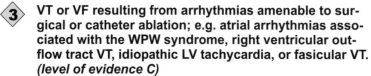

7. Patients with coronary artery disease, LV dysfunction and prolonged QRS duration in the absence of spontaneous or inducible sustained or nonsustained VT who are undergoing coronary bypass surgery. *(level of evidence B)*

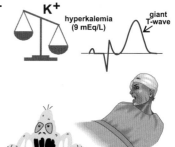

8. NYHA Class IV drug-refractory congestive heart failure in patients who are not candidates for cardiac transplantation. *(level of evidence C)*

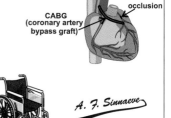

A. F. Sinnaeve

Abbreviations : LV = left ventricle ; MI = myocardial infarction ; NYHA = New York Heart Association ; VF = ventricular fibrillation ; VT = ventricular tachycardia ; WPW = Wolff-Parkinson-White syndrome (pre-excitation syndrome) ;

Note : NYHA Class 4 : patients who should be at complete rest, confined to bed or chair, any physical activity brings discomfort and symptoms occur at rest.

Figure 2.05

INDICATIONS FOR ICD THERAPY- 6

An important ICD indication is based upon the duration of the QT interval ! So, let us review some basic facts about the QT interval...

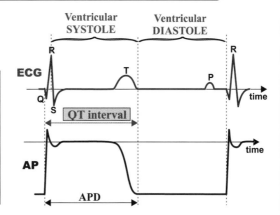

QT is the duration of the electrical signal from the start of QRS to the end of the T wave, nearly coinciding with the mechanical ventricular systole and basically corresponding to the duration of the myocardial action potential (AP).
The duration of the normal QT interval is 400 ms (± 40 ms) at a rate of 60 bpm. Since the QT interval depends upon the rate, the measured interval has to be corrected to determine whether it is normal or not.

RULE OF THUMB :
The normal QT interval is equal or shorter than half the preceding RR interval.

BAZETT's FORMULA

$$\text{Corrected : QTc (in ms)} = \frac{\text{measured QT interval (in ms)}}{\sqrt{\text{RR interval (in s)}}}$$

The configuration of the myocardial action potential with its five phases is governed by ionic currents through the membranes of the myocardial cells. The involved ions are mainly sodium (Na^+), potassium (K^+) and calcium (Ca^{++}).

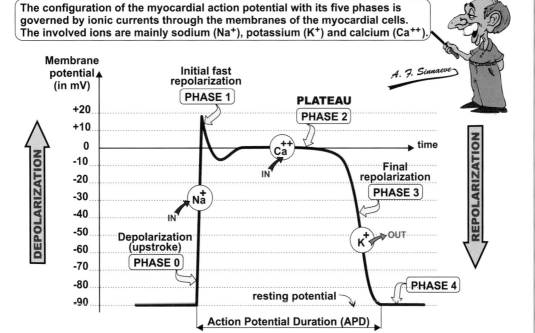

The ionic currents flow through a lot of "channels" in the cell membranes. They all have their typical characteristics and open and close at different membrane potentials. Some of the important ionic currents that influence APD are reviewed on the next page.

Abbreviations : AP = action potential; APD = Action potential duration; Ca = calcium; K = potassium; Na = sodium; s = seconds ; ms = milliseconds

Figure 2.06

INDICATIONS FOR AN ICD - 7

Repolarization is like emptying a barrel. It goes faster the more is going out and the less is flowing in !

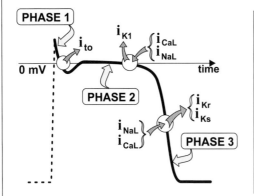

The repolarization process :

Phase 1 : initial fast repolarization by i_{to}, mainly carried by a transient outward potassium current

Phase 2 : the plateau phase is a "fine tuning" between i_{CaL}, a depolarizing inward calcium current (L : long-lasting), i_{NaL} a small sustaining inward sodium current and a repolarizing outward potassium current i_{K1}

Phase 3 : the final repolarization is mostly due to the combined action of the repolarizing outward potassium currents i_{Kr} and i_{Ks} (r : rapid ; s : slow) and the depolarizing inward currents i_{NaL} and i_{CaL} (L : long-lasting)

In search of an equilibrium for voltage-dependent currents

Normal repolarization is the result of a fine balance between repolarizing currents (making the cell more negative) and depolarizing currents (making the cell more positive). An imbalance will result in an abnormal AP that may cause arrhythmias.

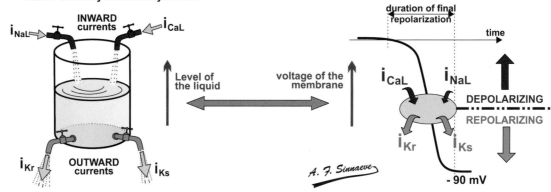

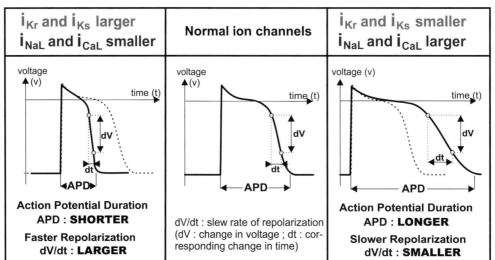

i_{Kr} and i_{Ks} larger i_{NaL} and i_{CaL} smaller	Normal ion channels	i_{Kr} and i_{Ks} smaller i_{NaL} and i_{CaL} larger
Action Potential Duration APD : **SHORTER** Faster Repolarization dV/dt : **LARGER**	dV/dt : slew rate of repolarization (dV : change in voltage ; dt : corresponding change in time)	Action Potential Duration APD : **LONGER** Slower Repolarization dV/dt : **SMALLER**

i_{Kr} : rapid outward repolarizing potassium current
i_{Ks} : slow outward repolarizing potassium current
i_{CaL} : long-lasting inward depolarizing calcium current

i_{NaL} : long-lasting inward depolarizing sodium current
i_{K1} : repolarizing outward potassium current
i_{to} : transient outward current (mainly potassium)

Figure 2.07

Gene mutations may cause either a gain or a loss in function of the important ion channels influencing the repolarization process and thus the action potential duration (APD). This is the basis of Long QT, Short QT and Brugada syndromes.

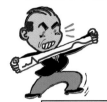

INDICATIONS FOR AN ICD - 8

THE LONG QT SYNDROME (LQTS)

CATEGORIES
1. **Congenital LQTS** due to hereditary defects of ion channels reponsible for the repolarization process.
2. **Acquired LQTS** as a result of electrolyte disturbances or QT-prolonging drugs impairing the repolarization process.

GENOTYPES of CONGENITAL LQTS
- ♥ *Malfunction of ion channels* can express itself either as a gain or loss of function.
- ♥ *Prolongation of the APD* (and hence of the QT interval) may be due to
  ★ decreased function of the channels for the repolarizing i_{Kr} or i_{Ks}
  ★ increased function of the channels for the depolarizing i_{NaL} or i_{CaL}

A. F. Sinnaeve

PHENOTYPES of CONGENITAL LQTS :

- ❈ **ROMANO - WARD** syndrome : ● Only cardiac arrhythmias
  ● Autosomal dominant
- ❈ **JERVELL - LANGE NIELSEN** syndrome ● Cardiac arrhythmias and deafness
  ● Autosomal recessive
- ❈ **ANDERSEN - TAWIL** syndrome : ● Ventricular arrhythmias
  ● Periodic paralysis & facial/skeletal dysmorphism

| \
CHANNELOPATHY - GENETICS OF THE LQTS			
LQTS type	Aberrant GENE	ION CHANNEL MALFUNCTION	% LQTS INCIDENCE
Romano-Ward			
LQT 1	KCNQ1 (KVLQT1)	i_{Ks} (loss)	50 %
LQT 2	KCNH2 (HERG)	i_{Kr} (loss)	45 %
LQT 3	SCN5A	i_{NaL} (gain)	3 - 4 %
LQT 4	ANK2		< 1 %
LQT 5	KCNE1	i_{Ks} (loss)	< 1 %
LQT 6	KCNE2	i_{Kr} (loss)	< 1 %
Andersen-Tawil	KCNJ2	i_{K1} (loss)	< 1 %
Jervell - Lange Nielsen	KCNQ1 (KVLQT1)	i_{Ks} (loss)	< 1 %

ST segment and T wave in hereditary LQTS

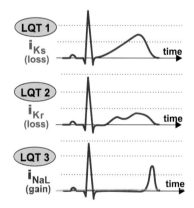

i_{Kr} : rapid outward repolarizing potassium current
i_{Ks} : slow outward repolarizing potassium current
i_{CaL} : long-lasting inward depolarizing calcium current
i_{NaL} : long-lasting inward depolarizing sodium current

"Genotype" refers to the hereditary information i.e. the exact genetic makeup or particular set of (malfunctioning) genes.
"Phenotype" represents the actual physical properties or specific manifestations (ECG, sudden cardiac death, ...). Patients with the same genotypic mutation of K-channels can be phenotypically different due to environmental conditions or the influence of other (modifying) genes.

Figure 2.08

30

Let me tell you about the possible deadly consequences of the LQTS !

LQTS (long QT syndrome)
→ EAD (early afterdepolarization)
→ TdP (torsades de pointes)
→ VF (ventricular fibrillation)
→ **SD** (sudden death)

INDICATIONS FOR AN ICD - 9

THE LONG QT SYNDROME AS A SOURCE OF ARRHYTHMIAS

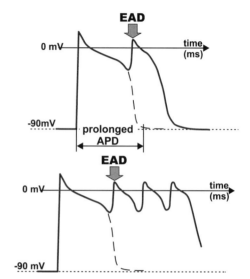

EARLY AFTERDEPOLARIZATIONS (EAD)

* EADs originate during the phase 2 (plateau) or phase 3 (final repolarization) of the action potential.
* EADs are frequently found with prolonged action potential durations (as with LQTS) when Ca channels can partly be re-activated (note that Ca currents are depolarizing).
* EADs often occur with slow heart rates and usually following an extrasystole (i.e. after a compensatory pause).

TORSADES DE POINTES (TWISTING OF THE POINTS)

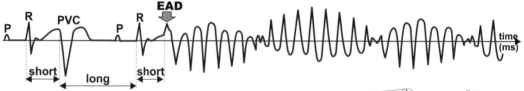

TORSADES DE POINTES (TDP) IS A FORM OF POLYMORPHIC VT ASSOCIATED WITH LQTS

The ECG pattern of TdP shows a continuous undulation of the QRS complexes around the isoelectric line.

The ventricular rate is very fast at 200 to 250 bpm

TdP may be transient and terminate spontaneously (only syncope) or may degenerate into ventriclar fibrillation (VF) leading to sudden death (SD)

TdP are often induced by an early after depolarization (EAD) after a compensatory pause following a premature ventricular complex (PVC)

TdP is sustained by a reentry mechanism that is made possible by dispersion

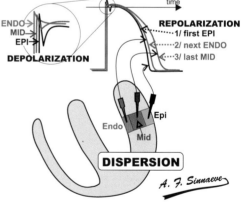

Dispersion or difference of the action potential duration (APD) occurs even in the normal heart. The epicardial APD is the shortest !

Abbreviations : APD : action potential duration ; EAD : early afterdepolarization ; Endo : endocardial layer ; Epi : epicardial layer ; Mid : middle myocardial tissue ; LQTS : long QT syndrome ; PVC : premature ventricular complex ; TdP : torsades de pointes (F) or twisting of the points (E) ;

Figure 2.09

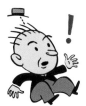

INDICATIONS FOR AN ICD - 10

LQTS - CLINICAL SYMPTOMS & TRIGGERS OF CARDIAC EVENTS

1 **Sudden syncope** is largely related to exercise or emotion
"Fight, flight, fright syncopes" in children or young adolescents are often due to LQTS

2 * **Adrenergic stimuli** may provoke TdP in patients with LQTS associated with loss of function of the potassium channels (i_{Ks} with LQTS1 and i_{Kr} with LQTS2).
* In LQTS1 and LQTS2 adrenergic stimulation increases transmural dispersion during repolarization and hence the chances for malignant rhythm disturbances.
* Beta-blockers are useful in both LQTS1 and LQTS2 !

☑ With *LQTS1*, rhythm disturbances mainly occur during sports, especially swimming

  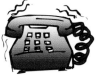

Adrenergic stimulation increases i_{Ks}, shortens action potential duration (APD) but increases the dispersion (affecting epicardial and endocardial cells).

☑ With *LQTS2*, rhythm disturbances are often triggered by auditory stimuli such as telephones, alarm clocks,...

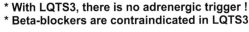

Adrenergic stimulation also increases i_{Ks}, and increases the dispersion (by increasing the repolarization duration in the mid or M cells of the myocardium).

3 For *LQTS3* patients with sodium channel malfunction (i_{NaL}), symptoms mostly occur at rest or during the night.

* With LQTS3, there is no adrenergic trigger !
* Beta-blockers are contraindicated in LQTS3

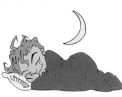 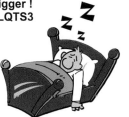 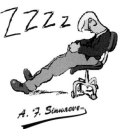

A. F. Sinnreve

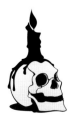

* For 10% of patients, sudden death is the first and tragic symptom !

* LQTS1 and LQTS2 patients have more cardiac events than LQTS3 patients. However, benign cardiac symptoms such as palpitations, syncope and epileptiform insults degenerate more easily in sudden death in LQTS3 patients !

Abbreviations : LQTS = long QT syndrome ; TdP = torsades de pointes ; i_{Kr} = rapid outward repolarizing potassium current ; i_{Ks} = slow outward repolarizing potassium current ; i_{NaL} = long-lasting inward depolarizing sodium current .

Figure 2.10

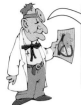

The Brugada syndrome was only recently described (1992).
It is an important cause of sudden death in patients with a *structurally normal heart.*

INDICATIONS FOR AN ICD - 11

THE BRUGADA SYNDROME (BS)

CHARACTERISTICS :

1 The Brugada syndrome (BS) is characterized by ST-segment elevation in the right precordial leads (V1 - V3) and is often associated with a right bundle branch block (RBBB) pattern on the surface ECG.

2 BS is genetically determined and most likely autosomal dominant.

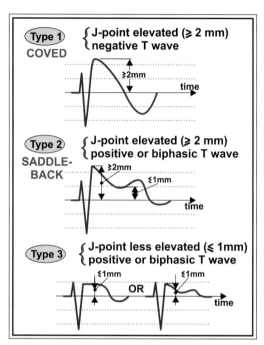

Type 1 COVED	J-point elevated ($\geq$ 2 mm) negative T wave
Type 2 SADDLE-BACK	J-point elevated ($\geq$ 2 mm) positive or biphasic T wave
Type 3	J-point less elevated ($\leq$ 1mm) positive or biphasic T wave

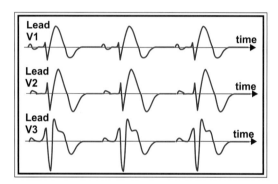

Lead V1 — time
Lead V2 — time
Lead V3 — time

Only *type 1 is directly diagnostic* for BS ! Type 2 and 3 are considered significant if there is a conversion to type 1, spontaneously or during administration of class I A/C antiarrhythmic drugs (flecainide, etc.). Controversy exists about the evaluation and therapy of the asymptomatic patient with a type 1 pattern but no positive family history of sudden cardiac death. To stratify the risk in patients with type 1 pattern, three major factors have been suggested: typical ECG pattern in the basal state, a history of syncope, and inducible VT/VF during EPS. However, the indication and usefulness of an EPS is debatable.
In patients with a type 2 or 3 pattern, a pharmacological test is indicated in the presence of symptoms or of familial history.

Sometimes the BS is intermittent or even concealed.
It can be emphasized by a high placement of the right precordial electrodes (one intercostal space higher), or it can be revealed by IV administration of Ajmaline (not available in the USA), Flecainide or Procainamide.

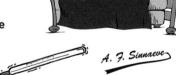

Before flecainide
V2 — time
After flecainide
V2 — time

Sudden death in patients with BS mostly occurs at night when the heart rhythm is very low (low rates enhance rhythm disturbances).

Although fever increases the heart rate, it is remarkable that fever amplifies the expression of BS (because Na channels are temperature dependent and inactivate faster at higher temperature).

A. F. Sinnaeve

Abreviations : EPS : electrophysiologic study ; IV = intravenous ; Na = sodium ; RBBB = right bundle branch block ; VF = ventricular fibrillation ; VT = ventricular tachycardia ;

Figure 2.11

INDICATIONS FOR AN ICD - 12

When is the implantation of an ICD necessary ?

THE BRUGADA SYNDROME (2)

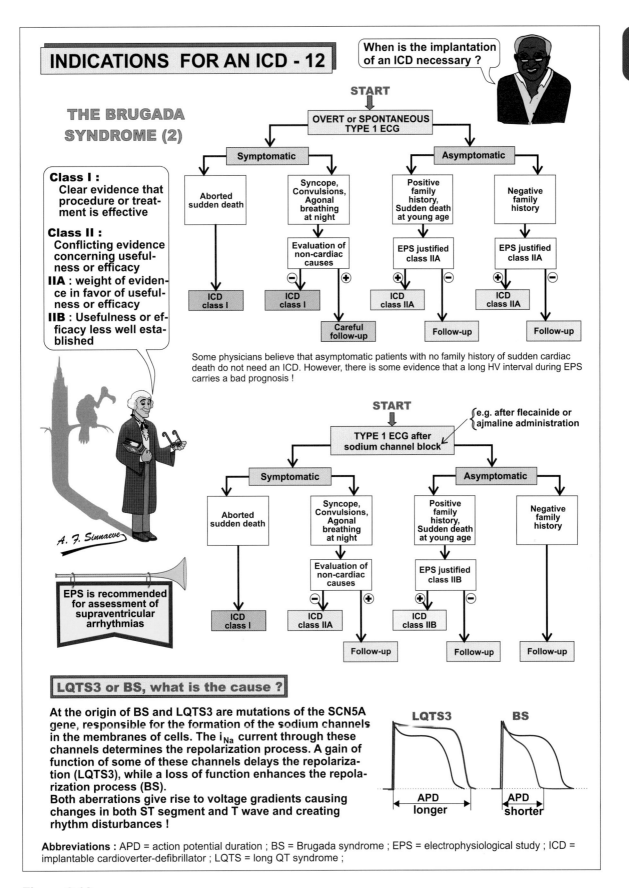

Class I :
Clear evidence that procedure or treatment is effective

Class II :
Conflicting evidence concerning usefulness or efficacy

IIA : weight of evidence in favor of usefulness or efficacy

IIB : Usefulness or efficacy less well established

EPS is recommended for assessment of supraventricular arrhythmias

A. F. Sinnaeve

START

OVERT or SPONTANEOUS TYPE 1 ECG

Symptomatic

Aborted sudden death → ICD class I

Syncope, Convulsions, Agonal breathing at night → Evaluation of non-cardiac causes → (−) ICD class I / (+) Careful follow-up

Asymptomatic

Positive family history, Sudden death at young age → EPS justified class IIA → (+) ICD class IIA / (−) Follow-up

Negative family history → EPS justified class IIA → (+) ICD class IIA / (−) Follow-up

Some physicians believe that asymptomatic patients with no family history of sudden cardiac death do not need an ICD. However, there is some evidence that a long HV interval during EPS carries a bad prognosis !

START

TYPE 1 ECG after sodium channel block — e.g. after flecainide or ajmaline administration

Symptomatic

Aborted sudden death → ICD class I

Syncope, Convulsions, Agonal breathing at night → Evaluation of non-cardiac causes → (−) ICD class IIA / (+) Follow-up

Asymptomatic

Positive family history, Sudden death at young age → EPS justified class IIB → (+) ICD class IIB / (−) Follow-up

Negative family history → Follow-up

LQTS3 or BS, what is the cause ?

At the origin of BS and LQTS3 are mutations of the SCN5A gene, responsible for the formation of the sodium channels in the membranes of cells. The i_{Na} current through these channels determines the repolarization process. A gain of function of some of these channels delays the repolarization (LQTS3), while a loss of function enhances the repolarization process (BS).
Both aberrations give rise to voltage gradients causing changes in both ST segment and T wave and creating rhythm disturbances !

LQTS3 — APD longer

BS — APD shorter

Abbreviations : APD = action potential duration ; BS = Brugada syndrome ; EPS = electrophysiological study ; ICD = implantable cardioverter-defibrillator ; LQTS = long QT syndrome ;

Figure 2.12

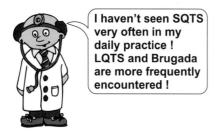

I haven't seen SQTS very often in my daily practice ! LQTS and Brugada are more frequently encountered !

INDICATIONS FOR AN ICD - 13

THE SHORT QT SYNDROME (SQTS)

In the SQTS the QT interval is shorter than 300 ms. The T wave is symmetrical and has a large magnitude.

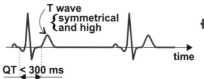

T wave symmetrical and high

QT < 300 ms

time

❁ SQTS supposes intrinsic aberrations of the ion channels that are involved in the repolarization process. A shortened QT interval due to fever, hypercalcemia, hyperkalemia, acidosis or digitalis are not to be confused with SQTS.

❁ SQTS patients do not have structural heart disease, but often have a family history of syncope and sudden death (SQTS is possibly the cause of sudden infant death syndrome SIDS). Palpitations and episodes of atrial fibrillation as well as atrial flutter are frequently seen in SQTS patients, even in very young patients.

❁ SQTS is caused by a gain in function of the i_{Kr} and i_{Ks} channels, making the repolarization process very fast and the action potential duration very short. This gain of function is due to mutations of the KCNQ1 gene (responsible for i_{Ks}) and/or the KCNH2 gene (responsible for i_{Kr}).

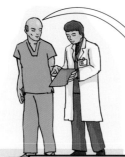

It isn't very difficult ! It is all about the repolarization process ! This is what you should remember : there are two kinds of ionic currents, some are depolarizing while the others are repolarizing. And according to the abnormal gene, there may be a gain or a loss of function...

SUMMARY of CHANNELOPATHY

GENE	IONIC-CURRENT	FUNCTION OF CHANNEL	SYNDROME
SCN5A	i_{Na} (depolarizing)	function loss ⬇	* Brugada * Conduction-disturbances
		function gain ⬆	* LQTS 3
KCNQ1	i_{Ks} (repolarizing)	function loss ⬇	* LQTS 1
		function gain ⬆	* inherited AF * SQTS
KCNH2 (HERG)	i_{Kr} (repolarizing)	function loss ⬇	* LQTS 2
		function gain ⬆	* SQTS

A. F. Sinnaeve

Abbreviations : AF : atrial fibrillation ; LQTS : long QT syndrome ; SQTS : short QT syndrome ; i_{Na} current of sodium ions ; i_{Ks} : slow current of potassium ions ; i_{Kr} : rapid current of potassium ions ;

Figure 2.13

ARVD/C is a new condition recently recognized.
The clinical challenge is how to identify individuals with ARVD/C who have mild or minimal structural abnormalities of the right ventricle.

INDICATIONS FOR ICD THERAPY - 14

ARRHYTHMOGENIC RIGHT VENTRICLE DYSPLASIA / CARDIOMYOPATHY (ARVD/C)

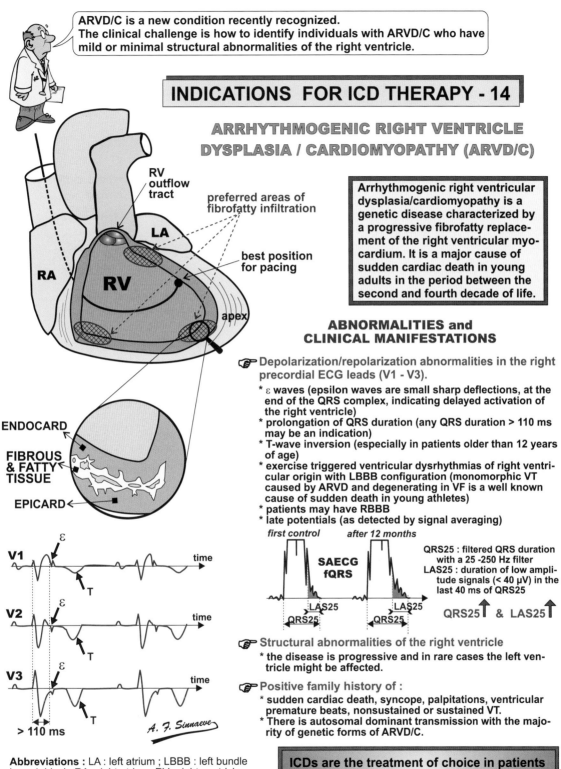

RV outflow tract

preferred areas of fibrofatty infiltration

best position for pacing

LA

RA

RV

apex

ENDOCARD

FIBROUS & FATTY TISSUE

EPICARD

Arrhythmogenic right ventricular dysplasia/cardiomyopathy is a genetic disease characterized by a progressive fibrofatty replacement of the right ventricular myocardium. It is a major cause of sudden cardiac death in young adults in the period between the second and fourth decade of life.

ABNORMALITIES and CLINICAL MANIFESTATIONS

☞ Depolarization/repolarization abnormalities in the right precordial ECG leads (V1 - V3).

* ε waves (epsilon waves are small sharp deflections, at the end of the QRS complex, indicating delayed activation of the right ventricle)
* prolongation of QRS duration (any QRS duration > 110 ms may be an indication)
* T-wave inversion (especially in patients older than 12 years of age)
* exercise triggered ventricular dysrhythmias of right ventricular origin with LBBB configuration (monomorphic VT caused by ARVD and degenerating in VF is a well known cause of sudden death in young athletes)
* patients may have RBBB
* late potentials (as detected by signal averaging)

first control   *after 12 months*

SAECG
fQRS

LAS25   LAS25
QRS25   QRS25

QRS25 : filtered QRS duration with a 25 -250 Hz filter
LAS25 : duration of low amplitude signals (< 40 µV) in the last 40 ms of QRS25

QRS25 ↑ & LAS25 ↑

☞ Structural abnormalities of the right ventricle

* the disease is progressive and in rare cases the left ventricle might be affected.

☞ Positive family history of :

* sudden cardiac death, syncope, palpitations, ventricular premature beats, nonsustained or sustained VT.
* There is autosomal dominant transmission with the majority of genetic forms of ARVD/C.

V1   ε   time   T

V2   ε   time   T

V3   ε   time   T

> 110 ms

A. F. Sinnaeve

Abbreviations : LA : left atrium ; LBBB : left bundle branch block; RA : right atrium; RV : right ventricle; RBBB : right bundle branch block ; SDC : sudden cardiac death; VF : ventricular fibrillation; VT : ventricular tachycardia; fQRS : filtered QRS ; SAECG : signal averaged ECG ; endocard : endocardial (inner) layer of the heart muscle ; epicard : epicardial (outer) layer of the heart muscle ;

ICDs are the treatment of choice in patients with syncope, cardiac arrest, documented VT and positive family history of SDC.
Possible problems : low endocardial signals and increased pacing thresholds.

Figure 2.14

OK, I know the two catecholamines norepinephrine and epinephrine (or adrenaline as the Europeans say) and I know their role in the regulation of the heart by the adrenergic or sympathetic nervous system... But how can they generate a VT or VF ?

INDICATIONS FOR ICD THERAPY - 15

CATECHOLAMINERGIC POLYMORPHIC VENTRICULAR TACHYCARDIA (CPVT)

Some distinguishing features of CPVT have been pointed out :

1. A direct relation between adrenergic activation (physical or emotional stress) and the onset of arrhythmias.

2. Absence of structural cardiac abnormalities.

3. An unremarkable resting ECG (with the exception of sinus bradycardia and the presence of "U" waves in some patients).

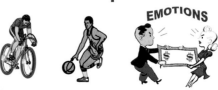

4. A typical pattern of "bidirectional" VT with an alternating 180° QRS-axis on a beat-to-beat basis
(or an irregular polymorphic VT without QRS vector alternans in some patients).

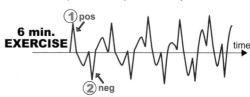

Molecular mechanisms of CPVT arrhythmogenesis

CPVT is caused by mutations of cardiac ryanodine (RyR2) and calsequestrin (CASQ2) genes. Both genes affect the amount of Ca^{++} released from the sarcoplasmatic reticulum during adrenergic stimulation. The elevated intracellular Ca^{++} levels (Ca^{++} overload) may cause delayed afterdepolarizations (DAD) which may initiate arrhythmias.

A. F. Sinnaeve

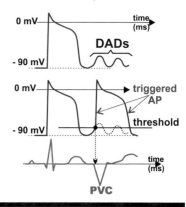

PART OF MYOCARDIAL CELL WITH Ca-CHANNELS

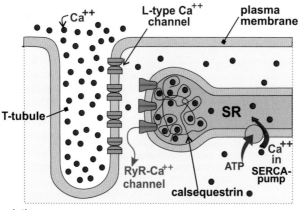

CPVT is an genetically determined arrhythmogenic disease characterized by ventricular tachycardia, syncope and sudden cardiac death. Antiadrenergic treatment with beta-blockers is the first therapy for patients with CPTV. However, in most cases an ICD is recommended.

Abbreviations :
ATP : adenosine triphosphate (universal energy carrier) ; DAD : delayed afterdepolarization ; SCD : sudden cardiac death; SR : sarcoplasmic reticulum ; SERCA : sarco/endoplasmic reticulum Ca-pump (pump for Ca uptake by the SR) ; RyR : ryanodine receptor (for Ca-induced Ca release of the SR) ; L-type : long lasting Ca channel (opening induced by depolarization of the membrane; the Ca inflow through these channels triggers the RyR channels) ; VF/VT : ventricular fibrillation/tachycardia;

Figure 2.15

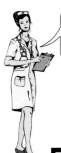

HCM is a disorder of the myocardium characterized by excessive myocardial hypertrophy, with predilection for the interventricular septum.
There is a broad heterogeneity in disease causing genetic mutations (10 genes are known so far) and in phenotypic expression, treatment and prognosis.

INDICATIONS FOR ICD THERAPY - 16

HYPERTROPHIC CARDIOMYOPATHY (HCM)

* Myopathy is muscle degeneration. In hypertrophic cardiomyopathy (HCM) the ventricular wall is abnormally thick and the cavity is small or very small.
* HCM is an inherited myocardial disorder with an autosomal dominant trait.
* HCM is usually associated with microscopic evidence of myocardial fiber disarray.

NORMAL **HCM**

aligned fibers   disordered fibers

Possible responses to exercise in patients with HCM

NORMAL BP

HYPOTENSION during exercise

HYPOTENSION during exercise

ABNORMAL BP during recovery

ABNORMALITIES and CLINICAL MANIFESTATIONS

☞ Short, plump, hypertrophic myocardial fibers in apparent disarray, interspersed with loose intercellular connective tissue in the involved areas of the myocardium.

☞ SCD may occur without warning signs or symptoms, as the initial disease manifestation, and may be triggered by vigorous exercise or competitive sports activity.
SCD is more common in children.

☞ Severe left-ventricular hypertrophy (echocardiography may even show wall thickness of >30 mm).

☞ Family history of premature SCD.

☞ Unexplained syncope, sustained and non-sustained VT (24h Holter).

☞ Abnormal exercise/rest blood pressure pattern.

☞ Obstructive subaortic pressure gradient and mitral regurgitation : since the LV outflow tract is narrowed by HCM, a very rapid initial outflow (venturi effect) is created and part of the mitral leaflets is drawn against the septum (systolic anterior motion or SAM). This SAM not only obstructs the outflow, but causes mitral regurgitation.

A. J. Sinnicova

ICD implantation is considered the most effective and reliable treatment option and has been recommended in HCM patients at high risk of sudden death.

Abbreviations :
RA : right atrium; RV : right ventricle; SCD : sudden cardiac death; VF : ventricular fibrillation; VT : ventricular tachycardia;

Figure 2.16

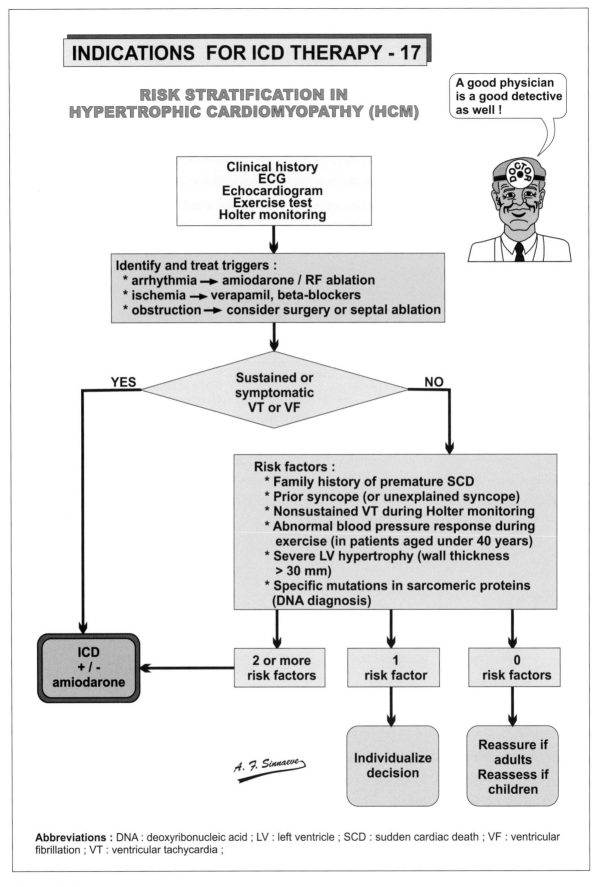

INDICATIONS FOR ICD THERAPY - 17

RISK STRATIFICATION IN HYPERTROPHIC CARDIOMYOPATHY (HCM)

A good physician is a good detective as well !

Clinical history
ECG
Echocardiogram
Exercise test
Holter monitoring

Identify and treat triggers :
* arrhythmia → amiodarone / RF ablation
* ischemia → verapamil, beta-blockers
* obstruction → consider surgery or septal ablation

Sustained or symptomatic VT or VF

YES   NO

Risk factors :
* Family history of premature SCD
* Prior syncope (or unexplained syncope)
* Nonsustained VT during Holter monitoring
* Abnormal blood pressure response during exercise (in patients aged under 40 years)
* Severe LV hypertrophy (wall thickness > 30 mm)
* Specific mutations in sarcomeric proteins (DNA diagnosis)

ICD + / - amiodarone

2 or more risk factors

1 risk factor

0 risk factors

A. F. Sinnaeve

Individualize decision

Reassure if adults
Reassess if children

Abbreviations : DNA : deoxyribonucleic acid ; LV : left ventricle ; SCD : sudden cardiac death ; VF : ventricular fibrillation ; VT : ventricular tachycardia ;

Figure 2.17

ICD HARDWARE

① The lithium-SVO battery
* Chemistry
* Construction & discharge characteristics
* Voltage delay

② Capacitors
* The HV system - an overview
* Physical principles
* Definitions and units
* Charging - a model with elastic membrane
* Exponential charging via a resistor
* Exponential charging and time constant
* Charging and discharging
* How a pacing pulse is formed
* High voltage (HV) pulse - definition of tilt
* HV shock - monophasic vs biphasic
* Energy content of a pulse
* Energy and falling rocks
* Energy or volt as a parameter for pulses
* Electrolytic capacitors
* Charging time
* The HV charging circuit - parts 1, 2, 3 and 4

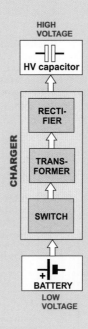

③ Leads and electrodes - some technical aspects
* Single vs dual defibrillation coils
* Epicardial and ancillary defibrillation electrodes
* Coaxial vs multiluminal leads ; current distribution of coils
* Lead connections
* The new ISO four-pole connector

Figure 3.00

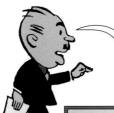

THE LITHIUM - SVO BATTERY - 1

Why don't we use the proven lithium-iodine battery as in a pacemaker ?

The battery in a pacemaker has only to deliver a rather small current.
But the battery in an ICD has also to provide high-current pulses for defibrillation (via capacitor charging).

The ICD presents a significant challenge to meet all the requirements :
* A lot of charge has to be stored in a small volume (i.e. a very high charge density is needed)
* A large maximum current rating (up to 3A) is required
* A long shelf life is essential (no loss of charge or self-discharge by internal leakage is allowed)
* A high reliability and safety are essential

There is no iodine in this cell. The cathode consists of silver vanadium oxide ($Ag_2V_4O_{11}$)
Although the construction is different, the electrochemical principles are still the same !
The lithium anode loses electrons (i.e. oxidation) while the cathode absorbs electrons (i.e. reduction) ...

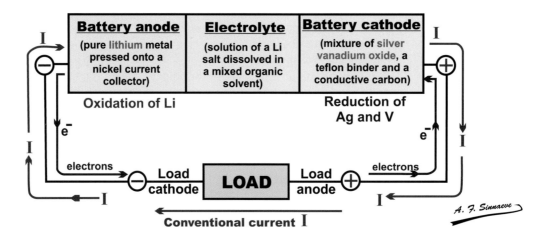

♥ The cell discharge (i.e. reduction of the silver and the vanadium) takes place in multiple steps. As a consequence, the Li/SVO cell has a distinctive discharge curve with two regions of nearly constant voltage, one at 3.2 V and one at 2.6 V. These two regions are joined by a region of sloping voltage, and the voltage also slopes downward after the 2.6 V plateau.

♠ The reduction of silver to its metallic state increases the conductivity of the cathode during the depletion of the battery. Hence, the decline in voltage is not caused by an increase in cell resistance in general and the cell's current delivery capability is retained throughout the discharge process.

♦ Initially the internal resistance of the battery decreases (from beginning of life until middle of life), then increases towards the end of life.

♣ The battery is enclosed in a stainless steel container which is hermetically sealed. This case is connected to the battery anode (i.e. the negative pole).

Figure 3.01

THE LITHIUM - SVO BATTERY - 2

For a large current capability, a large surface area of the electrodes is necessary. Therefore a folded construction or a flattened coil is used so that both sides of the electrodes are active !

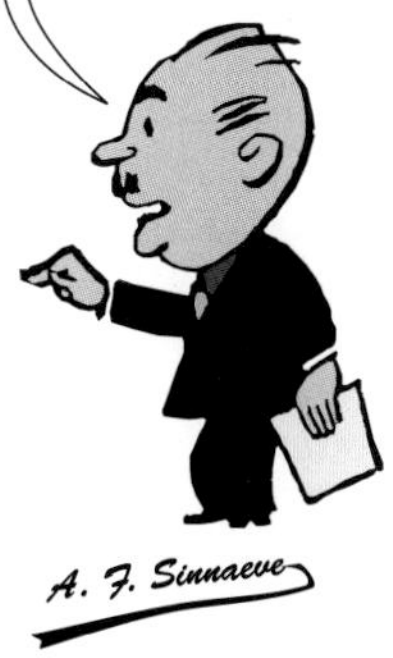

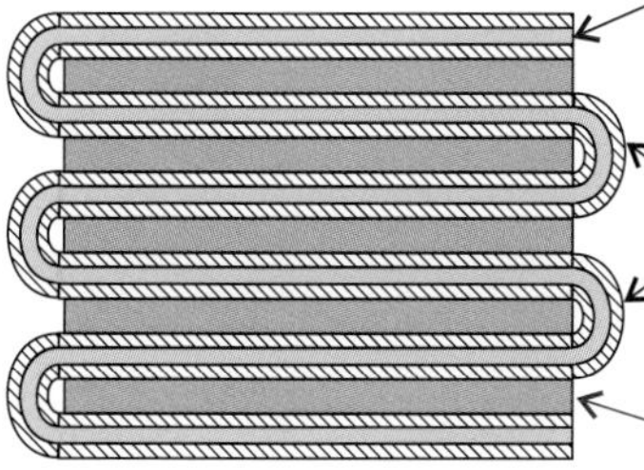

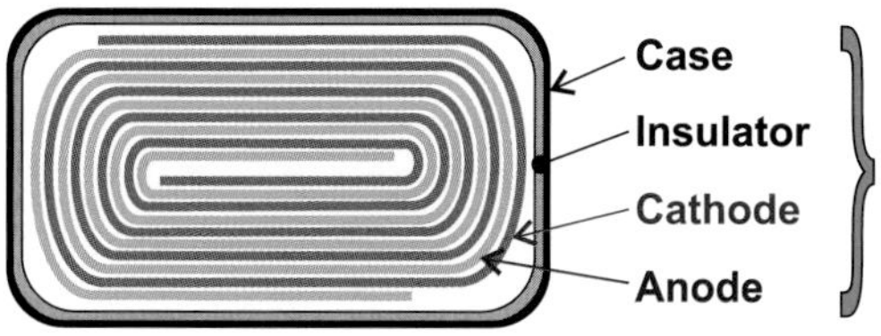

Medtronic : flattened coil construction
(The separator, which is situated between the anode and cathode, is not shown for clarirty)

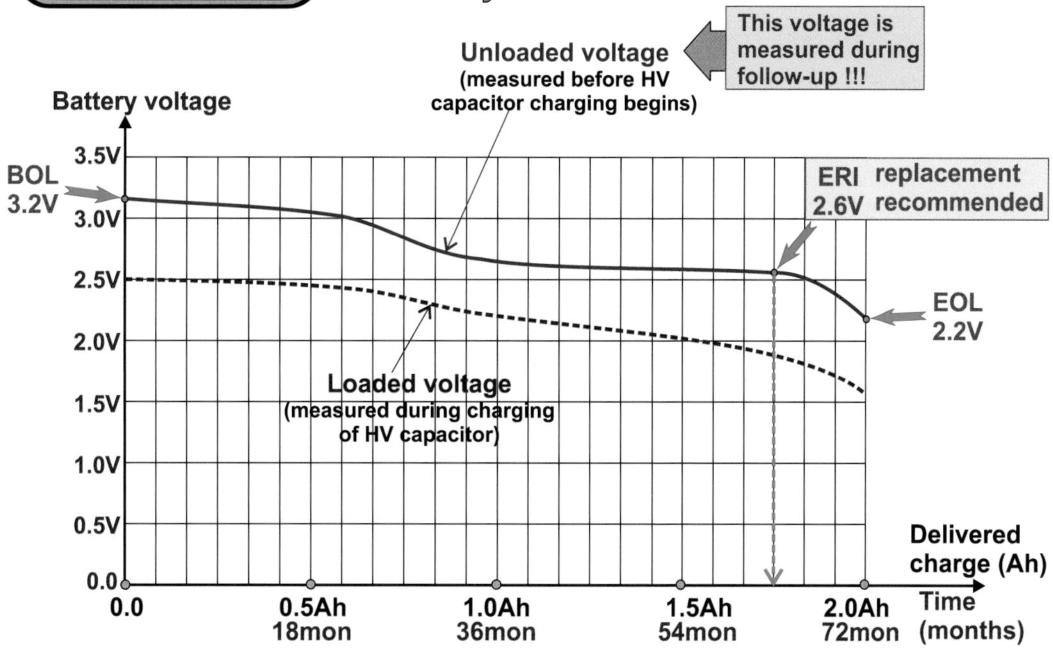

BOL (Beginning of Life)
ERI (Elective Replacement Indicator) : battery voltage at which replacement of the device (ICD) is recommended. ERI does not alter the device operation in any way.
EOL (End of Life) : battery voltage indicating urgent need of generator replacement because of erratic function of the ICD may occur at low battery voltage.

Abbreviations : Ah = ampere-hour = historical measure for charge delivered by a battery ; Ag = (argentum) = silver ; Li = lithium = light metal of the alkaline group ; V = vanadium ; O = oxygen

Figure 3.02

42

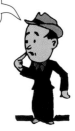

Can someone tell me what *"voltage delay"* means and how it influences the charging time of the HV capacitor ?

THE LITHIUM - SVO BATTERY VOLTAGE DELAY

That's a rather technical question, but you will understand it ! It is all about the complicated chemical reactions in the cathode pellets.

(1) During cell discharge, the reduction of vanadium in the cathode occurs in discrete steps, creating discrete plateaus at 3.2 V and 2.6 V in the unloaded voltage of the battery. During the second step (when the vanadium reduces from valence state IV to III) a chemical buildup on the cathode takes place if the battery hasn't been pulsed for more than 3 months (i.e. hasn't been used to charge the HV capacitor).

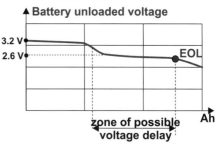

(2) The chemical buildup on the cathode increases the internal resistance of the battery and causes a substantial voltage drop (larger than the usual voltage drop over the internal resistance).

Since the loaded battery voltage with chemical buildup is much lower than normal, the charging time of the HV capacitor will be a lot longer and delivery of the shock will be delayed !

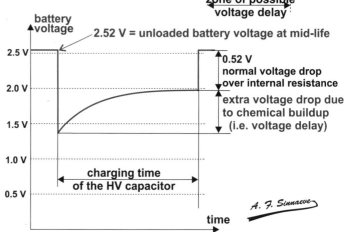

(3) Fortunately the chemical buildup on the cathode disappears when the battery delivers a larger current for some time. The large voltage drop at the start of the charging normalizes when the HV capacitor becomes fully charged. A succeeding charging cycle does not show a voltage delay !

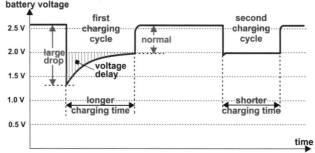

To avoid voltage delay the frequency of HV capacitor reforming should be driven up when the second voltage plateau is reached (e.g. from every 3 months to every month)

The normal voltage drop over the internal resistance of the battery depends on the current needed by the charger : e.g. if the charger takes 2 A from the battery and the internal resistance of the battery is 0.26 Ω, then the voltage drop will be 0.26 x 2 = 0.52 V (Ohm's law).
It is normal to go from 2.52 V to 2.0 V while charging the HV capacitor. During the entire charging cycle, the loaded battery voltage stays at 2 V if everything is OK. When the chemical buildup around the cathode of the battery is dispersed, the loaded battery voltage returns to the normal value of 2 V (i.e. a drop of 0.52 V).

Abbreviations : EOL = end-of-life ; HV = high voltage ; SVO = silver-vanadiumoxide

Figure 3.03

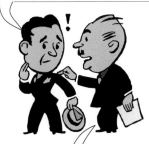

What's all the fuss about high voltage (HV) capacitors ? What are they and what's their purpose ? Do we really need them in our ICDs ?

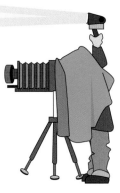

CAPACITORS - 1

Yes, they are indispensable in ICDs ! They are just like those used in the flash of photographers when taking some snapshots ! They too need an HV capacitor. Conventional pacing is often called low-voltage therapy and defibrillation high-voltage therapy. But don't panic, it's not difficult at all. I'll explain it to you...

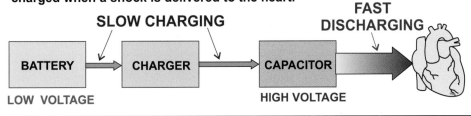

- ✿ A battery can produce enough charge to deliver a lot of shocks (or a lot of flashes). However, a battery cannot deliver a large quantity of charge all at once, while an ICD (as well as a flash) requires delivery in a very short time.
- ✿ A battery has a fixed low voltage. A shock for defibrillation (or a sudden flash) requires a much higher voltage.
- ✿ The HV capacitor is slowly charged toward a high voltage and very rapidly discharged when a shock is delivered to the heart.

SLOW CHARGING — FAST DISCHARGING

BATTERY → CHARGER → CAPACITOR → (heart)

LOW VOLTAGE   HIGH VOLTAGE

A. F. Sinnaeve

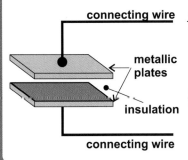

connecting wire

metallic plates

insulation

connecting wire

- ❋ A capacitor is like a reservoir. It is a device that is able to store electricity (i.e. an electric charge). The ability of a capacitor to store an electric charge is called "capacitance"

- ❋ A capacitor is an electronic component that consists of two conducting surfaces called plates (e.g. a metal such as aluminum) which are separated by insulating material called the dielectric (e.g. dry air or plastic)

Abbreviations : HV = High Voltage
From ELECTRICITY : CHARGE = an electric charge on a metallic surface is caused by a surplus (-) or a lack (+) of electrons (i.e. small particles of an atom). A charge of 1coulomb corresponds to 6.242×10^{18} electrons.

Figure 3.04

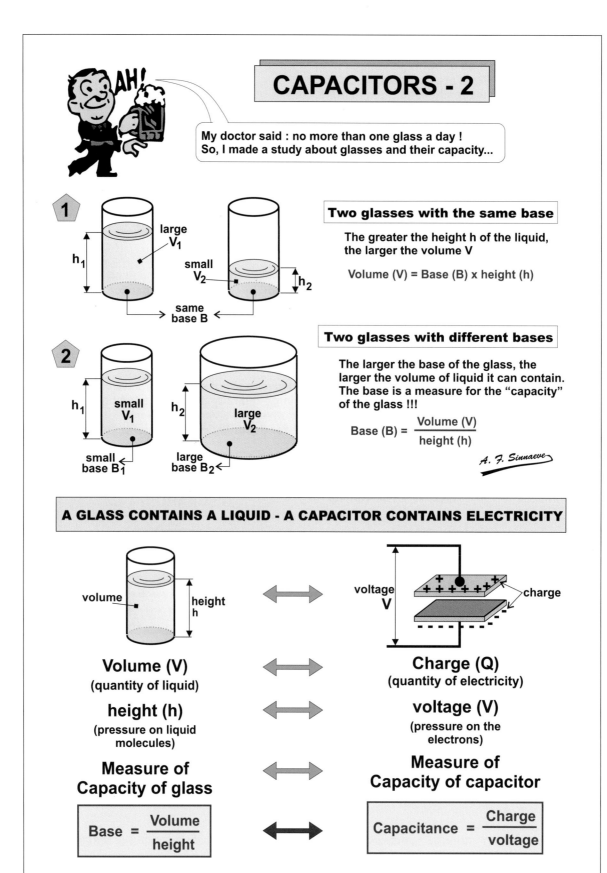

Figure 3.05

CAPACITORS - 3

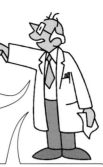

Capacitors are very important in ICDs ! We already know :
1. A **capacitor** consists of two conducting surfaces, separated by an insulating material.
2. The **capacitance** is the ability of such a device to store an electric charge.

A capacitor is charged by removing some charge (a quantity of electrons) from one plate and placing it on the other. The redistribution of the charge might be done by a battery (source) pumping electrons from one side to the other...
The amount of charge (Q) pumped is proportional to the battery's voltage (V) and the constant of proportionality is the capacitance (C).

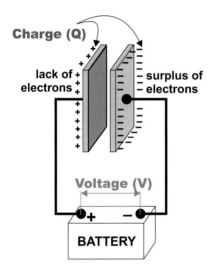

Charge (Q)

lack of electrons

surplus of electrons

Voltage (V)

BATTERY

CHARGE = CAPACITANCE x VOLTAGE

$$Q = C.V$$

$$\text{CAPACITANCE} = \frac{\text{CHARGE (coulomb)}}{\text{VOLTAGE (volt)}}$$

$$C = \frac{Q}{V}$$

THERE IS A SPECIAL UNIT OF CAPACITANCE

The SI unit of capacitance is the **FARAD (F)**. A capacitor has a capacitance of 1 farad (1F) when a voltage of 1 volt (1V) creates charge of 1 coulomb or 1ampere x 1 second (1C = 1 As)

$$1F = \frac{1C}{1V}$$

The farad is a large unit for everyday use. Commonly used are :

microfarad - symbol μF ; $1\ \mu F = 10^{-6}\ F$

nanofarad - symbol nF ; $1\ nF = 10^{-9}\ F$

picofarad - symbol pF ; $1\ pF = 10^{-12}\ F$

A. F. Sinnaeve

Figure 3.06

CAPACITORS - 4

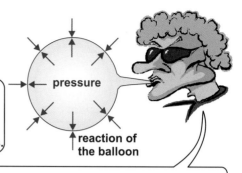

The more I blow, the more the pressure builds up in the balloon. But as the balloon is inflated, a tension is created in its wall trying to deflate the balloon. When the reaction of the balloon becomes equal to the maximum pressure of my lungs, the inflation stops.

Let's look at a simple model to understand the charging of a capacitor.

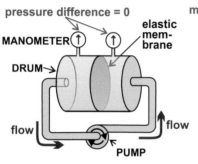

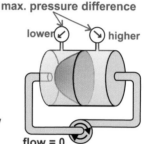

A drum is divided in 2 parts by an impermeable elastic membrane. A small rotating pump pumps the air from the left compartment to the right.

At the start, both compartments have an equal volume and there is no pressure difference between them. Since there is not yet any reaction force of the membrane, a substantial airflow moves from the left to the right.

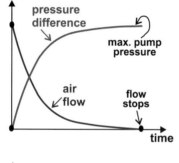

While the pressure difference between the two compartments is increasing, the membrane deforms and develops a reaction opposing to the pressure. These reaction tries to push back the air and therefore decreases the airflow.

When the pressure difference equals the maximum pressure of the pump, the deformation of the membrane is also maximum and the airflow stops.

The charging of a capacitor is done in the same way ! But it is a battery pumping electrons from one side to the other. Since the membrane is impermeable, the air flow is transient. The electron flow is also transient because the dielectric is an insulator.

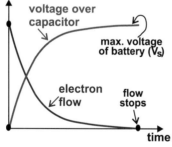

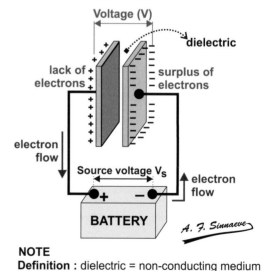

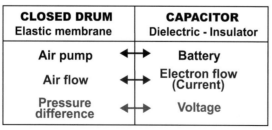

CLOSED DRUM Elastic membrane	CAPACITOR Dielectric - Insulator
Air pump	⟷ Battery
Air flow	⟷ Electron flow (Current)
Pressure difference	⟷ Voltage

NOTE
Definition : dielectric = non-conducting medium between capacitor plates

Figure 3.07

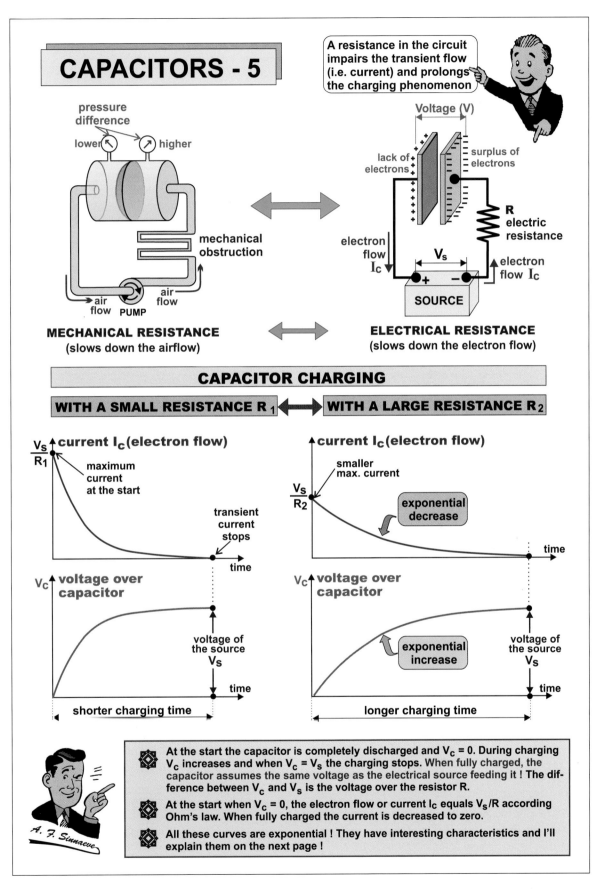

Figure 3.08

We know that the charging time of a capacitor depends upon its capacitance C and the total resistance R in the circuit !

The product τ = R.C is called the time constant.
The course of an exponential curve is determined by RC !

The time constant refers to the rate of change of charging. It indicates the amount of time required to change a value by 63.2%.

CAPACITORS - 6

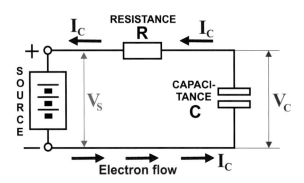

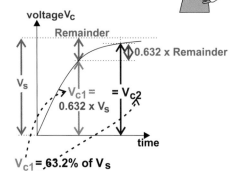

V_{c1} = 63.2% of V_s
Remainder = 100 - 63.2% = 36.8%
V_{c2} = 63.2 + (0.632 x 36.8) = 86.4% of V_s
etc.

time	V_c (% of V_s)	I_c (% of V_s/R)
t = 1RC	63.2%	36.8%
t = 2RC	86.4%	13.6%
t = 3RC	95.0%	4.98%
t = 4RC	98.1%	1.83%
t = 5RC	99.3%	0.07%

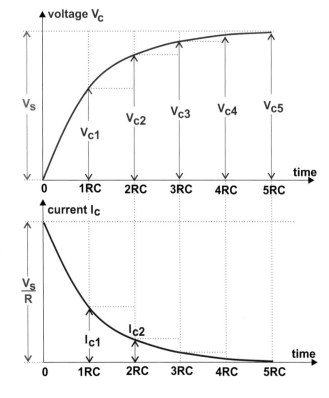

For all practical purposes, we may accept that a capacitor is completely charged after a time of 5RC.

e.g. : A capacitor of 100 μF is charging via a resistor of 20 kΩ
The time constant (= R.C) is :
$100 \times 10^{-6} \times 20 \times 10^{3}$ = 2 sec
The charging time (= 5RC) is then :
5 x 2 s = 10 sec

A. F. Sinnaeve

NOTE : τ **=** Greek letter tau (equivalent to the letter t)

Abbreviations : Vs = voltage of the source; Vc = voltage over the capacitor; Ic = charging current in the circuit; τ = RC = time constant; t = time; μF = microfarad = 10^{-6}F;

Figure 3.09

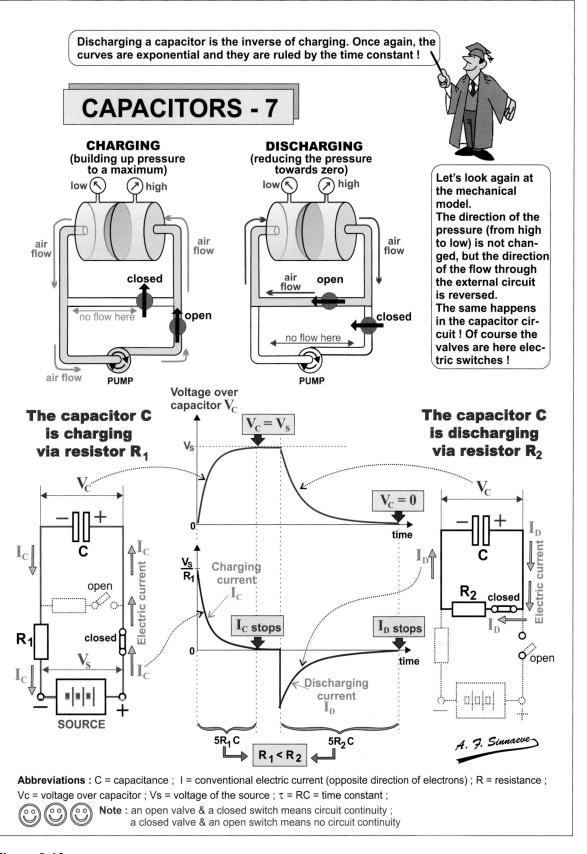

Discharging a capacitor is the inverse of charging. Once again, the curves are exponential and they are ruled by the time constant !

CAPACITORS - 7

CHARGING
(building up pressure to a maximum)

DISCHARGING
(reducing the pressure towards zero)

Let's look again at the mechanical model.
The direction of the pressure (from high to low) is not changed, but the direction of the flow through the external circuit is reversed.
The same happens in the capacitor circuit ! Of course the valves are here electric switches !

The capacitor C is charging via resistor R_1

The capacitor C is discharging via resistor R_2

$V_C = V_S$

$V_C = 0$

$R_1 < R_2$

Abbreviations : C = capacitance ; I = conventional electric current (opposite direction of electrons) ; R = resistance ; Vc = voltage over capacitor ; Vs = voltage of the source ; τ = RC = time constant ;

Note : an open valve & a closed switch means circuit continuity ; a closed valve & an open switch means no circuit continuity

Figure 3.10

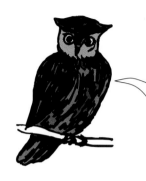

CAPACITORS - 8

Now, you should be able to understand how the output pulse of a simple pacemaker is formed.
The output capacitor of the pacemaker charges through an internal resistance R_{ch} and discharges through the heart R_p. Of course, the resistance R_p is much smaller than the charging resistance R_{ch}.

Slowly charging the output capacitor C_o via the high resistance R_{ch} while switch S is open.

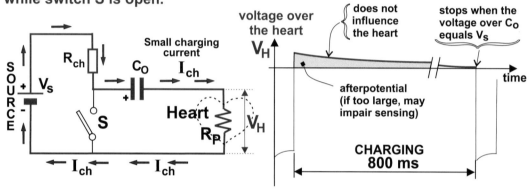

Quick discharge when switch S is closed. Only the small pacing resistance R_P limits the current; the source voltage V_s determines the amplitude.

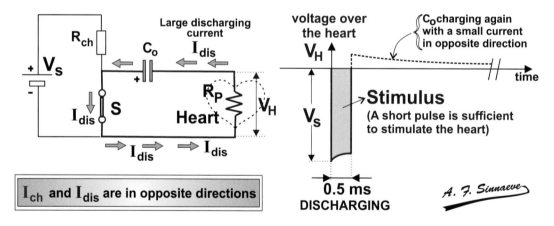

I_{ch} and I_{dis} are in opposite directions

NOTE 1: the discharging stops long before the voltage over the output capacitor C_o becomes zero or the current through the heart becomes zero, i.e. the discharging is truncated ! The rest of the charge stays in the capacitor

NOTE 2: the switch is controlled by the timing mechanism of the pacemaker.

NOTE 3: sensing of heart activity by the pacemaker prevents closing the switch S while the charge remains on the capacitor.

Abbreviations : C_o = output capacitor of the pacemaker; R_{ch} = charging resistance; R_p = pacing resistance; S = electronic switch; V_s = source voltage (may be less than the battery voltage)

Figure 3.11

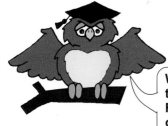

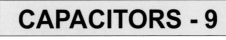

CAPACITORS - 9

When delivering a pulse to a patient by discharging a capacitor, the voltage always drops exponentially.
For a pacemaker, the pulse duration is very short and the DROOP or the voltage difference between leading and trailing edge is normally small.
The discharging time of the high voltage capacitor of an ICD is much longer and hence a much larger TILT may occur.

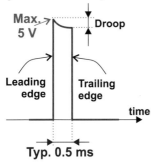

Low voltage pacemaker pulse

Max. 5 V
Droop
Leading edge
Trailing edge
time
Typ. 0.5 ms

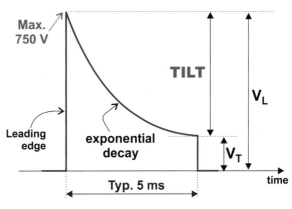

High voltage pulse of an ICD

Max. 750 V
TILT
V_L
Leading edge
exponential decay
V_T
time
Typ. 5 ms

By definition we have :

$$\text{TILT in \%} = \frac{V_L - V_T}{V_L} \cdot 100\%$$

NOTE that tilt, pulse duration and resistance are always coupled

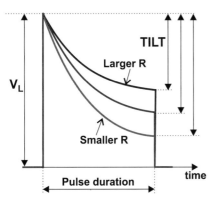

TILT
Larger R
V_L
Smaller R
Pulse duration
time

With fixed pulse duration : a smaller resistance between the high voltage electrodes results in a larger tilt.

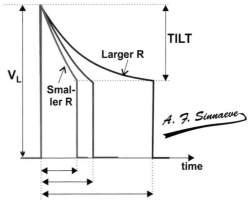

TILT
Larger R
V_L
Smaller R
time

A. F. Sinnaeve

With fixed tilt : a smaller resistance between the high voltage electrodes results in a shorter pulse duration.

Abbreviations : V_L = voltage at the start of the pulse (leading edge) ; V_T = voltage at the end of the pulse (trailing edge) ; R = resistance between the two high voltage electrodes ; V = volt ;

Note : droop and tilt describe the same phenomenon. However, droop is usually reserved for pacemakers.

Figure 3.12

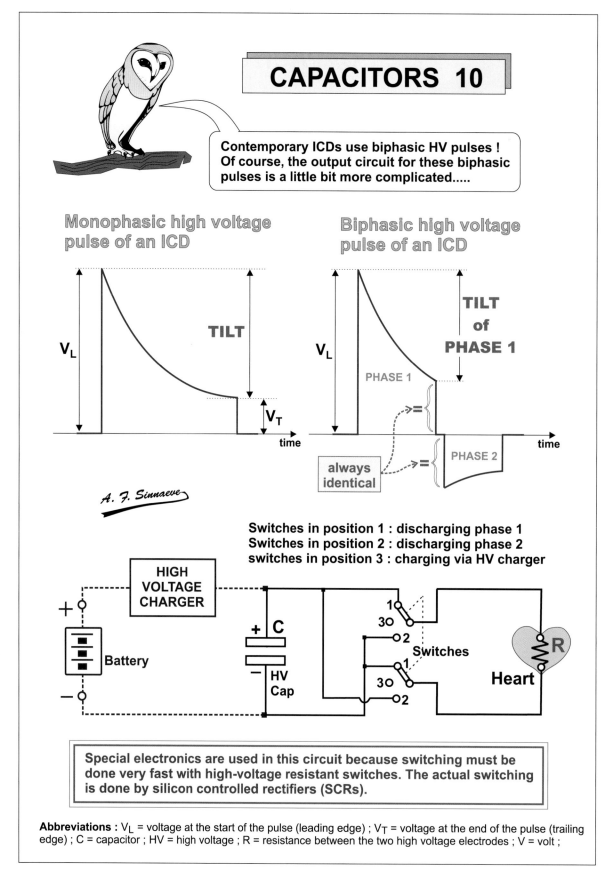

CAPACITORS 10

Contemporary ICDs use biphasic HV pulses !
Of course, the output circuit for these biphasic
pulses is a little bit more complicated.....

Monophasic high voltage pulse of an ICD

V_L

TILT

V_T

time

Biphasic high voltage pulse of an ICD

V_L

TILT of PHASE 1

PHASE 1

always identical

PHASE 2

time

A. F. Sinnaeve

Switches in position 1 : discharging phase 1
Switches in position 2 : discharging phase 2
switches in position 3 : charging via HV charger

HIGH VOLTAGE CHARGER

+

Battery

−

+ C

− HV Cap

1
3
2

1
3
2

Switches

R

Heart

Special electronics are used in this circuit because switching must be done very fast with high-voltage resistant switches. The actual switching is done by silicon controlled rectifiers (SCRs).

Abbreviations : V_L = voltage at the start of the pulse (leading edge) ; V_T = voltage at the end of the pulse (trailing edge) ; C = capacitor ; HV = high voltage ; R = resistance between the two high voltage electrodes ; V = volt ;

Figure 3.13

CAPACITORS 11

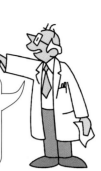

Yes, it's me again. I have to say something about ENERGY !
A capacitor is charged by removing some charge from one plate and placing it on the other. Of course, some energy is needed to displace this charge and it is stored as a potential energy in the capacitor. When the capacitor is discharged, this energy is delivered to the resistances of the discharging circuit and converted into heat !

> **The energy stored in a capacitor is directly proportional to its capacitance and directly proportional to the square of the voltage.**

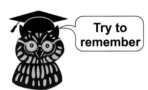 **Try to remember**

$$W = \frac{C.V^2}{2}$$

W = energy in joule (J)

C = capacitance in farad (F)

V = voltage in volt (V)

EXAMPLE :

A capacitor of 120µF is initially charged to 200V. It delivers a pulse which is truncated at a tilt of 65%. What is the energy delivered to the patient ?

Solution :

The tilt is 200V x 0.65 = 130V
At the end of the pulse the voltage is still 200V - 130V = 70V

Energy at the start $W_1 = \dfrac{120.10^{-6} \times 200^2}{2}$ = 2.4 joule

Energy at the end $W_2 = \dfrac{120.10^{-6} \times 70^2}{2}$ = 0.3 joule

Delivered to the patient : 2.4J - 0.3J = 2.1J

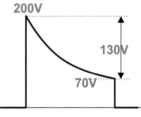

* The total available energy in the charged capacitor is only delivered to the heart if the capacitor is completely discharged i.e. for a pulse duration longer than 5RC.
* Since pulses are always truncated, the energy delivered to the patient is smaller than the maximum available energy !
* The smaller the tilt of the pulse, the larger the difference between the available energy and the energy delivered to the patient.

Abbreviations : RC = timeconstant of the circuit with C = high voltage capacitor and
R = shocking resistance between high voltage electrodes

A. F. Sinnaeve

Figure 3.14

54

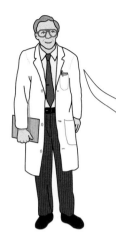

WHO IS AFRAID OF FALLING ROCKS ?

Energy and work are expressed in joule. It takes about one joule of energy to lift an apple approximately three feet.
Do you realize that defibrillators may administer a lot of energy to your patient and that shocks are not harmless !??

1kg

An external defibrillator can deliver shocks of 50 to 400 joule

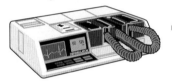

**300 joule is the energy of a block of concrete with a mass of 1 kilogram falling from a height of ca. 30 meter !!!
You better put on your helmet...**

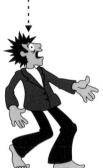

An implantable defibrillator can deliver shocks of 0.5 to 35 joule

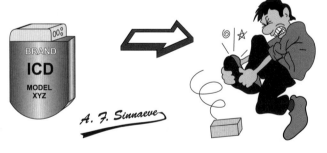

**20 joule corresponds to a block of concrete with a mass of 1 kilogram falling of a height of ca. 2 meter !!!
It still hurts when you got it on your toes...**

A. F. Sinnaeve

Figure 3.15

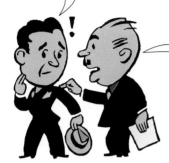

I always use volts for programming of pacemakers and I feel comfortable with this method ! Why should I learn now about energy and joules for the programming of ICDs ?

CAPACITORS 12

Well, the electrical dosage for defibrillation or cardio-version has traditionally been denominated in units of energy, i.e. joules (J) or watt.seconds (Ws). That comes from the well known external defibrillators.
There is only one reason for this practice ! And it isn't difficult to understand. I'll explain it to you.

The normal pacemaker pulse is *nearly* a constant voltage pulse :

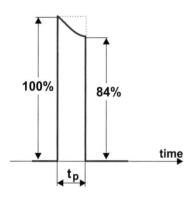

* The geometric surface area of electrodes for contemporary pacing systems is rather small and therefore its total pacing resistance is basically high.
* The pulse duration is very short and the output capacitor of the pacemaker cannot discharge much.

Example :

For an output capacitor C_o = 4.7 µF and a pacing resistance R_p of 600 Ω, the time constant of the circuit is C_oR_p = 600 x 4.7x10^{-6} = 2.82 ms and after a pulse duration t_p of 0.5 ms the voltage is decreased to 84% of the leading edge.

The HV pulse of an ICD is *not at all* a constant voltage pulse :

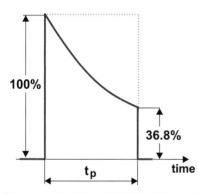

* The surface areas of HV defibrillation electrodes are a lot larger than those for pacing and therefore the load on the lead is small (typical 50 Ω).
* The pulse duration is long and that makes a large tilt.

Example :

For an HV capacitor of 120 µF and lead load of 50 Ω, the time constant is $C_{HV}.R_L$ = 120 x10^{-6} x 50 = 6 ms. If the pulse duration t_p = 6 ms, the voltage at the end of the pulse is decreased to 36.8% of the leading edge and the tilt will be 63.2%.

A. F. Sinnaeve

 An actual pacing stimulus approximates a constant voltage pulse. Hence, the threshold for cardiac pacing determined with such a pulse is also expressed in volt.

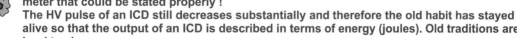 In the first external defibrillators, the voltage at the end of the high voltage pulse dropped to zero, since no truncation was used. The delivered energy in joules was the only parameter that could be stated properly !
The HV pulse of an ICD still decreases substantially and therefore the old habit has stayed alive so that the output of an ICD is described in terms of energy (joules). Old traditions are hard to change.

Evidently, the strength-duration curve for the defibrillation threshold can be expressed in terms of voltage and pulse duration.

Figure 3.16

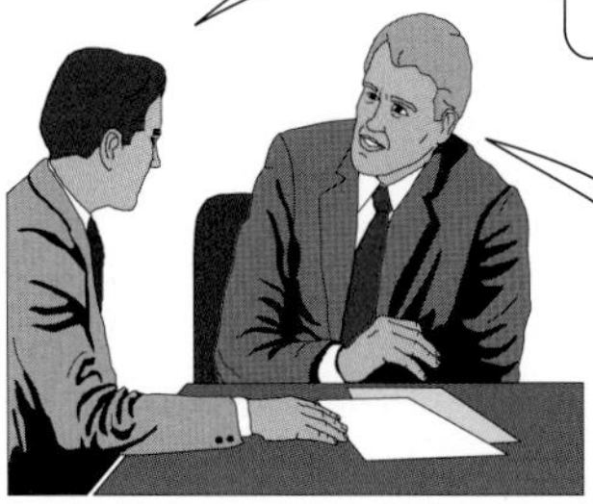

Can you explain why a capacitor needs maintenance ? What is dielectric deformation ? And what is leaking ?

CAPACITORS 13

Well, deformation is not the right word... Electrolytic capacitors are used in ICDs and they need some maintenance to prevent their dielectric from deforming. Let me explain !

Capacitors used in ICDs exhibit unique characteristics ! A combination of high voltage, high capacitance and small case size confines the choice to aluminum electrolytic capacitors.

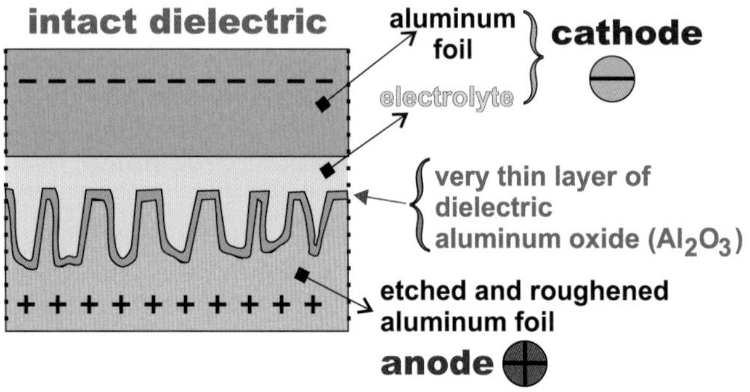
intact dielectric
aluminum foil
electrolyte
cathode
very thin layer of dielectric aluminum oxide (Al_2O_3)
etched and roughened aluminum foil
anode

The dielectric is a very thin layer of aluminum oxide. It is formed on the surface of the anode by an electrolytic process.
By etching and roughing the foil of the anode, its contact surface and therefore its capacitance can be multiplied many times.
The dielectric film is formed by oxidation and the thickness of the film is proportional to the oxidation voltage.

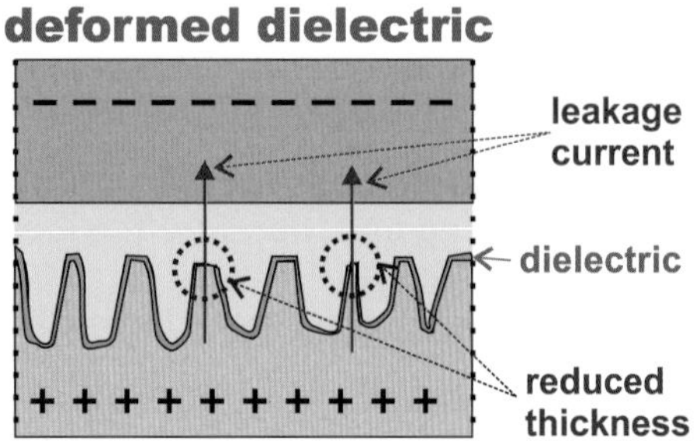
deformed dielectric
leakage current
dielectric
reduced thickness

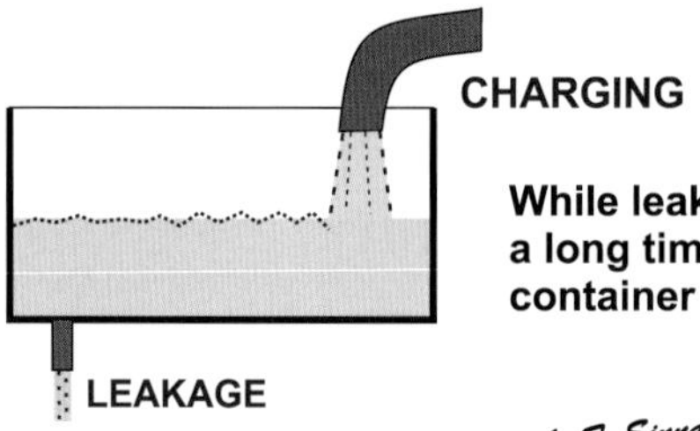
CHARGING
LEAKAGE

While leaking, it takes a long time before the container is full !!!

A. F. Sinnaeve

DEFORMING is a problem of the oxide layer.

With a low voltage (or the absence of voltage) across the terminals of the capacitor, the thickness of the aluminum oxide layer is slowly reduced due to normal chemical reactions within the capacitor. And so, when a higher voltage is applied, leakage current increases and performance declines as it takes longer to charge up the capacitor to the high voltage.

CAPACITOR MAINTENANCE is the solution to the problem

* Capacitor maintenance consists of the periodic charging of the high voltage capacitor (HV cap) in order to keep the dielectric intact so as to mitigate leakage.
* In older ICDs capacitor maintenance (*reforming* or charging) was done manually from the programmer; in contemporary ICDs it is automatically performed at regular intervals of 1 to 6 months (programmable in 1 month intervals).
* If arrhythmia detection charges the HV capacitor to or above the maintenance voltage, the maintenance timer is reset.
* The software in some ICDs (e.g. St Jude) auto-adjusts capacitor reforming to 1 month when the battery voltage reaches 3.05 volt in order to avoid "voltage delay" of the battery.

Figure 3.17

CAPACITORS 14

While the high voltage capacitor is charging, it is important to keep its charging time as short as possible so as to quickly treat the underlying dangerous ventricular tachyarrhythmia requiring shock therapy. There are three causes for a prolonged charging time : (1) Deforming of the capacitor's dielectric (2) Increased internal resistance of the battery and the associated decrease of voltage (3) An occasional component malfunction of the charger, capacitor, etc.

Charging the HV capacitor is like filling a tub !

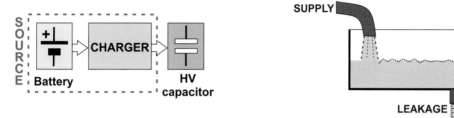

The time to fill the tub lengthens when the leakage is increased and when the supply is reduced. In the same way, the charging time of the capacitor lengthens when the leakage through the dielectric increases or when the supply voltage is reduced.

① **PROLONGED CHARGING TIME DUE TO INADEQUATE MAINTENANCE (REFORMING) OF THE HV CAPACITOR !**

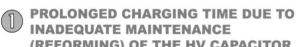

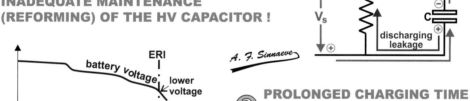

A. F. Sinnaeve

② **PROLONGED CHARGING TIME DUE TO A LOWER VOLTAGE OF THE BATTERY (CLOSE TO ERI)**

In contemporary ICDs the charging time is measured and stored in the memory after a shock and also after automatic reforming. Consequently these charging times must be evaluated during follow-up.

Charge times in excess of 12 seconds merit close attention and frequent follow-up, and those in excess of 15 seconds merit generator replacement !

IF THE CHARGING TIME IS TOO LONG

1. Check the automatic reforming function (is it an older type ?)
2. Verify the condition of the HV capacitor (when was the last full charging or reform performed ? every 90 days at BOL and every 30 days near ERI !)
3. Verify the condition of the battery (check the voltage; ERI ?)
4. If still in doubt, perform a manual reform and dump the charge into the internal test load. Try again after 10 minutes. If the charging is still too long while the battery is OK, there might be malfunction of the charger or the capacitor. Contact the manufacturer if the charging time remains too long (more than 15 seconds).

Abbreviations : HV = high voltage ; BOL = begin of life ; ERI = elective replacement indicator ;

Figure 3.18

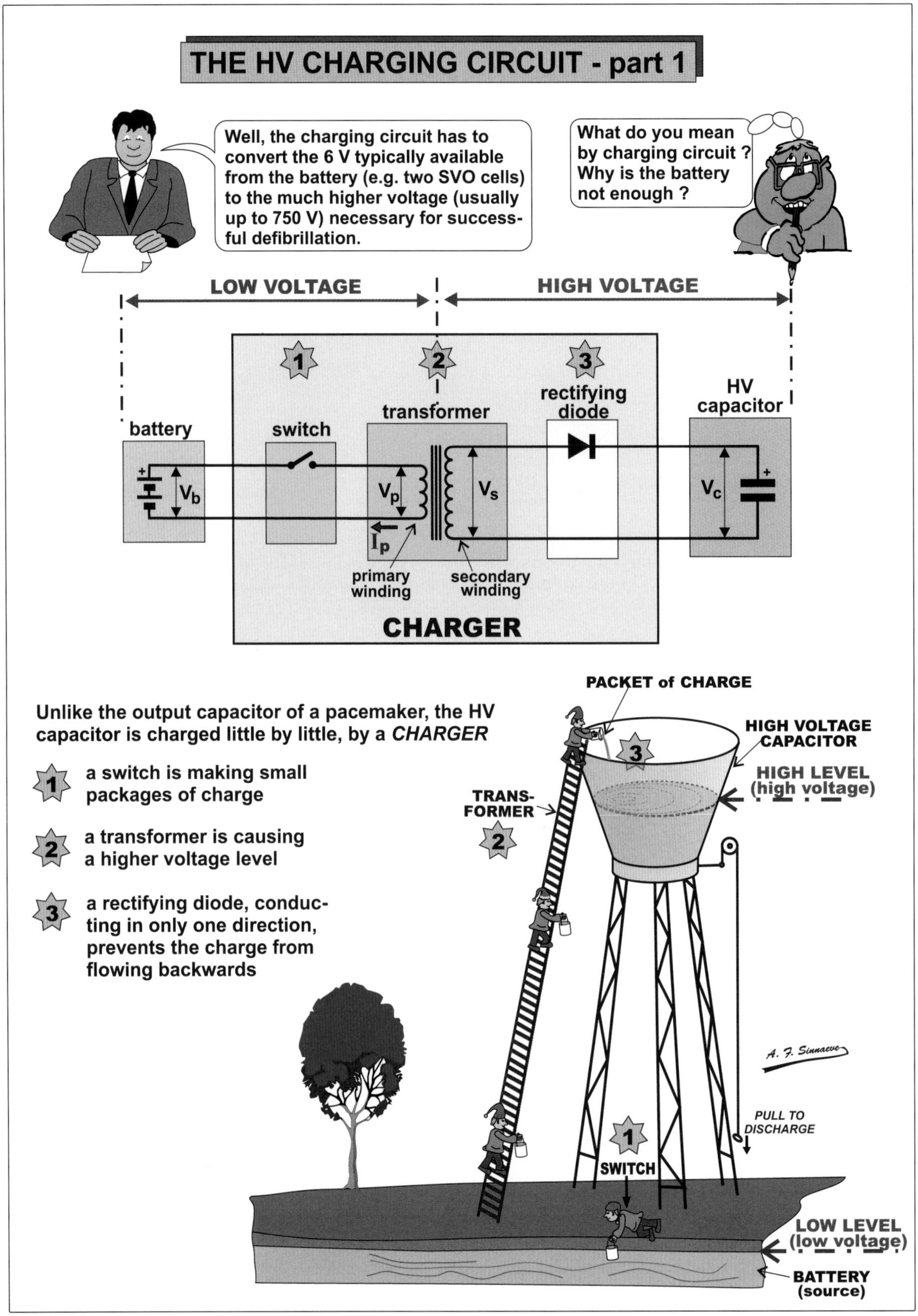
THE HV CHARGING CIRCUIT - part 1
Well, the charging circuit has to convert the 6 V typically available from the battery (e.g. two SVO cells) to the much higher voltage (usually up to 750 V) necessary for successful defibrillation.
What do you mean by charging circuit ? Why is the battery not enough ?
LOW VOLTAGE
HIGH VOLTAGE
1
2
3
battery
switch
transformer
rectifying diode
HV capacitor
Vb
Vp
Vs
Vc
Ip
primary winding
secondary winding
CHARGER
Unlike the output capacitor of a pacemaker, the HV capacitor is charged little by little, by a CHARGER
1 a switch is making small packages of charge
2 a transformer is causing a higher voltage level
3 a rectifying diode, conducting in only one direction, prevents the charge from flowing backwards
PACKET of CHARGE
HIGH VOLTAGE CAPACITOR
HIGH LEVEL (high voltage)
TRANS-FORMER
PULL TO DISCHARGE
SWITCH
LOW LEVEL (low voltage)
BATTERY (source)
A. F. Sinnaeve

Figure 3.19

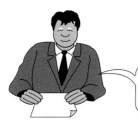

THE HV CHARGING CIRCUIT - part 2

First, let me explain how the small packages of charge are generated by periodically connecting the battery to the primary windings of the transformer ! Then, I will describe how the transformer works.

1 SWITCH

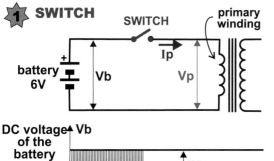

The switching is actually done by a transistor controlled by a high-frequency oscillator (e.g. 50 kHz). The central microprocessor turns on the oscillator after a tachycardia (for which a shock is indicated) is detected and turns it off when the HV capacitor attains the desired voltage for the programmed energy.

The voltage of the battery (Vb) remains constant, but the voltage on primary winding of the transformer (Vp) changes between zero (when the switch is open) and Vb (when the switch is closed).

Each time the switch closes, a current (Ip) flows through the primary winding and some energy from the battery is stored in the magnetic field in the transformer. The current Ip changes almost linear with time while the transformer is "charged up" with magnetic energy.

2 TRANSFORMER — HOW TO CONVERT A LOW VOLTAGE INTO A HIGH VOLTAGE

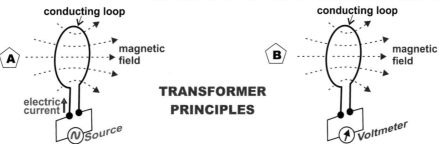

TRANSFORMER PRINCIPLES

When an electric current flows through a circuit loop it generates a magnetic field (proportional to the current : a changing current creates a changing magnetic field).

When a changing magnetic field spreads through a circuit loop, it induces a voltage in the loop. No voltage induction occurs if the magnetic field remains constant !
The induced voltage can be multiplied by putting a number of loops (windings) in series !

A transformer has two windings. An alternating current (I_{AC}) in winding # 1 creates a changing magnetic field. That varying field induces an electric voltage in winding # 2.

Figure 3.20

This is as tough as putting socks on a rooster !

THE HV CHARGING CIRCUIT - part 3

2 TRANSFORMER cont'd

To optimize the energy transfer between the windings, both are wrapped around a ferrous core (concentrating the magnetic field).

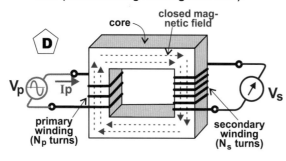

The induced voltage is proportional to the turns ratio : the more turns in coil # 2, as compared to coil # 1, the higher the voltage induced in coil # 2.

$$V_s = \frac{N_s}{N_p} \cdot V_p$$

e.g. if Ns = 100.Np, the secondary voltage Vs is 100 times larger than the primary voltage Vp.

Vp = primary voltage (input) ; Np = number of turns in primary winding ; Vs = secondary voltage (output) ; Ns = number of turns in secondary winding

The induced voltage in the secondary winding (Vs) also depends upon the rate of change of the current through the primary winding (Ip). The faster the rate of change of Ip, the higher the induced voltage Vs. When the switch is disconnecting the battery from the primary winding, the primary current (Ip) is dropping very fast to zero and a very high voltage is induced in the secondary winding.

A. F. Sinnaeve

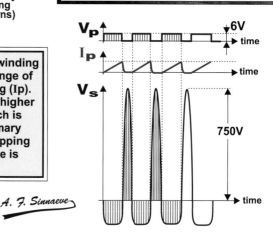

3 RECTIFYING DIODE

A transformer only operates with alternating voltages (AC). That's why the constant voltage (DC) of the battery is chopped by the switch. However, since a DC voltage is needed for defibrillation, the HV capacitor has to contain also a DC voltage. Therefore, a rectifying diode is used to reconvert the alternating voltage from the secondary winding of the transformer into a unidirectional DC voltage !

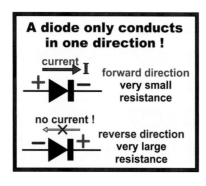

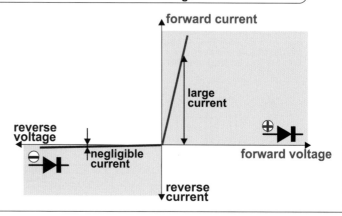

Figure 3.21

THE HV CHARGING CIRCUIT - part 4

3 RECTIFYING DIODE cont'd

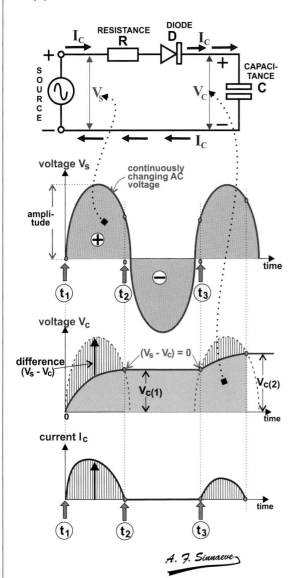

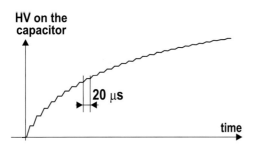

A. F. Sinnaeve

HV on the capacitor

20 µs

time

Electric current is always governed by Ohm's law !

$$I_C = \frac{(V_S - V_C)}{R}$$

t₁ At the start $V_S = 0$ V and $V_C = 0$ V , hence current $I_C = 0$

t₁→t₂ At first the source voltage V_S increases faster than the capacitor voltage V_C, thus the difference $(V_S - V_C)$ increases and so does the current I_C.
The current I_C charges the capacitor, building up V_C.

t₂ After a short time the source voltage V_S starts to decrease while the capacitor voltage V_C is still rising. When the difference becomes zero $(V_S - V_C = 0)$, the current stops.

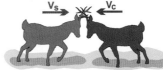

Equally strong : No passage !

t₂→t₃ When V_S becomes smaller than V_C (or negative), the diode is reversely polarized and blocks. Since no more current can flow, the capacitor voltage $V_{C(1)}$ remains constant.

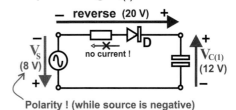

Polarity ! (while source is negative)

t₃ As soon as V_S rises above V_C , I_C starts again and the capacitor voltage is further building up.

The HV capacitor charges little by little ! Each voltage step is a bit smaller than the preceding step. To obtain a charge of 30 J, as much as 250,000 steps may be needed. The higher the needed high voltage (HV) the longer the charging time.

Figure 3.22

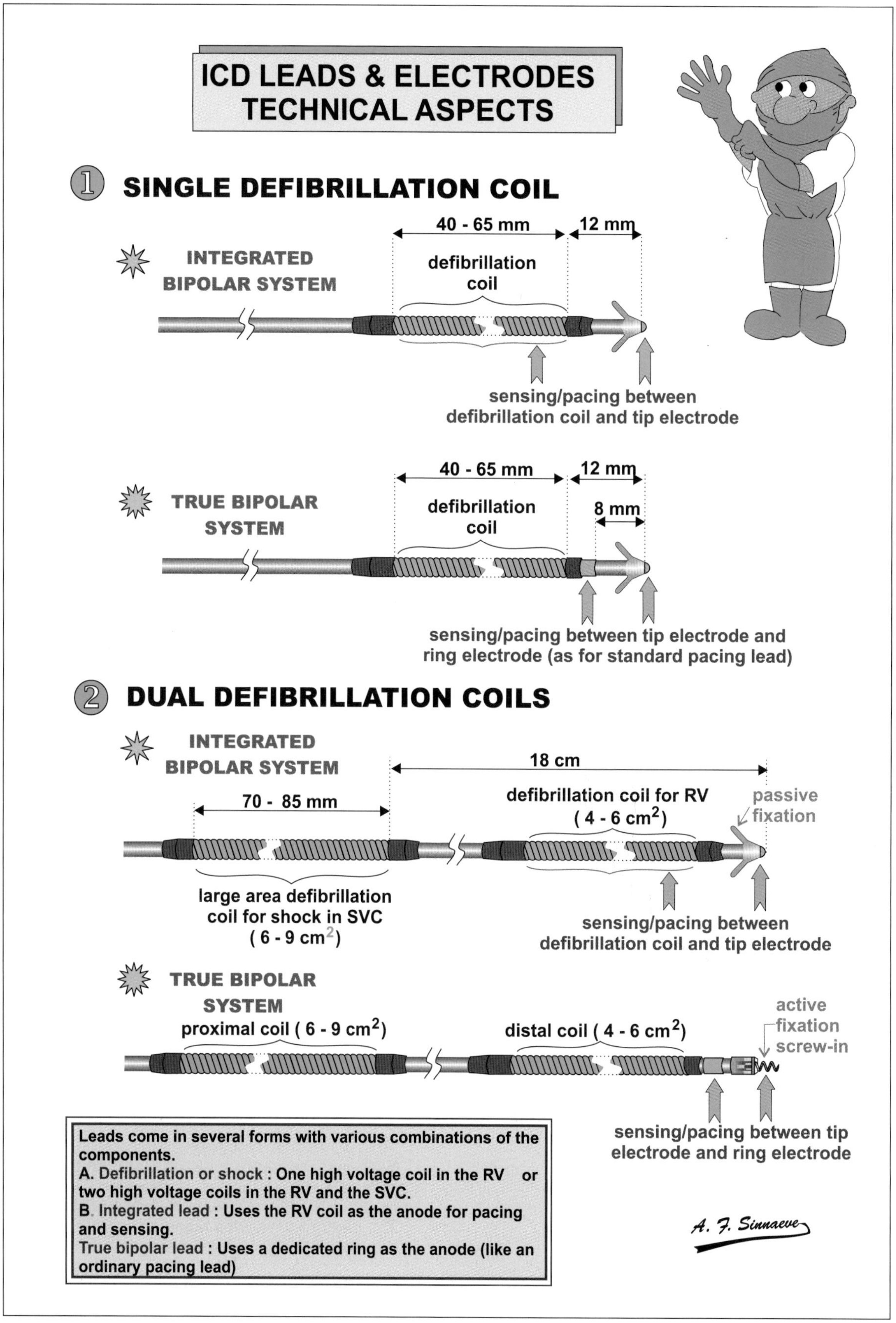
ICD LEADS & ELECTRODES
TECHNICAL ASPECTS
① SINGLE DEFIBRILLATION COIL
INTEGRATED BIPOLAR SYSTEM
40 - 65 mm
12 mm
defibrillation coil
sensing/pacing between defibrillation coil and tip electrode
TRUE BIPOLAR SYSTEM
40 - 65 mm
12 mm
defibrillation coil
8 mm
sensing/pacing between tip electrode and ring electrode (as for standard pacing lead)
② DUAL DEFIBRILLATION COILS
INTEGRATED BIPOLAR SYSTEM
18 cm
70 - 85 mm
defibrillation coil for RV (4 - 6 cm²)
passive fixation
large area defibrillation coil for shock in SVC (6 - 9 cm²)
sensing/pacing between defibrillation coil and tip electrode
TRUE BIPOLAR SYSTEM
proximal coil (6 - 9 cm²)
distal coil (4 - 6 cm²)
active fixation screw-in
sensing/pacing between tip electrode and ring electrode
Leads come in several forms with various combinations of the components.
A. Defibrillation or shock : One high voltage coil in the RV or two high voltage coils in the RV and the SVC.
B. Integrated lead : Uses the RV coil as the anode for pacing and sensing.
True bipolar lead : Uses a dedicated ring as the anode (like an ordinary pacing lead)
A. F. Sinnaeve

Figure 3.23

ICD LEADS & ELECTRODES TECHNICAL ASPECTS - 2

EPICARDIAL DEFIBRILLATION PATCHES & THEIR POSITIONING

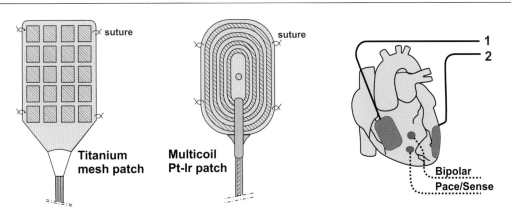

Titanium mesh patch

Multicoil Pt-Ir patch

1
2

Bipolar Pace/Sense

ANCILLARY DEFIBRILLATION ELECTRODES

A third epicardial patch

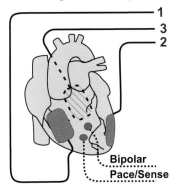

1
3
2

Bipolar Pace/Sense

Subcutaneous Patch

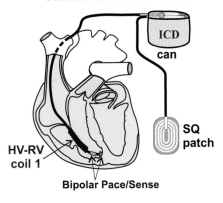

ICD can

SQ patch

HV-RV coil 1

Bipolar Pace/Sense

Single SVC lead

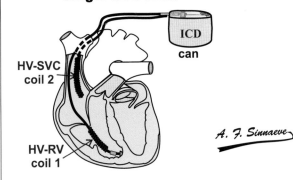

ICD can

HV-SVC coil 2

HV-RV coil 1

A. F. Sinnaeve

Subcutaneous Array

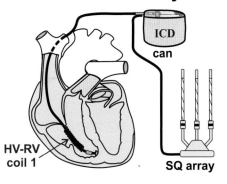

ICD can

HV-RV coil 1

SQ array

Figure 3.24

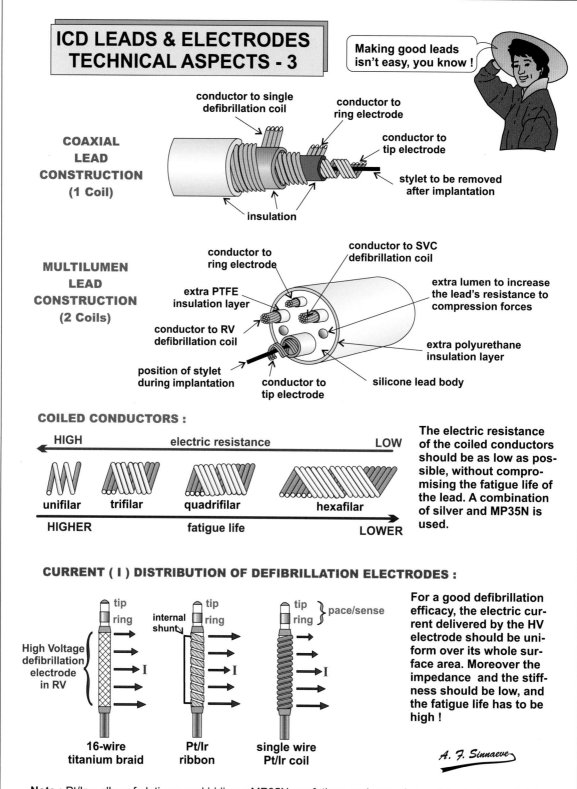

ICD LEADS & ELECTRODES TECHNICAL ASPECTS - 3

Making good leads isn't easy, you know !

COAXIAL LEAD CONSTRUCTION (1 Coil)

conductor to single defibrillation coil
conductor to ring electrode
conductor to tip electrode
stylet to be removed after implantation
insulation

MULTILUMEN LEAD CONSTRUCTION (2 Coils)

conductor to ring electrode
conductor to SVC defibrillation coil
extra PTFE insulation layer
extra lumen to increase the lead's resistance to compression forces
conductor to RV defibrillation coil
extra polyurethane insulation layer
position of stylet during implantation
conductor to tip electrode
silicone lead body

COILED CONDUCTORS :

HIGH ← electric resistance → LOW

unifilar   trifilar   quadrifilar   hexafilar

HIGHER   fatigue life → LOWER

The electric resistance of the coiled conductors should be as low as possible, without compromising the fatigue life of the lead. A combination of silver and MP35N is used.

CURRENT (I) DISTRIBUTION OF DEFIBRILLATION ELECTRODES :

tip
ring
internal shunt
tip
ring
tip
ring } pace/sense

High Voltage defibrillation electrode in RV

I   I   I

16-wire titanium braid   **Pt/Ir ribbon**   **single wire Pt/Ir coil**

For a good defibrillation efficacy, the electric current delivered by the HV electrode should be uniform over its whole surface area. Moreover the impedance and the stiffness should be low, and the fatigue life has to be high !

A. F. Sinnaeve

Note : Pt/Ir = alloy of platinum and iridium ; MP35N = a fatigue and corrosion resistant alloy containing nickel, chromium and molybdenum ; PTFE = teflon (poly-tetra-fluor-ethylene)

Figure 3.25

LEAD CONNECTIONS

Connecting an ICD may be rather complicated ! Apart from the international standards, older connections are still used and therefore adapters may be needed. Manufacturers use different arrangements on their ICDs and the physician has to work very carefully.

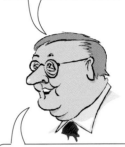

AAMI - ISO STANDARDS :

IS-1 connection (Pace/Sense)

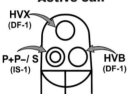

connector pin (cathode)
sealing rings
insulation
1.59
5.08
3.23
connector ring (anode)
2 coaxial helix conductors

DF-1 connection (High Voltage)

1.25
5.08
3.23
all dimensions are in mm

SOME EXAMPLES

**MEDTRONIC
Single chamber ICD
Active can**

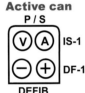

HVX (DF-1)
P+P-/ S (IS-1)
HVB (DF-1)

Medtronic nomenclature :

HV = high voltage (shock electrode)
HVA = A for active (active or hot can)
HVB = B for bottom (coil in RV)
HVX = X for extra (coil in SVC)

HVX & HVA have always the same polarity
HVB < HVA means active can is positive while RV coil is negative

All defibrillation systems contain either 2 or 3 HV defibrillation electrodes (not leads!!!)
One HV defibrillation electrode must always be in the RV.
One ancillary HV electrode may be on a separate intravascular lead, normally positioned in the SVC

**GUIDANT
Dual chamber ICD
Active can**

P / S

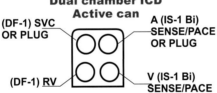

V A   IS-1
− +   DF-1
DEFIB

**ST JUDE MED
Dual chamber ICD
Active can**

(DF-1) SVC OR PLUG
A (IS-1 Bi) SENSE/PACE OR PLUG
(DF-1) RV
V (IS-1 Bi) SENSE/PACE

**Older Arrangement
Dual chamber ICD
Without active can**

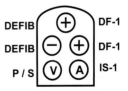

DEFIB   +   DF-1
DEFIB   − +   DF-1
P / S   V A   IS-1

✿ * With the advent of biphasic defibrillation waveforms and the "hot can", a defibrillation lead with either a single RV coil or 2 coils (RV and SVC) will work satisfactorily in virtually all patients. Additional leads were useful in the past but with current technology they are rarely needed to achieve an acceptable defibrillation threshold.

✿ * The pacing/sensing part of a defibrillation lead can be replaced if there is a problem such as undersensing while keeping the defibrillation coils active. The IS-1 pin of the pacing/sensing part of the defibrillation lead is capped and a new separate pacing/sensing pacemaker lead is inserted into the IS-1 port of the header.

✿ * DF-1 ports that are not utilized must be plugged !!!

✿ * Normal polarity : the HV defibrillation coil in the RV is traditionally negative while the hot can and all ancillary HV electrodes (SVC coil and SQ patch or array) are positive. *A. F. Sinnaeve*

Abbreviations : AAMI = Association for the Advancement of Medical Instrumentation ; ISO = International Organization for Standardization ; HV = high voltage ; RV = right ventricle ; SVC = superior vena cava ; SQ = subcutaneous ;
Note for Medtronic : P+P-/S = bipolar pacing and sensing (P+ is the ring electrode; P- is the tip electrode)

Figure 3.26

NEW ISO STANDARD for a FOUR-POLE CONNECTOR

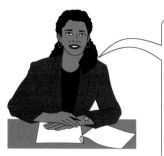

A new "International Standard" for a 4-pole defibrillator and pacemaker connector system is developed by a group of experts from a variety of manufacturers.
The new connector will have *several advantages* :
1. The proposed connector will reduce pocket bulk by eliminating lead bifurcations/trifurcations and reducing header size.
2. High and low voltage functions are combined into a single connector on defibrillator leads.
3. Seals are located in the pulse generator header rather than on the lead connector, providing fresh seals with every pulse generator replacement.
4. Features will allow for single setscrew lead fixation or for passive (tool-less) retention.

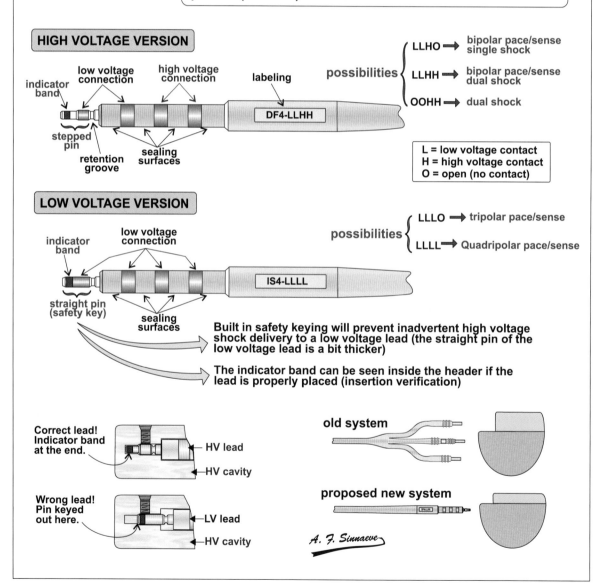

Figure 3.27

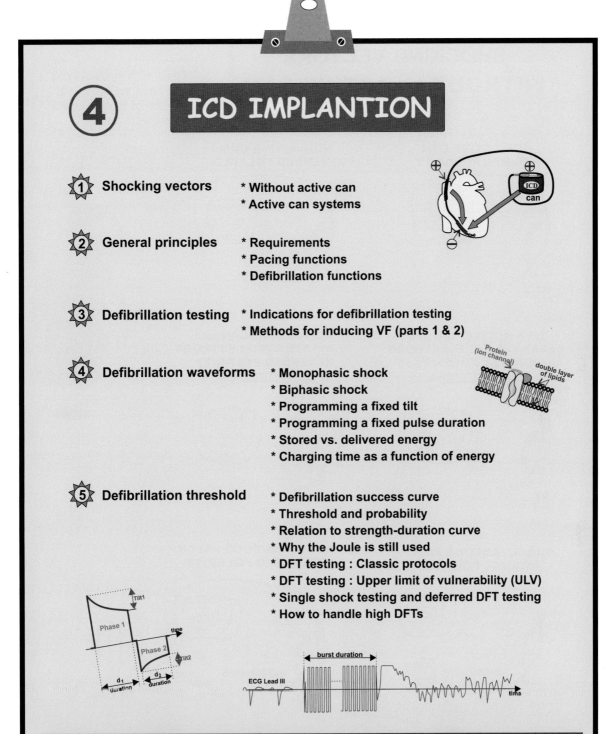

4 ICD IMPLANTION

1 Shocking vectors

* Without active can
* Active can systems

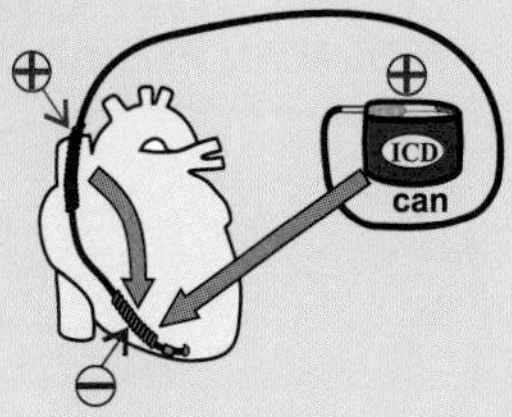

2 General principles

* Requirements
* Pacing functions
* Defibrillation functions

3 Defibrillation testing

* Indications for defibrillation testing
* Methods for inducing VF (parts 1 & 2)

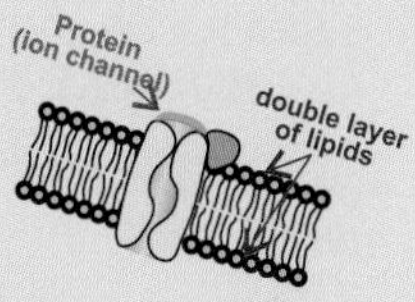

4 Defibrillation waveforms

* Monophasic shock
* Biphasic shock
* Programming a fixed tilt
* Programming a fixed pulse duration
* Stored vs. delivered energy
* Charging time as a function of energy

5 Defibrillation threshold

* Defibrillation success curve
* Threshold and probability
* Relation to strength-duration curve
* Why the Joule is still used
* DFT testing : Classic protocols
* DFT testing : Upper limit of vulnerability (ULV)
* Single shock testing and deferred DFT testing
* How to handle high DFTs

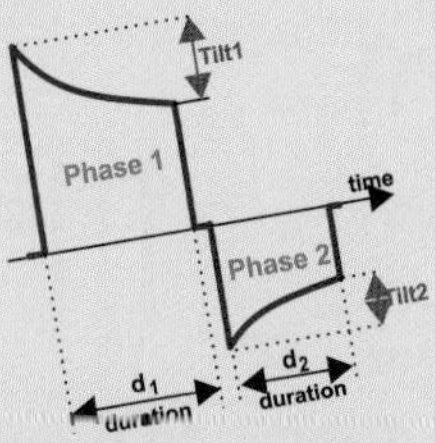

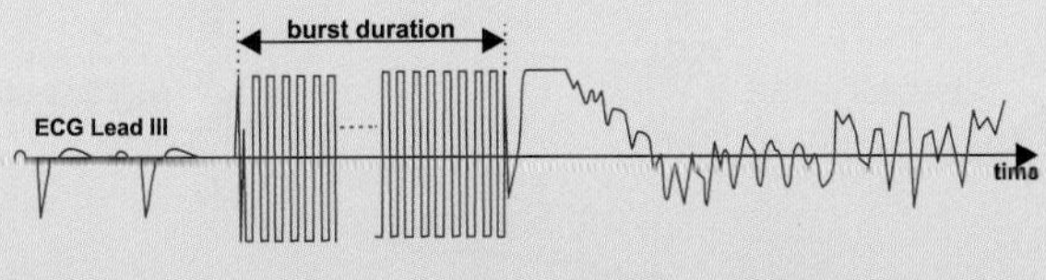

Figure 4.00

68

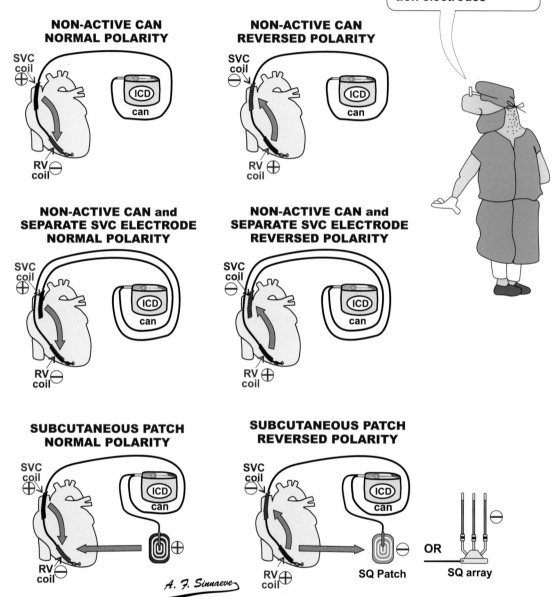

SHOCKING VECTORS WITHOUT AN ACTIVE CAN

Older ICD systems did not have an active can as one of the defibrillation electrodes

NON-ACTIVE CAN NORMAL POLARITY

NON-ACTIVE CAN REVERSED POLARITY

NON-ACTIVE CAN and SEPARATE SVC ELECTRODE NORMAL POLARITY

NON-ACTIVE CAN and SEPARATE SVC ELECTRODE REVERSED POLARITY

SUBCUTANEOUS PATCH NORMAL POLARITY

SUBCUTANEOUS PATCH REVERSED POLARITY

A. F. Sinnaeve

Abbreviations : HV = high voltage; RV = right ventricle; SVC = superior vena cava; SQ = subcutaneous

Figure 4.01

SHOCKING VECTORS
ACTIVE CAN SYSTEMS

Biphasic waveforms have lowered the defibrillation energy significantly. Furthermore the use of the can as an active defibrillation electrode (active or hot can), preferably implanted on the left side, has almost eliminated the need for subcutaneous patches or arrays, which were used more commonly in the past with older technology. These ancillary electrodes are still used when a high defibrillation threshold (DFT) is encountered. Fortunately this is very uncommon.

Also changing polarity may be worth trying in the setting of a high DFT, but this manipulation does not consistently help. Note that polarity can be reversed by reprogramming !

ACTIVE CAN NORMAL POLARITY

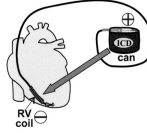

ACTIVE CAN REVERSED POLARITY

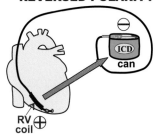

ACTIVE CAN NORMAL POLARITY

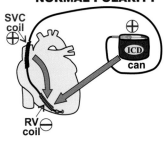

ACTIVE CAN REVERSED POLARITY

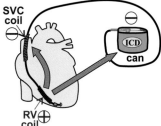

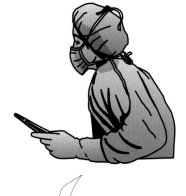

ACTIVE CAN and SEPARATE SVC ELECTRODE

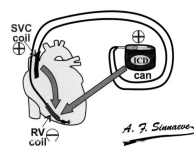

A. F. Sinnaeve

ACTIVE CAN and ANCILLARY SQ PATCH

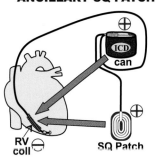

Abbreviations : DFT = defibrillation threshold ; RV = right ventricle ; SVC = superior vena cava ; SQ = subcutaneous ;

Figure 4.02

ICD IMPLANTATION - part 1 : REQUIREMENTS

Expertise in electrophysiology according to the guidelines :

* Due to the downsizing of ICDs, pectoral implantation by electrophysiologists has become routine. However, acute testing and management of ICDs require a lot of expertise !
* Skilled technical support personnel (engineer, technician, EP-trained cardiovascular nurse) are necessary.
* The operator must be familliar with the indications and the official guidelines for ICD (and pacemaker) implantation !

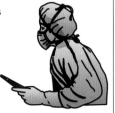

HRS, AHA, ACC, etc.

Access to the patient's complete chart :

* Indication for ICD
* Medications
* Allergies
* Laboratory tests (INR, blood group, ...)
* Latest 12-lead ECG and chest X ray

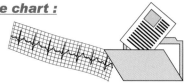
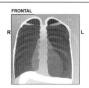

FRONTAL

R   L

The presence of the right ICD, leads, technical manual, and programmer should be checked before starting the procedure !

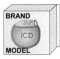
BRAND
ICD
MODEL
Sterile ICD

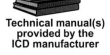
Technical manual(s) provided by the ICD manufacturer

Sterile magnets

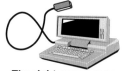
The right programmer with sterile head

Sterile leads & subcutaneous arrays or patches

Required equipment

* Physiologic recorders for monitoring the ECG, blood pressure, oxygenation and respiration are necessary. Recorders are also used to document and evaluate electrophysiologic variables.

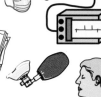
ECG machine

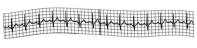

* Two functional external defibrillators (preferably with biphasic waveform) should always be available during defibrillation testing.

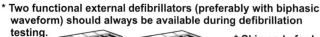

* Skin pads for backup defibillation should be put on the patient before the start of the procedure.

ICD
pad
pad

* Imaging equipment (fluoroscopy) is obligatory for positioning of the leads

* Oxygen

* A "crash cart" for emergencies is mandatory

* Antibiotics

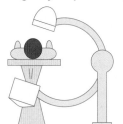

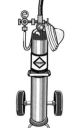

A. F. Sinnaeve

* Equipment for anesthesia is essential (during defibrillation threshold testing and if a subcutaneous electrode patch or array may be necessary)

Figure 4.03

ICD IMPLATATION - part 2 : PACING FUNCTION

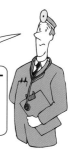

Contemporary ICDs are capable of treating not only life-threatening ventricular arrhythmias, but also bradyarrhythmias with dual chamber pacing and even congestive heart failure with biventricular pacing.
Positioning of the defibrillation lead must satisfy the need for optimal pacing, sensing and defibrillation.

Measure, verify and adjust !

Use a Pacemaker System Analyzer (PSA) or programmer to measure pacing thresholds and signals (atrial and ventricular). The programmer or PSA also measures the pacing impedance.

ACCEPTABLE VALUES AT INITIAL IMPLANTATION	Atrial	Ventricular
Voltage threshold (at 0.5ms pulse duration)	≤ 1.5V	≤ 0.5-1.0 V
Bipolar endocardial signal	≥ 2.0 mV	≥ 5 mV
Pacing impedance (at 5V and 0.5ms)°	< 750 Ω	< 750 Ω
Slew rate (only measured if the amplitude is small)	—	≥ 0.75 V/s

° *Special high impedance leads will register a higher impedance (consult manufacturers notes)*

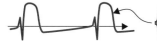

{ ST-segment shift recorded from tip electrode, due to current of injury, indicates good endocardial contact of RV. This ensures a low pacing threshold.

---

* Try pacing near threshold with deep respiration and coughing and look for eventual unstable position of the leads.
* Look at lateral or near lateral fluoroscopy to document the anterior position of the right ventricular lead and/or atrial lead if positioned in the right atrial appendage.
* If there is sensing when the ICD is placed in the subcutaneous tissue, reprogram to make sure that both channels are capable of pacing. The magnet in ICDs does not eliminate antibradycardia pacing. To confirm the pacing capability, the ICD can be temporarily programmed to the DOO mode.
* Pace A and V sequentially at 10V to rule out diaphragmatic stimulation
* Look for retrograde VA conduction at the time of implantation or later before hospital discharge.

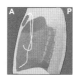

After connecting the leads to the ICD and placing it in the surgical pocket, retest the pacing thresholds, signal amplitude and pacing impedances using the ICD itself and the programmer.

MARKERS & INTRACARDIAC ELECTROGRAMS

Take simultaneous recordings of ECG with annotated markers and intracardiac electrograms. Document clean recordings free of interference that may be a sign of a lead or connection problem.

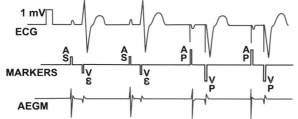

Appropriate ventricular sensing is crucial because the VF signals are variable and likely to be small !
Once the leads are connected, take a long rhythm strip to confirm appropriate sensing and amplitude of the ventricular electrogram on the recording paper.

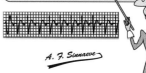

A. F. Sinnaeve

---

* Take a permanent chest X-ray soon after implantation for lead position and to rule out pneumothorax.
* Inspect by X-ray or fluoroscopy if the connector pin is well fixed.
* Interrogate the PM and reprogram if necessary; make a print-out for the patient's file.
* Document all implantation data in the patient's chart.

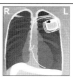

There is no need to perform ATP testing or low energy cardioversion for VT !

Figure 4.04

ICD IMPLATATION - part 3
DEFIBRILLATION TESTING

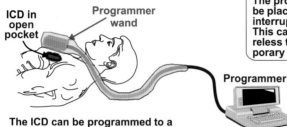

ICD in open pocket

Programmer wand

The testing procedure is performed with the ICD in the surgical pocket before closure of the wound. The device itself is used for testing defibrillation efficacy (device-based testing). The programmer wand must be placed over the ICD for uninterrupted telemetry. This can now be done with wireless telemetry with contemporary systems.

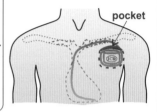

pocket

Programmer

The wand and its cable should be isolated from the patient by a sterile tubing (or the wand should be wireless).

The ICD can be programmed to a cutoff of 180 - 200 bpm and a ventricular sensitivity of 1.2 mV. Sensing VF potentials at 1.2 mV ensures VF sensing at the usual programmed sensitivity of 0.3 mV for long-term function. The first shock value is for testing. Subsequent shocks must be maximal ! A number of questions have to be answered. What is the best way to administer general anesthesia during shock delivery ? Is sensing of VF appropriate ? Is detection (diagnosis) appropriate ? Is VF converted with a given shock ? What is the charge time between device diagnosis and delivery of the shock ? What is the high voltage (HV) or shocking impedance of the system ? This is usually between 20 and 100 Ω at implantation. In the past, the only method for measuring shocking (HV) lead impedance in patients with an ICD was to deliver a low energy test shock. Measurements of shock (HV) impedance are now taken in most ICDs via painless, subthreshold pulses that do not capture the heart thereby eliminating the need to perform painful, high-voltage testing with a small shock before DFT testing.

INDUCTION OF VF

* A method has to be choosen, depending upon the manufacturer and the capabilities of the device and programmer.
    * *Shock on T-wave during vulnerable period*
    * *DC voltage (DC fibber - St Jude)*
    * *Burst of impulses - 50 Hz burst (Medtronic)*
      - V Fib burst (Guidant)
    * *External AC voltage*
* Check the pacing lead impedances by telemetry before inducing VF. Also test the defibrillation impedance with a manual test shock before VF induction (optional).

DETERMINATION OF DFT AND SAFETY MARGIN

* Defibrillation thresholds (DFTs) are determined by a sequence of repeated fibrillation - defibrillation trials. There are many protocols to establish DFT. The one shown below is probably one of the most popular DFT testing protocol.
  In most cases a "two-shock" protocol is used to verify that a measured safety margin of 10 J is guaranteed (i.e. the measured DFT is at least 10 J below maximum energy ouput of the ICD).

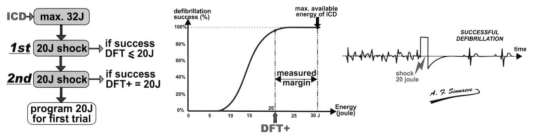

ICD → max. 32J

1st 20J shock → if success DFT ≤ 20J

2nd 20J shock → if success DFT+ = 20J

program 20J for first trial

defibrillation success (%)

max. available energy of ICD

measured margin

DFT+

SUCCESSFUL DEFIBRILLATION

time

shock 20 joule

A. F. Sinnaeve

* When fibrillation is redetected (unsuccessful first attempt) the next shock should be at the maximal output according to the programming sequence done before DFT testing (i.e. 32 J in the example).
* High DFTs require special attention (check the integrity of all connections; check position and fixation of epicardial patches; try repositioning of the lead and change polarity; add a SVC lead or deactivate the SVC electrode if a dual coil lead is used; use a subcutaneous array or patch).
* Abnormal HV impedance :
    - Too high : the lead is not secured or the lead is damaged ;
    - Too low : outer insulation has been damaged.
    If the problem cannot be corrected, the lead should be replaced.

Figure 4.05

INDICATIONS FOR DEFIBRILLATION TESTING

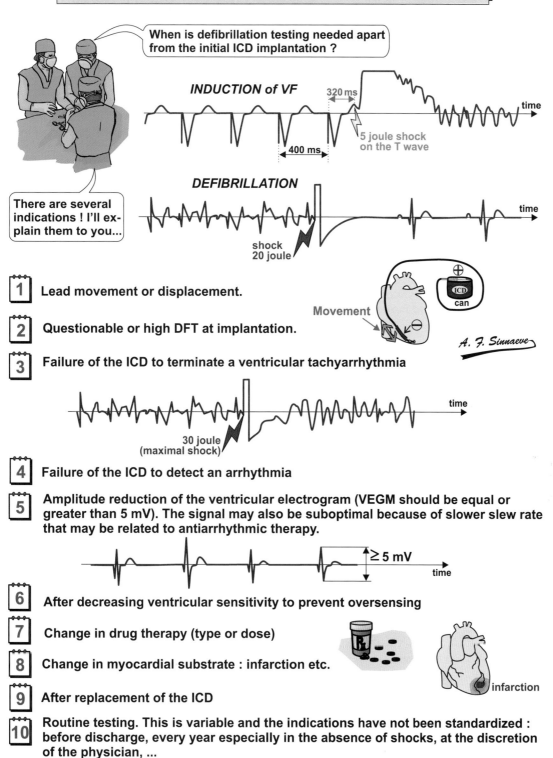

When is defibrillation testing needed apart from the initial ICD implantation ?

INDUCTION of VF

320 ms

400 ms

time

5 joule shock on the T wave

DEFIBRILLATION

time

shock 20 joule

There are several indications ! I'll explain them to you...

Movement

A. F. Sinnaeve

1 Lead movement or displacement.

2 Questionable or high DFT at implantation.

3 Failure of the ICD to terminate a ventricular tachyarrhythmia

time

30 joule (maximal shock)

4 Failure of the ICD to detect an arrhythmia

5 Amplitude reduction of the ventricular electrogram (VEGM should be equal or greater than 5 mV). The signal may also be suboptimal because of slower slew rate that may be related to antiarrhythmic therapy.

$\geq$ 5 mV

time

6 After decreasing ventricular sensitivity to prevent oversensing

7 Change in drug therapy (type or dose)

8 Change in myocardial substrate : infarction etc.

infarction

9 After replacement of the ICD

10 Routine testing. This is variable and the indications have not been standardized : before discharge, every year especially in the absence of shocks, at the discretion of the physician, ...

Abbreviations : *DFT = defibrillation threshold ; VEGM = ventricular electrogram ;*

Figure 4.06

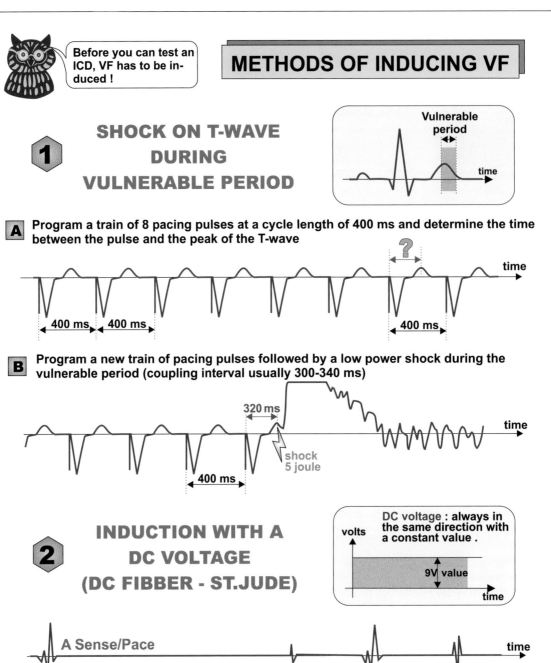

Before you can test an ICD, VF has to be induced !

METHODS OF INDUCING VF

1 SHOCK ON T-WAVE
DURING
VULNERABLE PERIOD

Vulnerable period

time

A Program a train of 8 pacing pulses at a cycle length of 400 ms and determine the time between the pulse and the peak of the T-wave

?

time

400 ms   400 ms   400 ms

B Program a new train of pacing pulses followed by a low power shock during the vulnerable period (coupling interval usually 300-340 ms)

320 ms

time

shock
5 joule

400 ms

2 INDUCTION WITH A
DC VOLTAGE
(DC FIBBER - ST.JUDE)

DC voltage : always in the same direction with a constant value .

volts

9V value

time

A Sense/Pace

time

Defib. Status

x   x x x   x   x x x   x   x
      F F F   F   F F F   F   F

time

DC Fibber   9V

V Sense/Pace

time

programmable 0.5 to 5.0 sec
recommended : 0.5 to 2.0 sec

A. F. Sinnaeve

Figure 4.07

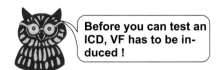

Before you can test an ICD, VF has to be induced !

METHODS OF INDUCING VF

3 ### INDUCTION WITH A
50 Hz burst (Medtronic)

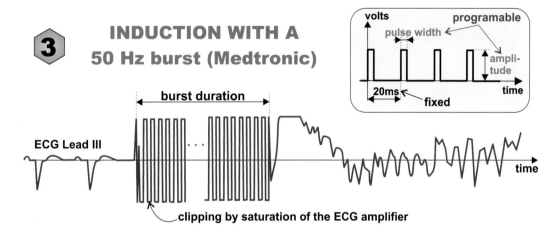

The repetition frequency of the pulses is fixed at 50 Hz thus fixing the cycle length at :

$$\frac{1}{50} \text{ sec} = 0.020 \text{ s} = 20 \text{ ms}$$

The pulse width is selectable (0.03; 0.06; 0.1; 0.2; ...; 1.6 ms) and so is the pulse amplitude (1; 2; ... ...6; 8 V). The 50 Hz burst is generated by the ICD as long as the "Burst Press & Hold" on the programmer is pressed.

4 ### INDUCTION WITH A
"V Fib" burst (GUIDANT)

Delivers high rate, high output pulses through the shocking electrodes at the command of the programmer.
Principally the same as the 50 Hz burst except that the amplitude and the pulse width are fixed while the cycle length is selectable (50 ms for V Fib Low or 30 ms for V Fib High).

5 ### EXTERNAL INDUCTION
WITH AC VOLTAGE

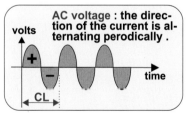

While using an external source to induce VF, the ICD has to be blinded from the induction so it doesn't detect it as an arrhythmia. After VF is induced, the ICD should be unblinded so it can detect VF and deliver therapy.

CL = cycle length = 20 ms (Europe)
or = 16.6 ms (USA)

WARNING Keep an external defibrillator (preferably 2) immediately available and on stand-by ! Before starting, make sure the batteries are loaded and the entire equipment is ready to use !!!

A. F. Sinnaeve

Figure 4.08

DEFIBRILLATION WAVEFORMS - 1

The exact mechanism by which electrical energy defibrillates the heart has not yet been determined.
The electrical shock is thought to electrically synchronize cells by either activation or, for cells in the refractory state, by extending refractoriness !

MONOPHASIC SHOCK

- The monophasic shock defibrillates by resynchronizing the myocardial cells in the large majority of ventricular cells (at least 60%, according to some studies even 90%).

- Recovered cells (i.e. those in electrical diastole) are stimulated while the action potential is extended for those cells that are already activated.

- The required voltage for this resynchronization is rather high, i.e. the defibrillation threshold with monophasic shocks is also high.

MEMBRANE OF A CARDIAC CELL

The double lipid layer of the cell membrane is an insulator and forms a capacitor with the conducting electrolytes at both sides. The intrinsic proteins are equivalent to a leakage resistance. Consequently, the cell membrane has a time constant $R_m \times C_m$ and will be charged exponentially if a constant current is applied. However, a HV pulse applied to cardiac tissue also sees an intercellular resistance R_i between cells. Therefore the total resistance is a combination of R_i and R_m.

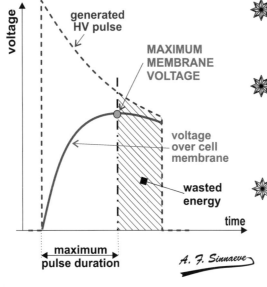

- The shock voltage is not constant but decreases exponentially because it is generated by discharging the HV capacitor. Therefore, the membrane voltage rises to a maximum and then decreases again.

- Obviously, at maximum membrane voltage, the largest number of cells are able to be captured. By extending the shock beyond this point, the decreasing voltage reduces the probability of successful defibrillation perhaps by interfering with the potential capture that was initiated at the peak.

- Obviously, if the pulse duration is too long a lot of energy is wasted (corresponding with the shaded area). Indirectly, this cuts down battery life since more energy is stored in the capacitor than strictly needed.

A. F. Sinnaeve

Abbreviations : HV = high voltage

Figure 4.09

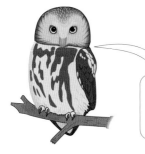

DEFIBRILLATION WAVEFORMS - 2

Biphasic waveforms have become the standard waveform for most (if not all) ICD pulse generators !
The effectiveness of the single capacitor biphasic waveform is superior to that of the previously used monophasic waveform !

BIPHASIC SHOCK

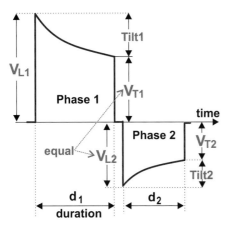

- ❖ The polarity of the pulse is reversed by simply switching the lead connections inside the ICD; therefore, the trailing edge of phase 1 always equals the leading edge of phase 2.

- ⌘ The function of phase 1 is identical to that of a monophasic shock i.e. to depolarize and/or extend the refractory periods of virtually all ventricular myocytes.

- ✳ The function of phase 2 is to remove residual charge on cells that were not "captured" (i.e. those without extension of refractory period). This "burping" diminishes the number of borderline stimulated cells, which would otherwise exhibit delayed activations capable to desynchronize the heart.

- ◈ The second phase also serves to remove charge from cells that were too close to the electrodes and hence were at least temporarily injured by the excessive fields.

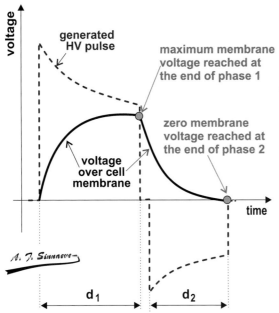

- ✴ The membrane should ideally attain its maximum possible voltage at the end of phase 1, while it should return to zero voltage at the end of phase 2.

- ✴ The defibrillation threshold and hence the pulse duration to reach maximum possible membrane voltage, depends upon the ICD type (value of HV capacitor), type and position of shocking electrodes (shock impedance) and the time constant of the cell membranes of the patient (medication).

- ✴ The time constant for mammalian cardiac tissue ranges between 2 and 5 ms. For typical values of 120 - 140 μF for the HV capacitor and a shock impedance of about 50 Ω, the duration of phase 1 is 4 - 5 ms and the duration of phase 2 is 2.5 - 3 ms.

Note : Time constant of mammalian cardiac tissue = time it takes for the voltage over the tissue to reach 63.2% of an available constant voltage (see Capacitors 6).
Abbreviations : V_L = voltage of leading edge (at the start of the shock); V_T = voltage of the trailing edge (at the end of the shock); d_1 = duration of phase 1; d_2 = duration of phase 2; HV = high voltage

Figure 4.10

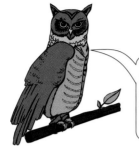

PROGRAMMING
DEFIBRILLATION WAVEFORMS - 1

Early investigators decided to truncate the exponentially decreasing waveform from the discharging HV capacitor at a time duration equal to one time constant which produced a 63.3% decay of the waveform voltage. This historical "accident" is probably responsible for the widespread acceptance of a 65% tilt of the waveforms used today.

PROGRAMMING A FIXED TILT

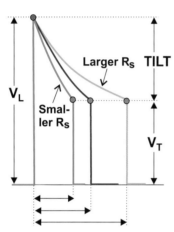

Energy at a given tilt remains constant regardless of pulse duration. The values of C_{HV}, V_L and V_T all remain constant at a given tilt (C_{HV} = the high voltage capacitor of the ICD).

The energy of all these waveforms is identical according to the formula :

$$W_{deliv} = \frac{C_{HV}}{2} \cdot (V_L^2 - V_T^2)$$

despite the variations of the pulse duration provided the tilt remains the same.

CONSTANT TILT = CONSTANT ENERGY !

The device delivers a constant energy by varying the pulse width as a function of the patient's shock resistance R_S. A smaller resistance between the high voltage electrodes results in a shorter pulse duration.

* Studies have shown that tilts between 40% and 65% are better than 80% tilts.
* Since the pulse duration is adapted automatically , it should be remembered that waveforms longer than 10 ms can actually re-fibrillate the heart !
* When a waveform is specified as fixed tilt, programming of the therapy is done in joules of delivered energy (peak voltage may be provided as a reference value)

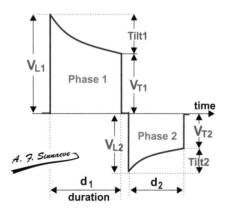

For all manufacturers $V_{L2} = V_{T1}$

MEDTRONIC (Marquis)
tilt 1 & tilt 2 are both fixed at 50%
durations d_1 & d_2 automatically adapted

GUIDANT (Vitality)
tilt 1 is fixed at 65%
duration d_1 is automatically adapted
duration $d_2 = 0.66 \times d_1$

ST. JUDE MEDICAL (Photon)
it is possible to program a fixed tilt at 42%, 50%, 60%, 65% (but a fixed pulse duration is also possible)

Abbreviations : C_{HV} = high voltage capacitor inside the ICD expressed in farad; HV = high voltage; Rs = shock resistance (typ. 50 Ω);V_L = voltage of the leading edge; V_T = voltage of the trailing edge of the HV pulse;

Figure 4.11

PROGRAMMING
DEFIBRILLATION WAVEFORMS - 2

To defibrillate the heart a minimum potential gradient or voltage is required. Therefore, energy as a measure of defibrillation "dosage" has fundamental limitations. Programming the HV shock by voltage and pulse duration takes some more time, but studies show that "tuned" waveforms can lower defibrillation thresholds !

PROGRAMMING A FIXED PULSE DURATION

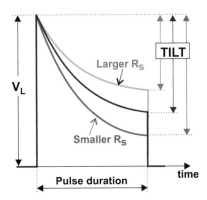

The device delivers an amount of energy that varies as a function of the patient's shock resistance R$_S$. A smaller resistance between the high voltage electrodes results in a larger tilt and the delivery of more energy.

Adjusting the pulse durations of both phase 1 and phase 2 (of a biphasic pulse), allows a fine tuning of the output according to the "burping" theory. This fine tuning results in the best defibrillation efficiency, i.e. the lowest defibrillation threshold.

* Avoiding long pulse durations (i.e. longer than 10 ms) that can re-fibrillate the heart is not longer a problem!
* When a waveform is specified as fixed pulse duration, programming of the therapy is done in volts (the available or stored energy corresponding to the peak voltage may be provided as a reference value)
* The use of short pulses with a small tilt and a high average voltage, extends the life time of the battery.

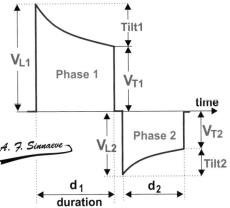

ST. JUDE MEDICAL (Photon) programmed as fixed pulse width

 The maximum voltage V$_{L1}$ (i.e. the leading edge of phase 1) is programmable from 50 to 800 V in 50 V increments

 The optimal pulse durations d$_1$ and d$_2$ depend upon the HV capacitor (changing with type of ICD), the shock resistance R$_S$ (changing with the electrodes) and the time constant of the heart (changing with the patient). Taking these parameters into account the manufacturer has published readily available tables with the calculated optimal values.

Abbreviations : HV = high voltage; Rs = shock resistance (typically 50 Ω);

Figure 4.12

80

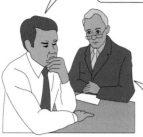

So, you claim that I'm not giving my patient a shock of 30 joule when the HV capacitor is charged to 30 joule !? That is shocking !

STORED AND DELIVERED ENERGY

That's right ! That's because the shock is always truncated and there always remains some charge in the HV capacitor.

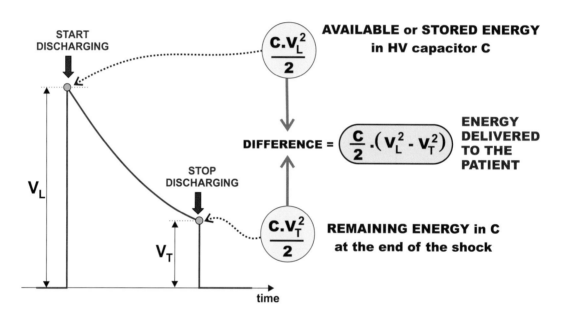

START DISCHARGING

$\dfrac{C \cdot V_L^2}{2}$ — AVAILABLE or STORED ENERGY in HV capacitor C

DIFFERENCE = $\left(\dfrac{C}{2} \cdot (V_L^2 - V_T^2) \right)$ — ENERGY DELIVERED TO THE PATIENT

STOP DISCHARGING

V_L

V_T

$\dfrac{C \cdot V_T^2}{2}$ — REMAINING ENERGY in C at the end of the shock

time

◆ The delivered energy is always smaller than the stored energy in the capacitor.

◆ When the shock waveform is of the "constant tilt" type the programmer usually displays the "delivered" energy !

◆ When the shock waveform is of the "constant duration" type the programmer can only display the stored energy and you do not know the exact amount of energy delivered to the patient !

Are you saying that I cannot guarantee the delivered energy to my patient when I program a shock of constant duration ? Isn't that dangerous ?

That's OK, provided that the duration of the shock is adequate and its voltage is high enough. Actually, it is the voltage that generates the force to change the status of the cardiac cells ! The high voltage (HV) is displayed on the programmer and the stored voltage can be seen as a quick control !

A. F. Sinnaeve

Figure 4.13

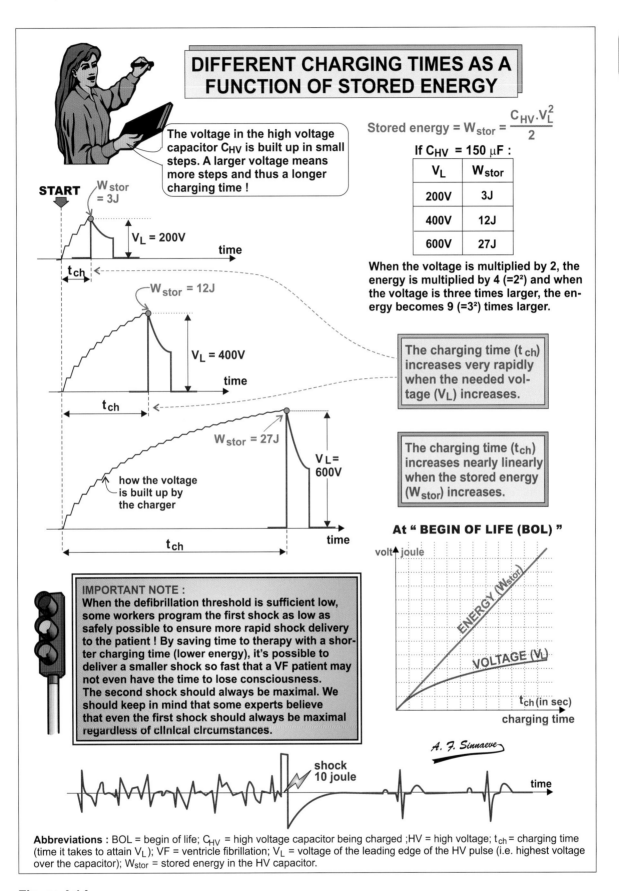

DIFFERENT CHARGING TIMES AS A FUNCTION OF STORED ENERGY

The voltage in the high voltage capacitor C_{HV} is built up in small steps. A larger voltage means more steps and thus a longer charging time !

Stored energy = W_{stor} = $\dfrac{C_{HV} \cdot V_L^2}{2}$

If C_{HV} = 150 µF :

V_L	W_{stor}
200V	3J
400V	12J
600V	27J

When the voltage is multiplied by 2, the energy is multiplied by 4 (=2²) and when the voltage is three times larger, the energy becomes 9 (=3²) times larger.

START
W_{stor} = 3J
V_L = 200V
time
t_{ch}

W_{stor} = 12J
V_L = 400V
time
t_{ch}

W_{stor} = 27J
V_L = 600V
how the voltage is built up by the charger
time
t_{ch}

The charging time (t_{ch}) increases very rapidly when the needed voltage (V_L) increases.

The charging time (t_{ch}) increases nearly linearly when the stored energy (W_{stor}) increases.

At " BEGIN OF LIFE (BOL) "

volt joule
ENERGY (W_{stor})
VOLTAGE (V_L)
t_{ch} (in sec)
charging time

IMPORTANT NOTE :
When the defibrillation threshold is sufficient low, some workers program the first shock as low as safely possible to ensure more rapid shock delivery to the patient ! By saving time to therapy with a shorter charging time (lower energy), it's possible to deliver a smaller shock so fast that a VF patient may not even have the time to lose consciousness. The second shock should always be maximal. We should keep in mind that some experts believe that even the first shock should always be maximal regardless of clinical circumstances.

A. F. Sinnaeve

shock 10 joule
time

Abbreviations : BOL = begin of life; C_{HV} = high voltage capacitor being charged ;HV = high voltage; t_{ch} = charging time (time it takes to attain V_L); VF = ventricle fibrillation; V_L = voltage of the leading edge of the HV pulse (i.e. highest voltage over the capacitor); W_{stor} = stored energy in the HV capacitor.

Figure 4.14

THE DEFIBRILLATION THRESHOLD (DFT) - 1

The electric forces acting upon the membranes of the many cardiac cells are never the same for all parts of the ventricles :
(a) In the area of the strongest field the shock is able to extend the action potentials of all cells.
(b) In the weaker field areas the shock can extend the action potentials of those cells in phase 3.
(c) In the weakest field areas the shock can only "pace" thus capturing excitable gaps.

These 3 effects interact with a process of traveling wavefronts (wavefront propagation and regeneration) that is fairly random. There are moment-to-moment variations in factors that are unknown and not controllable. Hence the defibrillation efficacy is best expressed as a dose-response (or defibrillation success) curve as a function of delivered energy.

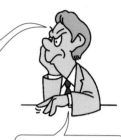

Yes, you're right ! It isn't easy at all...

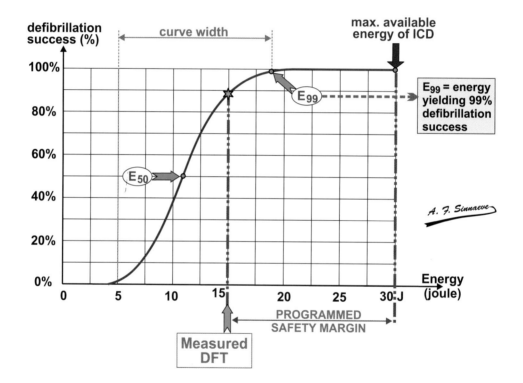

1. The defibrillation success curve is often characterized by particular points on the curve such as the energy associated with 50% or 99% likelihood of defibrillation (E_{50} and E_{99} respectively). The defibrillation success curve as a whole, is never clinically tested as too many shocks are needed to define such a curve.

2. E_{99} is a theoretical point that cannot be measured clinically.

3. Note that at E_{50}, a small increase in energy dose results in a large increase in the success rate as the E_{50} is on the steep portion of the curve.

Abbreviatons : DFT = defibrillation threshold (minimum amount of energy required for successful defibrillation).

Figure 4.15

THE DEFIBRILLATION THRESHOLD (DFT) - 2

There is still more trouble !!!

The probabilistic defibrillation success curve itself is not a constant !
Shifts in the defibrillation requirements may occur as a result of :
  1/ Changes in position of endocardial lead system
  2/ Prolonged fibrillation time (e.g. due to a longer charging time)
  3/ Progression of the underlying disease
  4/ Ischemia
  5/ Altered antiarrhythmic drug therapy
  6/ Other yet undefined factors

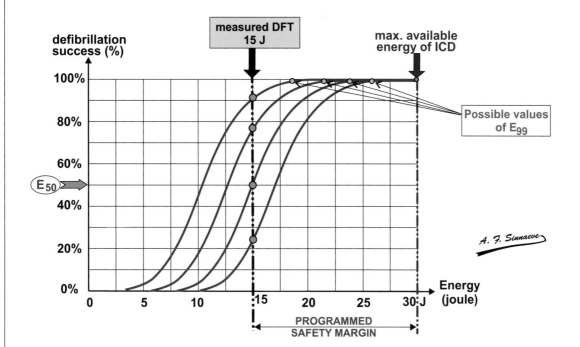

Note that these four curves are never clinically tested (too many defibrillations would be needed); they are derived from experimental work and help to understand the concepts of defibrillation.

The wider the plateau from E_{99} to the ICD output, the more favorable the situation because the success for defibrillation becomes better than 99% (close to 100%) at the maximum output of the ICD. The curve shifted most to the right represents the patient with the narrowest plateau on the summit of the curve : it is the least favorable situation where the success rate may be less than 100%.

A single DFT mesurement is not sufficient to determine how to program the ICD which has to provide an appropriate energy output to ensure virtually consistent defibrillation success. Since defibrillaton is a rather random process, it is unknown if the measured DFT is located at the bottom of a particular curve, or in the middle or close to the top : e.g. a measured DFT of 15 J may correspond to 25%, 50%, 78% or 91% depending on its exact position on the shifted defibrillation success curve.

Abbreviatons : DFT = defibrillation threshold (minimum amount of energy required for successful defibrillation).

Figure 4.16

THE DEFIBRILLATION THRESHOLD (DFT) - 3

The human heart's defibrillation requirements follow an average current law for both monophasic defibrillation shocks and the first phase of biphasic shocks. It has been shown that these requirements also obey the Weiss-Lapicque strength-duration (SD) curve which is defined by the rheobase current and the chronaxie duration. However, the response to very short or very long pulse durations may deviate from this rule due to some other effects. Due to the probabilistic nature of defibrillation, a SD curve is only valid for a specific percentage of success (e.g. 50%); a different % defibrillation success will produce a different SD curve.

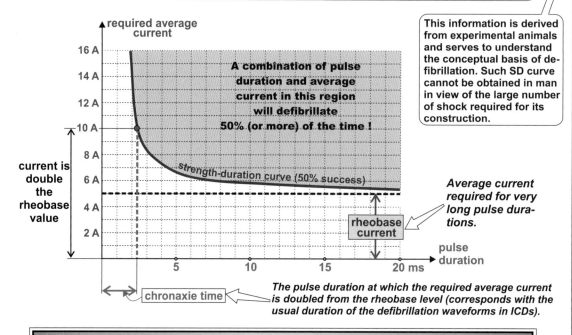

This information is derived from experimental animals and serves to understand the conceptual basis of defibrillation. Such SD curve cannot be obtained in man in view of the large number of shock required for its construction.

The pulse duration at which the required average current is doubled from the rheobase level (corresponds with the usual duration of the defibrillation waveforms in ICDs).

The rheobase currents in man are 2.3 - 5.6 A depending upon surface area and position of the shocking electrodes.
The chronaxie time for humans is about 3.2 ms (ranging from 2 to 4 ms in different animals)

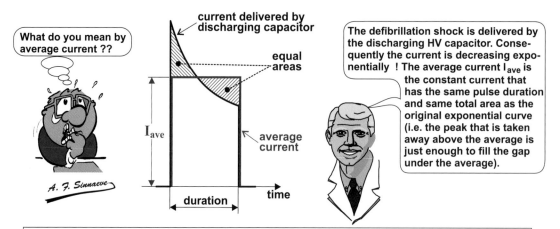

The defibrillation shock is delivered by the discharging HV capacitor. Consequently the current is decreasing exponentially ! The average current I_{ave} is the constant current that has the same pulse duration and same total area as the original exponential curve (i.e. the peak that is taken away above the average is just enough to fill the gap under the average).

Note : The shocking impedance between the high voltage electrodes is low (usually 50 ohm ; in rare occasions above 100 ohm). A initial voltage of 650 V will produce an initial current of 650V / 50Ω = 13A (ampere) at the start of the shock.

Figure 4.17

THE DEFIBRILLATION THRESHOLD (DFT) - 4

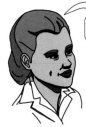

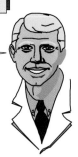

Dear colleague, why are the average current and the strength-duration curve so important to you ?

Well, the strength-duration curve is the basic rule of electrophysiology ! And it has some very important consequences :
1. An average current lower than the rheobase is unable to defibrillate.
2. Longer pulse durations may deliver more energy but are not necessarily more effective.

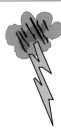

A monophasic shock or the first phase of a biphasic shock defibrillates by resynchronizing the myocardial cells. Recovered cells that are in electrical diastole are stimulated, while the action potential is extended for those cells that are already activated.
If the average current of a shock is lower than required by the strength-duration curve, some of the myocardial cells are not resynchronized and the fibrillation waves are not terminated or may restart after the shock.

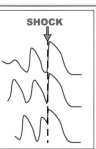

The delivered energy is given by :

$$E_{deliv} = \frac{C}{2} \cdot (V_L^2 - V_T^2)$$

If the high voltage capacitor C is discharged during a longer period of time, the minimum voltage V_T of the shock is lower and hence the delivered energy increases but the average current is also decreasing. If the average current is lower than the rheobase, VF will not be eliminated

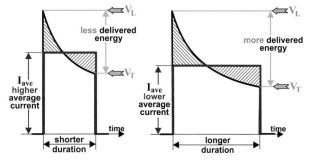

(or will stop and restart) : very long shock durations are not effective, even if they provide a large shock energy.
Hence the importance of a waveform of critical duration and voltage, to generate the optimal average current for defibrillation. Despite these considerations energy (J), which is an indirect measurement, remains the most important parameter to describe "defibrillation dose".

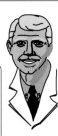

If the average CURRENT (in A) is the crucial factor for defibrillation, why do we use ENERGY (in J) ?

Well, It Is very hard for an ICD to measure current, especially a large average current ! However, the device can easily measure the V_L and V_T voltage on HV capacitor. Knowing the capacitance of the HV capacitor and these two voltages, the calculation of the delivered energy is easy ! All manufacturers measure and display energy. Just because it is traditional and technically more convenient...

A. F. Sinnaeve

Abbreviations : V_L = maximum voltage or voltage of the leading edge of the defibrillation shock ;
V_T = minimum voltage or voltage of the trailing edge of the defibrillation shock ;

Figure 4.18

THE DEFIBRILLATION THRESHOLD (DFT) - 5

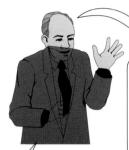

There are so many protocols to assess defibrillation efficacy that I am confused as what to use !

True, but two methods predominate : the single-energy success and the step-down protocols. Using one of these two methods would simplify testing of the DFT at the time of ICD implantation. For both protocols, the first shock is set at least 10 J below the maximal output of the ICD (often 20 J). If the first shock is successful, the same energy level can be repeated to establish the DFT+ (at 20 J for example). This is becoming a popular approach and after two successful 20 J shocks, the ICD can be programmed to 30 J (i.e. a threshold of 20 J plus a safety margin of 10J). The procedure is simple as it often involves only two shocks ! To be quite sure, the same energy level (20 J) can be repeated twice to establish the DFT++ and used for programming the ICD in the same way.

That's really easy to remember and the patient receives only two test shocks !

Yes, that's the reason why it is becoming popular and it works because of the high efficiency of contemporary ICDs. However, with this simple method, you are committed to program the ICD to deliver the maximum output for the first shock.
In the "step-down method", the shock energy is decreased with each trial until a shock fails to defibrillate. The DFT is the lowest energy level that achieves successful defibrillation. This method may allow programming of the first shock to a value less than the maximum output of the ICD !

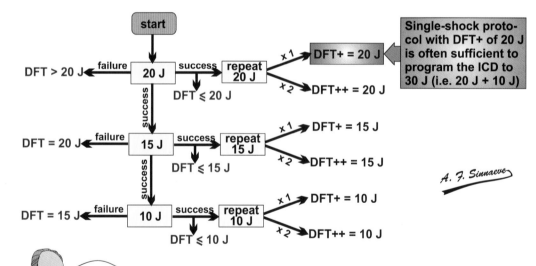

Single-shock protocol with DFT+ of 20 J is often sufficient to program the ICD to 30 J (i.e. 20 J + 10 J)

So, the magic number is still 10 J !?

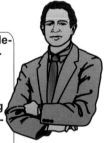

Yes, but there are many other protocols based on accurate determination of the DFT. I agree that accepting the "10 J" concept as a safety margin has simplified things.
Chronic DFTs for biphasic waveforms are stable in most patients, but increases that compromise defibrillation efficacy may occur in up to 15% of patients, particularly in the setting of chronic amiodarone therapy or acute ischemia. So, a safety margin of 10 J is necessary (and in some rare cases even not sufficient).

Figure 4.19

Professor, what do you think about other issues of DFT testing, such as the ULV method ?

DFT TESTING - OTHER ISSUES - 1

UPPER LIMIT OF VULNERABILITY (ULV)

The defibrillation (DFT) method is used most frequently because it is intuitive. When should alternative testing methods be considered ? Testing the upper limit of vulnerability (ULV) seems attractive because it can avoid inducing VF in very sick patients. ULV testing provides an accurate estimate of the probability of defibrillation success and is more reproducible than the step-down DFT method. The vulnerability method minimizes the risk related to VF or circulatory arrest such as intractable VF, cerebral hypoperfusion, and myocardial ischemia. Is it appropriate to defer DFT testing in critically ill patients ? I think so, but only for some selected patients.

! **DEFINITION**

The ULV is the weakest shock at which ventricular fibrillation (VF) is not induced when the shock is delivered during the vulnerable period. A shock on top of the T wave can only induce fibrillation if the energy is smaller than a critical value. If a higher energy is applied, VF cannot be induced !

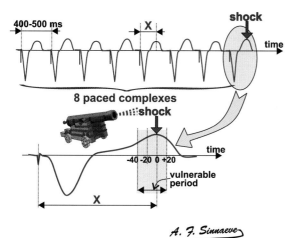

A. F. Sinnaeve

The timing of the peak of the vulnerable zone depends on the spatial relations between the shock field and the sequence of repolarization

* Right ventricular pacing is applied at cycle length 400 - 500 ms.
* All 12 surface ECG leads are inspected to select the lead with the latest-peaking monophasic T wave (with opposite polarity to the QRS).
* A shock is delivered on top of the T wave and if VF is not induced, subsequent shocks at the same energy level are given just before and just after the top. Using a dual-coil lead shocks are timed at -20, 0, +20 and +40 ms relative to the top. For single coil leads the shocks are timed at -40, -20, 0, and +20 ms. If no VF is induced, the procedure is repeated at a lower energy level.
* If only a safety margin is to be determined, a single scan with a 20 J shock may be used for a 30 or 35 J ICD. If no VF is induced at 20 J, the ICD can be programmed at a very safe 30 J.

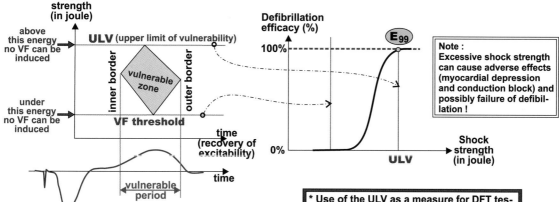

Note :
Excessive shock strength can cause adverse effects (myocardial depression and conduction block) and possibly failure of defibrillation !

* The ULV correlates closely with the DFT. Moreover its assessment is clinically safe, simple and highly reproducible.
* (ULV + 5 J) appears to be a good estimate for programming safely above E_{99} value.

* Use of the ULV as a measure for DFT testing minimizes the number of VF inductions with their associated risks.
* ULV avoids the need to program the ICD to maximum shock strength, thus reducing battery drainage and charging times.

Figure 4.20

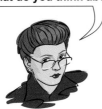

It seems that some physicians do not perform a DFT test at ICD implantation ! Others say a single shock of 14 - 15 J is sufficient to establish a defibrillation margin.
What do you think about that ?

DFT TESTING - OTHER ISSUES - 2

Well, I want to state first that DFT testing might be risky ! Induction of ventricular fibrillation, especially in very ill patients should be strictly limited.
However, a single-shock defibrillation safety-margin testing as well as deferred or delayed DFT testing are both strategies only to be considered in selected cases.
Before one abandons DFT testing in favor of simplified regimens, one must weigh the added morbidity from additional DFT shocks against the information gained.

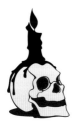

DFT testing is risky !!!
* Left atrial clot / AF without anticoagulation
* Recent cerebral anoxia
* Prolonged procedure, hypotension
* CRT implant in Class IV patients
* External defibrillation unreliable
* Adequate sedation or anesthesia unsafe
* Recent coronary stent

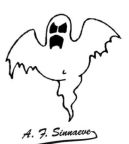

A. F. Sinnaeve

SINGLE SHOCK SAFETY-MARGIN TESTING

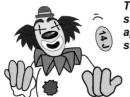

The evidence supporting this approach for a 14 - 15 J shock is good. Nevertheless, practice patterns with this approach are unknown. More data are required to standardize this method of testing

The LESS study (Low Energy Safety Study) showed that a single shock of 14 J was adequate for the termination of an induced VF in 91% of patients.

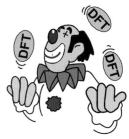

DEFERRED DFT TESTING

The indication for delayed testing is a contraindication to testing at implantation that has resolved by a month or two later.
This is probably done infrequently. It carries the risk that if testing is not done at the time of implantation, it is often not done at all. There is limited evidence for this approach but the available evidence is growing.

The most common reasons today to postpone DFT testing are atrial fibrillation with inadequate anticoagulation to ensure minimal risk of thromboembolism (because a shock can cause reversion to sinus rhythm), and cardiac resynchronization cases in which either the passive LV lead might be dislodged by shocks or the patient is in severe heart failure that may be improved after a month or two of cardiac resynchronization pacing when DFT testing may be considered.

NOTE 1 : Shocks are less effective for spontaneous VT/VF than induced VF even if DFT is low. Factors other than DFT determine success of shocks for spontaneous VT/VF (e.g. ischemia, autonomic tone).
NOTE 2 : Do not underestimate the importance of proper device programming. Empiric programming of antitachycardia pacing can terminate VT in many patients before shocks are necessary !

Abbreviations : AF = atrial fibrillation ; CRT = cardiac resynchronization therapy ; DFT = defibrillation threshold ; VF = ventricular fibrillation ; VT = ventricular tachycardia ;

Figure 4.21

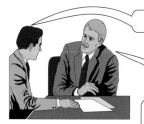

How do you handle high defibrillation thresholds ?

HOW TO HANDLE HIGH DFTs

Well, safety first ! Of course, since they guarantee lower DFTs, I always use biphasic shock waveforms and an active (hot) can system in the left infraclavicular region !

ONE Assess the integrity of all electrical connections manually and check the HV impedance of the defibrillation pathway (normally 20-100 ohm)

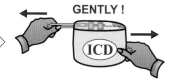
GENTLY !

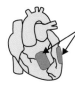
keep sufficient distance

TWO In epicardial systems : exclude the possibility that energy is shunted from the heart e.g. patches are too close or touching (lead impedance may be very low) and exclude patch crinkling and air or fluid under the patches (lead impedance may be too high).

THREE High DFTs are now rare with present technology. In patients with high DFTs, one must seek a better RV position and try to change the polarity of the shock (which does not always help)

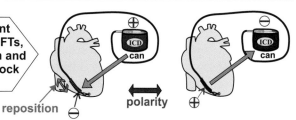
reposition   polarity

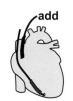
add   deactivate   OR

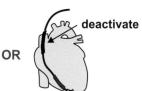

FOUR If a single-coil lead is in place, add an SVC lead.
If a dual-coil lead is in place, deactivate the SVC part.

FIVE Some ICDs (ST Jude) allow programmability of the waveform in terms of tilt or pulse duration. This may help and has to be done strictly according to the manufacturer's recommendations.

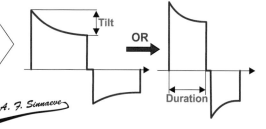
Tilt   OR   Duration

A. F. Sinnaeve

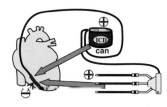

SIX Use an ancillary subcutaneous electrode array (or a SQ patch).

* A DFT+ of 25 J ? Try another shock ! If DFT++ = 25 J, it is reasonable to implant an ICD with a maximum output of 33-35 J (if necessary use a device with a high energy shock capability e.g. 40 J).
* Remember that a pneumothorax may cause a high HV shock impedance and that a retained inactive lead may shunt current away from the desired pathway and should be removed in this situation.
* In marginal cases follow-up testing should be considered several weeks after implantation especially in patients whose high DFT is related to previous amiodarone therapy.
* The addition of class III antiarrhythmic drugs (sotalol, dofetilide) may occasionally be useful to reduce the DFT.

Figure 4.22

SENSING and DETECTION

SENSING

* Sensing vs. detection - definitions
* Functional block diagram of the sening circuit
* What does the ICD see ?
* Sensing and sensitivity
* Dynamic sensitivity adjustment - 1 - Principle
* Dynamic sensitivity adjustment - 2 - Medtronic
* Dynamic sensitivity adjustment - 3 - Guidant (Boston Scientific)
* Dynamic sensitivity adjustment - 4 - St Jude Medical
* Dynamic sensitivity adjustment - 5 - St Jude Medical
* Oversensing of far-field R waves

DETECTION

* Detection criteria - parts 1 & 2
* Detection zones
* Sliding window for initial detection
* SJM Running average for initial detection - parts 1 & 2
* Overlapping VT/VF zones - parts 1 & 2
* Simultaneous counting in two zones - Guidant (Boston Scientific)
* Simultaneous counting in two zones - Medtronic
* Combined count detection

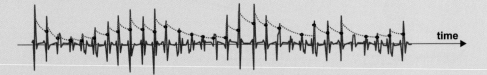

Figure 5.00

SENSING AND DETECTION

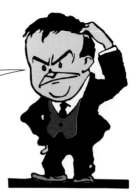

I've always thought that sensing and detection were synonymous, but obviously ICD people don't think so...!??

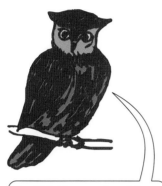

I will tell you about the problems of sensing and how to avoid them !

SENSING

* Sensing is always about the actual measurement of signals between two electrodes. The ventricular electrogram (VEGM) is a typical example of such a measurement.
* Sensing a signal is normally straightforward, but it can be hampered by external signals (problem of oversensing) or it can be complicated by the widely fluctuating amplitude of the VEGM during VF (problem of undersensing).
* Of course, the need for stable lead performance is mandatory to ensure reliable sensing.

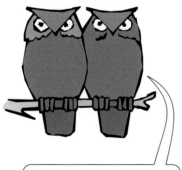

And we will teach you all about the algorithms and their problems.

A. F. Sinnaeve

DETECTION

* The device detects a tachyarrhythmia based upon sensing of the intrinsic cardiac activity and the fulfilment of some programmed detection criteria (algorithm).
* Detection is never a single nor an instantaneous measurement : it always involves the processing of the sensed signals during a circumscribed period of time.
* Detection algorithms have evolved from simple rate detection to complicated pattern recognition but their sensitivity as well as their specificity are still not 100%.

NOTE
SENSITIVITY is the capability to detect all rhythms that should be shocked
SPECIFICITY is the capability to reject all rhythms that should not be shocked

Figure 5.01

FUNCTIONAL BLOCK DIAGRAM OF THE SENSING CIRCUIT

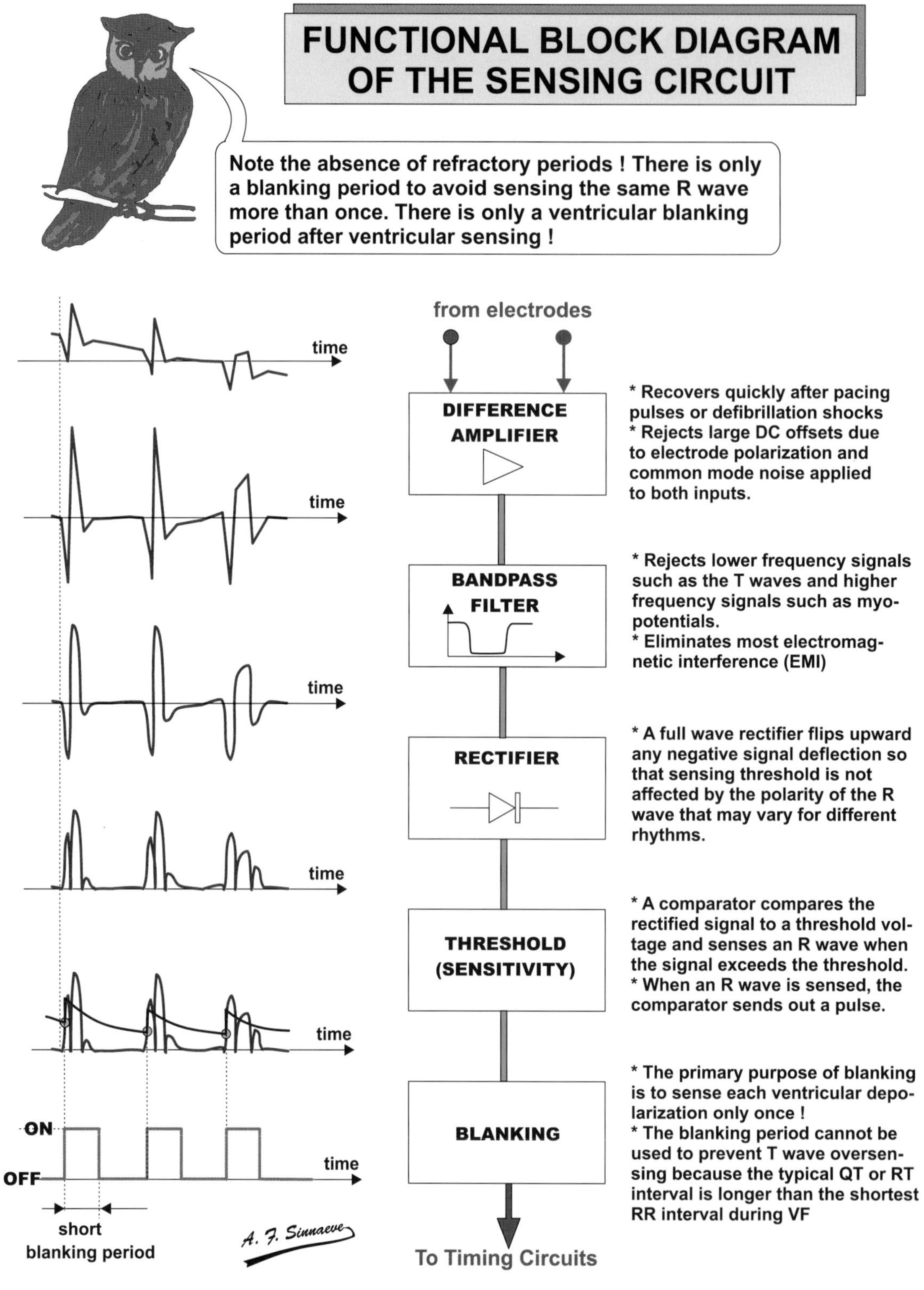

Figure 5.02

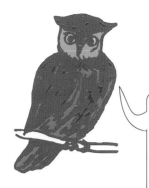

WHAT DOES THE ICD SEE ?

Near-field electrograms are recordings of the local bipolar ventricular electrogram. They represent the activation of the myocardium in the vicinity of the tip electrode.
Far-field electrograms may be recorded between shocking electrodes or between the RV coil and the active ICD can. They represent, more or less, the electrical activity of the whole heart.

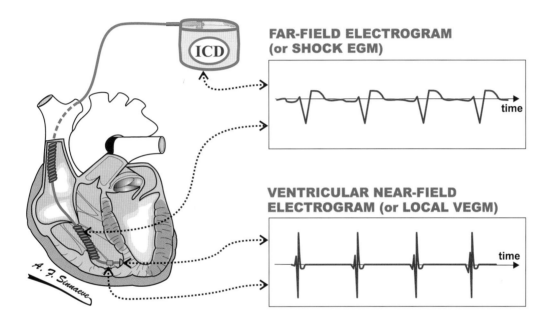

FAR-FIELD ELECTROGRAM (or SHOCK EGM)

VENTRICULAR NEAR-FIELD ELECTROGRAM (or LOCAL VEGM)

The near-field VEGM is the only one used by the ICD for arrhythmia detection (VT or VF). Due to the small surface area of the tip electrode and the small distance between tip and ring, the amplitude and the slew rate are a bit larger while the duration is shorter than the far-field VEGM.

The far-field VEGM may be stored to help the operator (not the device!!!) in the diagnosis of an event. This electrogram may show atrial activity to aid in arrhythmia identification. Moreover, the change in morphology of ventricular arrhythmias is often more obvious than in the near-field VEGM.

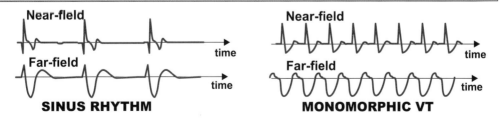

SINUS RHYTHM

MONOMORPHIC VT

ABBREVIATIONS : RV = right ventricle; VEGM = ventricular electrogram ; VF = ventricular fibrillation ; VT = ventricular tachycardia

Figure 5.03

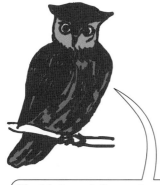

SENSING & SENSITIVITY

First let me tell you how to avoid missing too many of the low-amplitude fragmented ventricular signals during VF.

> The ability to sense small amplitude signals rapidly during ventricular fibrillation, while not oversensing T waves or noise in the absence of tachyarrhythmias, is essential for proper ICD function.
>
> The amplitude (as well as the rate) of the ventricular signals fluctuates markedly and chaotically during ventricular fibrillation (the amplitude of the signals usually diminishes to approximately 25% of the normal VEGM amplitude in sinus rhythm).

Basic Ventricular EGM in VF

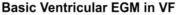

With fixed sensitivity a lot of low-amplitude fibrillatory electrograms may be missed

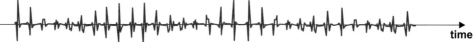

> **Automatic Gain Control (AGC) is a feedback system that attempts to keep the amplifier output signal amplitude constant for any input signal, i.e. the smaller the input signal, the greater the amplification (or gain).**

electronically modified waveform derived from the detected VEGM and processed by the sensing amplifier

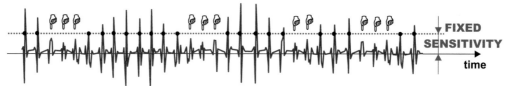

> **Auto-adjusting threshold or auto-adjusting sensitivity increases the sensitivity over time between ventricular events. After each sensed event the threshold is adjusted according to the amplitude of the measured VEGM and then decays with time producing a higher sensitivity.**

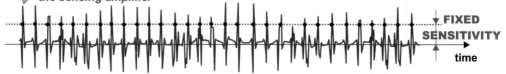

CHANGING THRESHOLD

A. F. Sinnaeve

ABBREVIATIONS : VEGM = ventricular electrogram

Figure 5.04

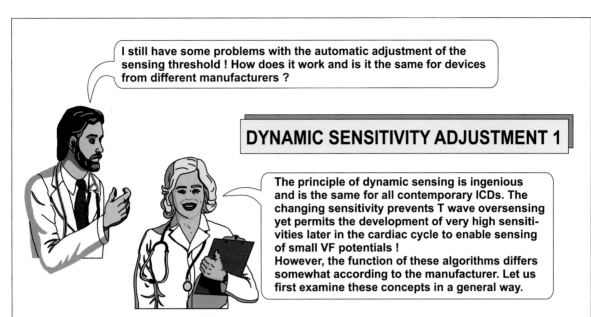

DYNAMIC SENSITIVITY ADJUSTMENT 1

I still have some problems with the automatic adjustment of the sensing threshold ! How does it work and is it the same for devices from different manufacturers ?

The principle of dynamic sensing is ingenious and is the same for all contemporary ICDs. The changing sensitivity prevents T wave oversensing yet permits the development of very high sensitivities later in the cardiac cycle to enable sensing of small VF potentials !
However, the function of these algorithms differs somewhat according to the manufacturer. Let us first examine these concepts in a general way.

When a ventricular event is sensed, the "peak value" of the signal is measured and a "threshold start" is determined as a percentage of this peak amplitude. After a short delay, the sensitivity starts to augment, i.e. the threshold decreases until another signal is sensed or the maximum sensitivity is reached. This delay is a blanking period to avoid double sensing of the VEGM.

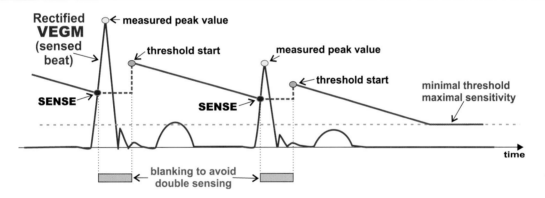

After a pacing pulse, the starting point of the sensitivity threshold is different from that initiated by sensing a spontaneous R wave. Immediately after a pacing pulse measurement of an R wave does not take place. Moreover, a longer ventricular blanking period is required after a ventricular paced beat to prevent sensing of wide QRS and T wave of paced beats.

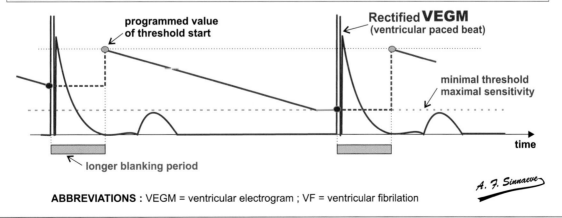

ABBREVIATIONS : VEGM = ventricular electrogram ; VF = ventricular fibrilation

Figure 5.05

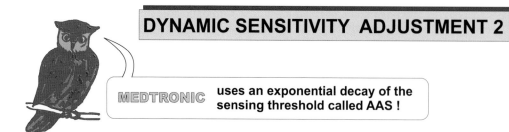

DYNAMIC SENSITIVITY ADJUSTMENT 2

MEDTRONIC uses an exponential decay of the sensing threshold called AAS !

① AUTO-ADJUSTING SENSITIVITY AFTER A SENSED VENTRICULAR EVENT

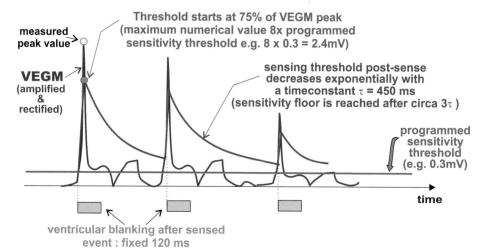

measured peak value

VEGM (amplified & rectified)

Threshold starts at 75% of VEGM peak (maximum numerical value 8x programmed sensitivity threshold e.g. 8 x 0.3 = 2.4mV)

sensing threshold post-sense decreases exponentially with a timeconstant τ = 450 ms (sensitivity floor is reached after circa 3τ)

programmed sensitivity threshold (e.g. 0.3mV)

time

ventricular blanking after sensed event : fixed 120 ms

② AUTO-ADJUSTING SENSITIVITY AFTER A PACED VENTRICULAR EVENT

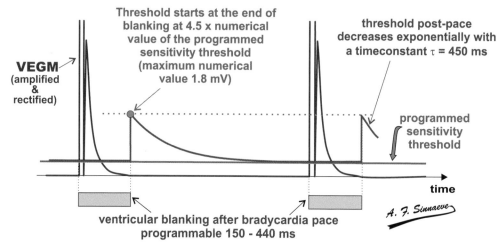

VEGM (amplified & rectified)

Threshold starts at the end of blanking at 4.5 x numerical value of the programmed sensitivity threshold (maximum numerical value 1.8 mV)

threshold post-pace decreases exponentially with a timeconstant τ = 450 ms

programmed sensitivity threshold

time

A. F. Sinnaeve

ventricular blanking after bradycardia pace programmable 150 - 440 ms

③ NOTE : After the end of a cardioversion or defibrillation charging period, the blanking period is 300 ms.
After delivered cardioversion or defibrillation therapy, the blanking period is 520 ms.

ABBREVIATIONS : AAS = auto-adjusting sensitivity ; VEGM = ventricular electrogram ;

Figure 5.06

DYNAMIC SENSITIVITY ADJUSTMENT 3

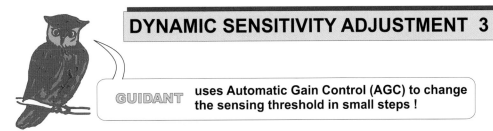

GUIDANT uses Automatic Gain Control (AGC) to change the sensing threshold in small steps !

① AUTOMATIC GAIN CONTROL AFTER A SENSED VENTRICULAR EVENT

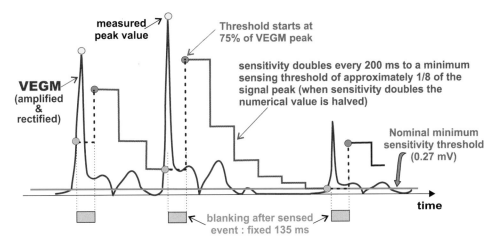

measured peak value

Threshold starts at 75% of VEGM peak

VEGM (amplified & rectified)

sensitivity doubles every 200 ms to a minimum sensing threshold of approximately 1/8 of the signal peak (when sensitivity doubles the numerical value is halved)

Nominal minimum sensitivity threshold (0.27 mV)

time

blanking after sensed event : fixed 135 ms

② AUTOMATIC GAIN CONTROL AFTER A PACED VENTRICULAR EVENT

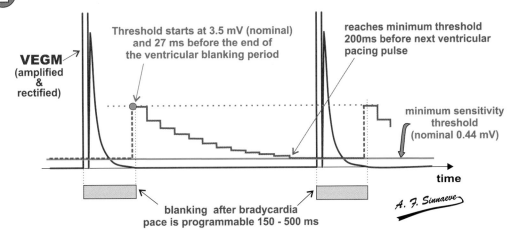

VEGM (amplified & rectified)

Threshold starts at 3.5 mV (nominal) and 27 ms before the end of the ventricular blanking period

reaches minimum threshold 200ms before next ventricular pacing pulse

minimum sensitivity threshold (nominal 0.44 mV)

time

A. F. Sinnaeve

blanking after bradycardia pace is programmable 150 - 500 ms

③ NOTE :

* The blanking period after a paced event can be fixed (programmable) or dynamic. If the dynamic option is enabled, the blanking period automatically shortens when the pacing rate increases.
* The minimum threshold and the threshold starting point after pacing can be programmed at three levels (most sensitive ; nominal ; least sensitive)
* The minimum sensitivity threshold after pacing is higher than that after sensing to avoid oversensing of afterpotentials, etc.

ABBREVIATIONS : AGC = automatic gain control; VEGM = ventricular electrogram ; VRP = ventricular refractory period;

Figure 5.07

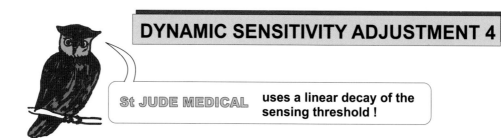

DYNAMIC SENSITIVITY ADJUSTMENT 4

St JUDE MEDICAL uses a linear decay of the sensing threshold !

① AUTO-ADJUSTING SENSITIVITY AFTER A SENSED VENTRICULAR EVENT

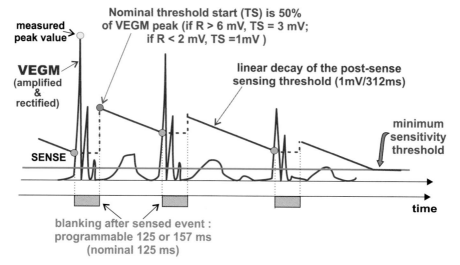

measured peak value

Nominal threshold start (TS) is 50% of VEGM peak (if R > 6 mV, TS = 3 mV; if R < 2 mV, TS =1mV)

VEGM (amplified & rectified)

linear decay of the post-sense sensing threshold (1mV/312ms)

minimum sensitivity threshold

SENSE

time

blanking after sensed event : programmable 125 or 157 ms (nominal 125 ms)

② AUTO-ADJUSTING SENSITIVITY AFTER A PACED VENTRICULAR EVENT

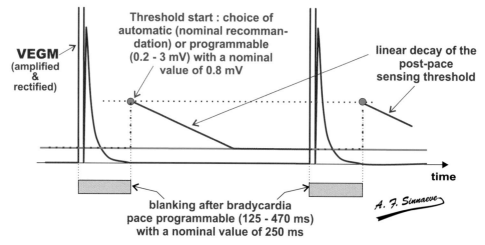

VEGM (amplified & rectified)

Threshold start : choice of automatic (nominal recommandation) or programmable (0.2 - 3 mV) with a nominal value of 0.8 mV

linear decay of the post-pace sensing threshold

time

blanking after bradycardia pace programmable (125 - 470 ms) with a nominal value of 250 ms

A. F. Sinnaeve

③ NOTE : If the "AUTO threshold start" is enabled, the threshold start will decrease as the pacing rate increases.

ABBREVIATIONS : R = R wave(peak of VEGM); TS = threshold start; VEGM = ventricular electrogram ;

Figure 5.08

In spite of ASC... oversensing of T waves has been reported on several occasions especially with long QT intervals.

DYNAMIC SENSITIVITY ADJUSTMENT 5

St JUDE MEDICAL

Oversensing of T waves may be caused by the automatic sensitivity control (ASC) that is decreasing the detection level too fast (i.e. increasing the sensitivity too quickly !).
This effect can be avoided easilly by proper programming the St Jude ICD.

 The nominal "threshold start" (TS) is 50% of the maximum peak amplitude sensed during the "sensed refractory period". However, TS may be programmed at 62.5%, 75% and 100%.

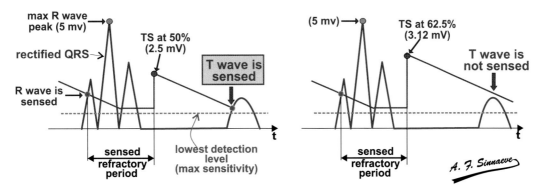

 The "Decay Delay" is the amount of time after the "Sensed Refractory period" that the sensitivity level of the device remains at the "Threshold Start" before beginning its decay (i.e. before the device begins to get more sensitive).

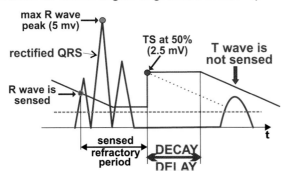

The ventricular decay delay is programmable : 0 (nominal), 30, 60, 95, 125, 190, 220 ms

AVOIDING T WAVE SENSING
The decay delay holds the sensitivity threshold at the starting value for a programmable amount of time (skips over the T wave)

Due to very low detection level at maximum sensitivity,oversensing of myopotentials may occur during pacing at a low rate when the sensing threshold decays towards its minimum value.

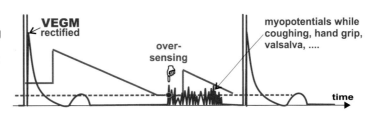

Figure 5.09

ICDs reject far-field signals in several ways !

OVERSENSING OF FAR-FIELD R WAVES

1. FF R wave sensing causes a typical alternation of atrial cycle length with long - short - long - short cycles !
2. The postventricular atrial refractory blanking period (PVAB) is similar to that used in pacemakers. Programming the PVAB carries the risk of atrial undersensing, especially atrial fibrillation. If this happens, the ICD underestimates the atrial rate of atrial fibrillation or flutter, causing inappropriate VT detection.
3. A decrease in baseline atrial sensitivity may control FF R wave sensing but it carries the risk of undersensing atrial fibrillation.
4. Algorithmic identification of the pattern of atrial and ventricular events as in the PR Logic system from Medtronic. The FF signal resides relatively close to the ventricular event and consequently creates alternating short and long atrial cycles recognizable by a device.
5. Some ICDs offer an automatic decrease in atrial sensitivity after a ventricular event so as to contain the FF signal. This is similar to the dynamic sensitivity used for ventricular sensing.
6. Sensing of FF R waves may cause the ICD to overestimate the atrial rate and may therefore inappropriately reject sensing of VT whenever there is consistent sensing of FF R waves. On the other hand, inconsistent sensing of FF R waves may cause inappropriate detection of SVT as VT.

Far-Field R wave sensing by atrial channel

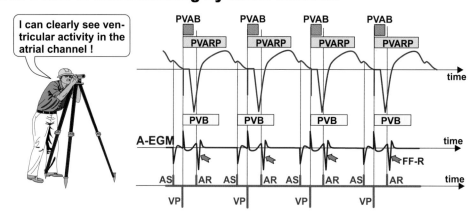

Far-field sensing eliminated by prolonging PVAB

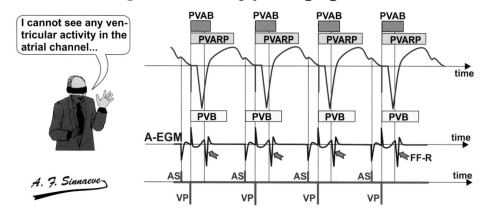

Abbreviations : AEGM = atrial electrogram; AS = atrial sensed event, AR = atrial sensed event during refractory period; PVAB = postventricular atrial blanking; PVARP = postventricular atrial refractory period; PVB = ventricular blanking after ventricular pace; VP = ventricular pace;

Figure 5.10

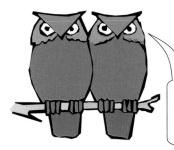

DETECTION CRITERIA 1

Detection should be prompt so that therapy is given before the patient develops syncope, before VEGM amplitude and slew rate deteriorate and before defibrillation thresholds rise.

 All contemporary ICDs use digital circuits, microprocessors and algorithms based on rate determination to detect VF. For detection of VF/VT they all use local or near-field VEGM from two closely spaced electrodes.

 Rate alone is still the most commonly used detection method for ventricular arrhythmias. The avoidance of inappropriate ICD shock for SVT is a challenging task ! Therefore, manufacturers have introduced several discrimination enhancements to reduce the false diagnosis of VF or VT produced by sinus tachycardia or SVT.

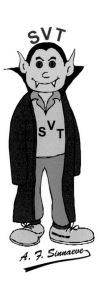

Discrimination enhancements to protect against inappropriate ventricular therapy triggered by SVT, may augment the specificity of the algorithms. This increase in specificity must not be at the expense of loss of sensitivity. One must not sacrifice sensitivity by trying to improve specificity aggressively with the use of algorithms that detect SVT and inhibit ventricular therapy. It is better to have an inappropriate shock for SVT than withhold therapy for a lethal ventricular tachyarrhythmia because of reduced sensitivity. Consequently such discrimination enhancements must be used and programmed very cautiously.

DISCRIMINATION ENHANCEMENTS
ARE NEVER USED IN THE VF ZONE

Modern ICDs are designed to withhold shocks for unsustained rapid and dangerous tachyarrhythmias. A confirmation algorithm looks for continuing tachycardia during and immediately after the charging of the capacitor. If the tachycardia has terminated, the charge is dissipated internally and not delivered to the patient. Systems with such a "second look" are called non-committed. A committed system delivers a shock regardless of tachycardia termination during charging of the capacitor.

Abbreviations : VEGM = electrogram ; VF = ventricular fibrillation ; VT = ventricular tachycardia ; SVT = supraventricular tachycardia ;

Figure 5.11

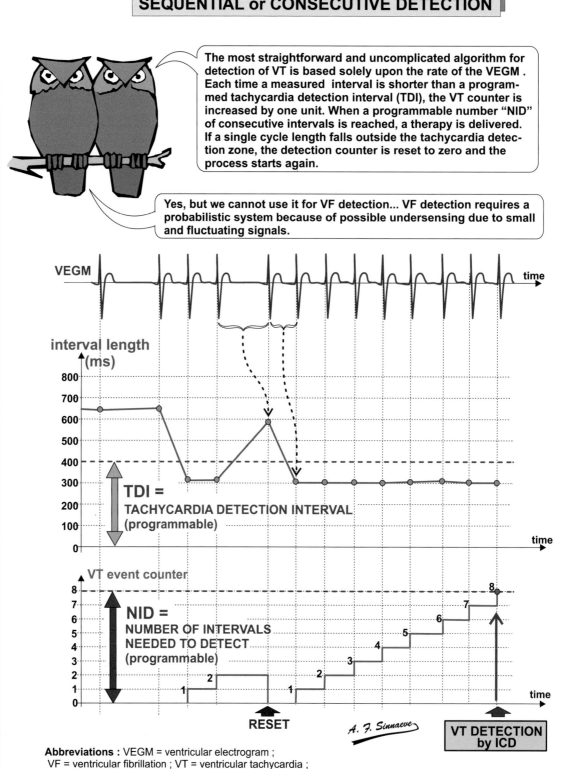

DETECTION CRITERIA 2
SEQUENTIAL or CONSECUTIVE DETECTION

The most straightforward and uncomplicated algorithm for detection of VT is based solely upon the rate of the VEGM . Each time a measured interval is shorter than a programmed tachycardia detection interval (TDI), the VT counter is increased by one unit. When a programmable number "NID" of consecutive intervals is reached, a therapy is delivered. If a single cycle length falls outside the tachycardia detection zone, the detection counter is reset to zero and the process starts again.

Yes, but we cannot use it for VF detection... VF detection requires a probabilistic system because of possible undersensing due to small and fluctuating signals.

VEGM ———— time

interval length (ms)

800
700
600
500
400
300
200
100
0
time

TDI =
TACHYCARDIA DETECTION INTERVAL (programmable)

VT event counter

8
7
6
5
4
3
2
1
0
time

NID =
NUMBER OF INTERVALS NEEDED TO DETECT (programmable)

RESET

A. F. Sinnaeve

VT DETECTION by ICD

Abbreviations : VEGM = ventricular electrogram ;
VF = ventricular fibrillation ; VT = ventricular tachycardia ;

Figure 5.12

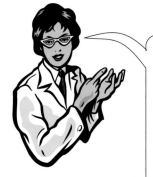

DETECTION ZONES

The first step in tachycardia detection involves measuring the cycle lengths (or rates) between consecutive ventricular depolarizations. Each detected cycle length or interval is assigned to an appropriate detection zone and counted. For tachycardia, the ICD makes a specific diagnosis when a given zone has accumulated the programmed number of appropriate cycle lengths so that the duration criterion is satisfied. Then the device initiates therapy for the arrhythmia according to the programmed sequence for this particular zone.

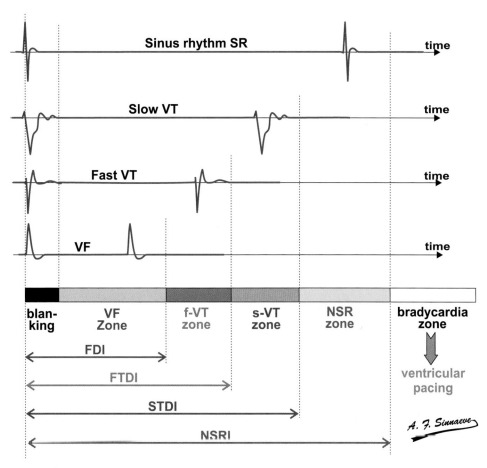

Abbreviations : f-VT = fast ventricular tachycardia
FDI = ventricular fibrillation detection interval
FTDI = fast ventricular tachycardia detection interval
NSRI = normal sinus rhythm interval
SR = sinus rhythm ; NSR = normal sinus rhythm ;
s-VT = slow ventricular tachycardia
STDI = slow ventricular tachycardia detection interval
VF = ventricular fibrillation ; VT = ventricular tachycardia

Figure 5.13

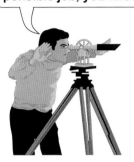

SLIDING WINDOW FOR INITIAL VF DETECTION

Amplitude and rate of the VEGM may fluctuate chaotically during VF. Missing one beat of this fast rhythm should not reset the VF counter and delay VF detection. An algorithm counting a number of consecutive cycles can be catastrophic ! A more sensitive algorithm for VF detection requires that only a percentage (for example 75 or 80%) of the intervals in a tachycardia be shorter than the fibrillation detection interval. Such an algorithm is known as "x out of y counting".

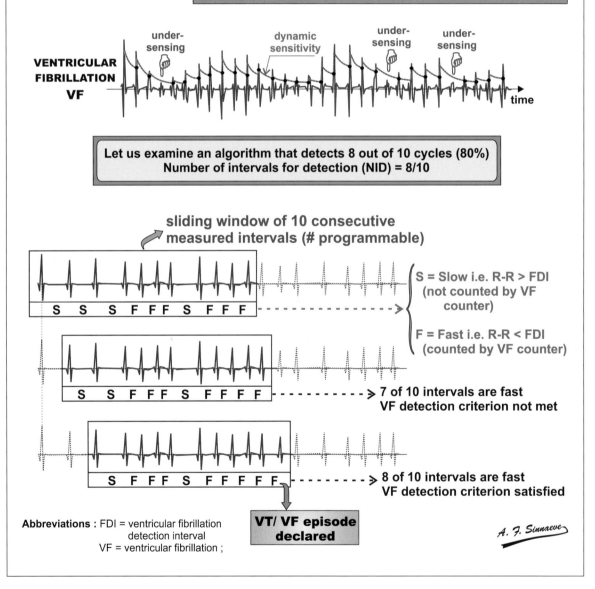

Let us examine an algorithm that detects 8 out of 10 cycles (80%)
Number of intervals for detection (NID) = 8/10

Abbreviations : FDI = ventricular fibrillation detection interval
VF = ventricular fibrillation ;

Figure 5.14

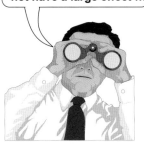

St JUDE's RUNNING AVERAGE FOR INITIAL DETECTION - part 1

I'm looking carefully for ventricular tachyarrhythmias and I'm using a special technique providing a smoothing effect on the detection so that 1 or 2 beat variations do not have a large effect ...

* The interval running average is determined by measuring the current interval in milliseconds plus the 3 prior intervals and dividing the sum by 4.
* When the current interval and the interval average are in the same zone, the interval is binned in that zone.
* When the current interval and the interval average are not classified in the same zone, the interval is binned in the faster zone (Always err on the safe side !)
* The interval is not binned (used for diagnostic counting) if either the interval or the interval average is classified in the "sinus zone".
* The ICD counts only the intervals that are binned !

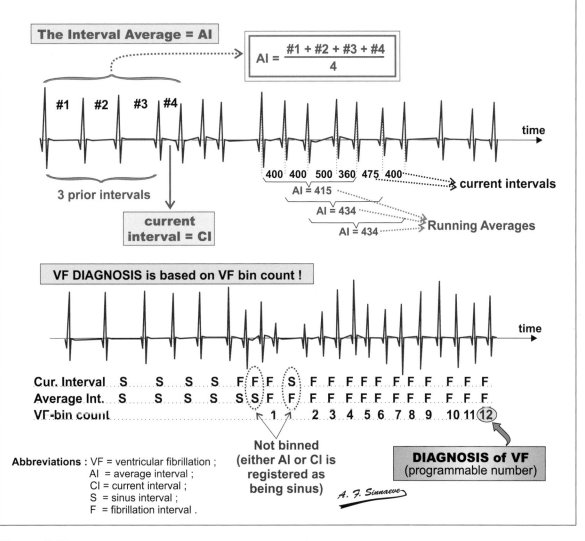

Figure 5.15

St JUDE's RUNNING AVERAGE FOR INITIAL DETECTION - part 2

It isn't very difficult, they said! But I am still thinking it over. I'm not convinced that it is easy...

INTERVAL DEFINITIONS

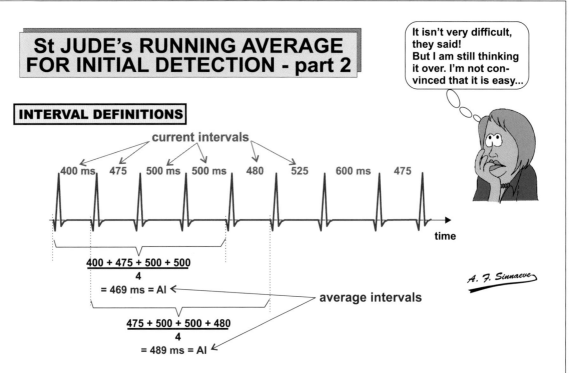

current intervals

400 ms   475   500 ms   500 ms   480   525   600 ms   475

time

$$\frac{400 + 475 + 500 + 500}{4}$$

= 469 ms = AI

average intervals

$$\frac{475 + 500 + 500 + 480}{4}$$

= 489 ms = AI

A. F. Sinnaeve

CURRENT INTERVAL (CI) : measures the time in ms between any two sensed events, paced events or combination

INTERVAL AVERAGE (AI) : the current interval (in ms) plus 3 prior intervals divided by 4 (this helps to provide a smoothing effect on detection, so that 1 or 2 beat variations don't have a large effect on detection)

BINNING RULES

✸ Binning is the proces of counting average intervals for rhythm diagnosis. Thus average intervals that are not binned, are discarded and not counted.

✸ When the current interval and the interval average are the same classification (e.g. both VF), the interval is binned in that zone.

✸ When current interval and interval average are not the same classification (e.g. VT and VF), the interval is binned in the faster zone (*always errs at the safe side !*).

✸ The interval is not binned if either the current interval or the interval average is classified as sinus (prevents 1 beat variation from impacting detection).

		CURRENT INTERVAL				
		Fib	Tach B	Tach A	Tach	Sinus
AVERAGE INTERVAL	Fib	Fib	Fib	Fib	Fib	Not Binned
	Tach B	Fib	Tach B	Tach B	N/A	Not Binned
	Tach A	Fib	Tach B	Tach A	N/A	Not Binned
	Tach	Fib	N/A	N/A	Tach	Not Binned
	Sinus	Not Binned	Not Binned	Not Binned	Not Binned	Sinus

N/A = not applicable (Tach stands for only 1 VT zone; Tach A & Tach B stand for 2 VT zones)

Figure 5.16

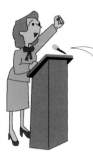

OVERLAPPING VT / VF zones - Part 1

You learned that we may program 3 tachycardia zones VF, f-VT and s-VT. But do you also know that the f-VT zone may overlap either the VF or VT zone ? Such an arrangement is used in Medtronic ICDs where VT diagnosis requires detection of consecutive ventricular intervals. The purpose of the algorithm is to provide ATP for rapid (relatively regular) VT that would otherwise be treated with a shock in the VF zone.

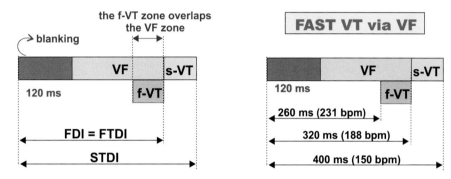

Detection follows VF rules. If the patient exhibits fast VT ordinarily in the VF zone (for which a shock is the only treatment), "fast VT via VF" can be programmed for more flexible alternative therapy.

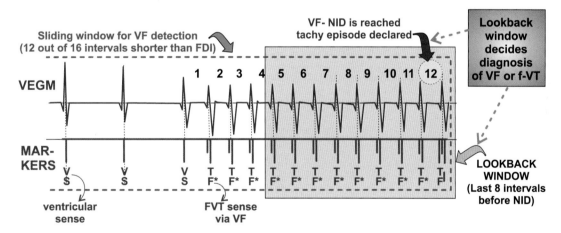

* If any of the intervals in the lookback window is shorter than the programmed range of intervals of the f-VT zone, the tachycardia episode is interpreted as VF.
* If all the 8 intervals in the lookback window are within the f-VT zone, the tachycardia episode is interpreted as f-VT. Then less aggressive therapy than a shock, such as ATP can be programmed for the f-VT.

Abreviations : ATP = antitachycardia pacing ; FDI = ventricular fibrillation detection interval ; NID = number of intervals needed to detect ; VEGM = ventricular electrogram ; VF = ventricular fibrillation ; VT = ventricular tachycardia ; f-VT = fast ventricular tachycardia ; s-VT = slow ventricular tachycardia ; FTDI = fast ventricular tachycardia detection interval ; STDI = slow ventricular tachycardia detection interval ;

A. F. Sinnaeve

Figure 5.17

OVERLAPPING VT / VF zones - Part 2

Here comes some more information about the other possibility. Remember that under certain circumstances, the overlapping zones in both "fast VT via VF" and "fast VT via VT" algorithms may merge during redetection of a tachycardia .

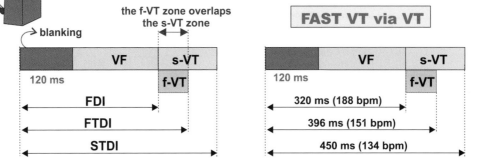

FAST VT via VT

If the patient exhibits two clinical VTs, both outside the VF zone, "fast VT via VT" has to be programmed to prevent misclassification of VF, and to offer a separate therapy regimen for each VT.

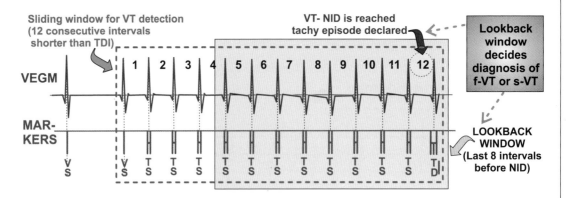

* If any of the intervals in the lookback window is shorter than FTDI or FDI, the tachycardia episode is interpreted as f-VT
* If all of the intervals in the lookback window are outside the VF zone and outside the f-VT zone, the tachycardia episode is interpreted as s-VT

MARKER SYMBOLS (MEDTRONIC)

ventr. pace	ventr. sense	FVT sense via VT	FVT sense via VF	VT sense	VF sense	FVT detection	VF detection	VT detection
V P	V S	T* F	T F*	T S	F S	T F	F D	T D

Abreviations : ATP = antitachycardia pacing ; FDI = ventricular fibrillation detection interval ; NID = number of intervals needed to detect ; VEGM = ventricular electrogram ; VF = ventricular fibrillation ; VT = ventricular tachycardia ; f-VT = fast ventricular tachycardia ; s-VT = slow ventricular tachycardia ; FTDI = fast ventricular tachycardia detection interval ; STDI = slow ventricular tachycardia detection interval ;

A. F. Sinnaeve

Figure 5.18

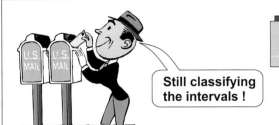

Still classifying the intervals !

SIMULTANEOUS COUNTING IN TWO ZONES VF & VT

GUIDANT

* Each zone has its own detection window.
* In the VF window all intervals are compared to the fibrillation detection interval (FDI) and classified fast (F) if they are shorter or slow (S) if they are longer than FDI. Only the fast (F) intervals are counted by the VF counter.
* In the VT window all intervals are compared to the tachycardia detection interval (TDI) and classified accordingly. Only the fast (F) intervals are counted by the VT counter.
* Intervals identified as fast (F) in a higher window (e.g. VF) are also classified as fast (F) in any lower window (e.g. VT).
* When 8 of 10 intervals are fast in any zone, the detection window of this zone is satisfied

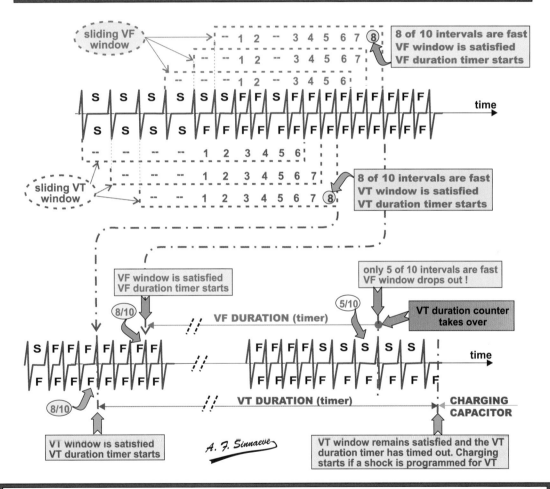

The **DURATION TIMER** (length of time) is programmable. It starts when the window of a particular zone has been satisfied and continues to elapse as long as the zone detection window remains satisfied (6/10 intervals). The duration timer ensures that the tachyarrhythmia remains sustained before initiating therapy. As a rule, the duration timing for VF should be shorter than that for VT.
NOTE : while a higher zone's duration timer (e.g. VF) is elapsing, it has precedence over a lower zone's duration timer (e.g. VT). The latter continues timing out in case the higher zone drops out.

Figure 5.19

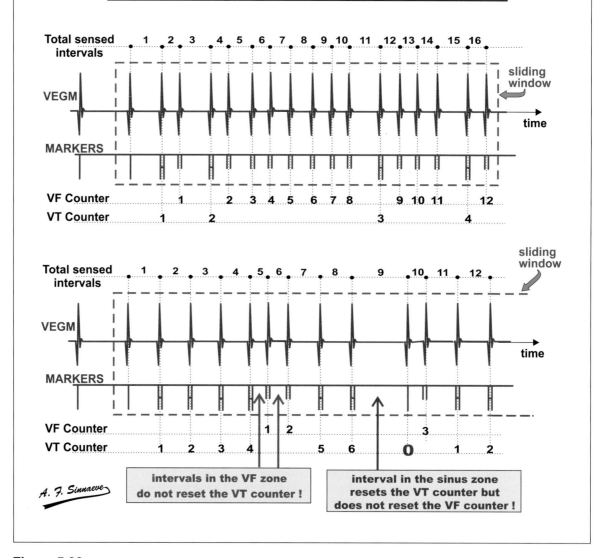

Figure 5.20

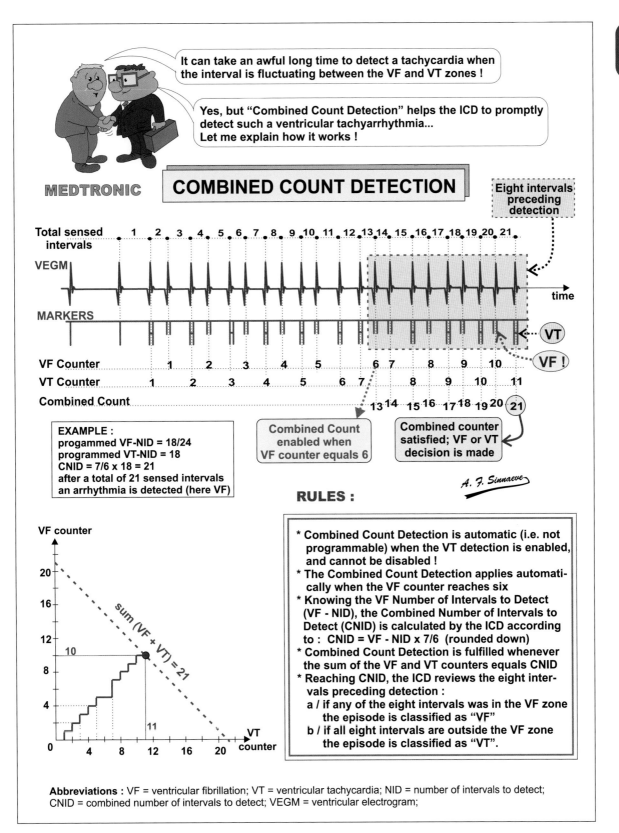

Figure 5.21

(6) SVT/VT DISCRIMINATION

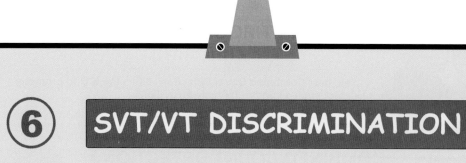

* Arrhythmia detection and discrimination :

    * General principles
    * Sensitivity and specificity

* Single chamber discriminators :

    * Summary of possibilities
    * The stability criterion
    * The onset criterion
    * Detection by EGM morphology :
        technical principles : 1 - 3
    * The Medtronic Marquis VR system parts 1 & 2
    * The St Jude Medical system
    * The Guidant (BS) system

* Dual chamber discriminators :

    * Summary of possibilities
    * Guidant Rhythm ID : parts 1 - 4
    * SJM Rate Branch algorithm : parts 1 - 6
    * Medtronic PR Logic : parts 1 - 5

* Duration-based features to override discriminators :

    * Guidant : Sustained duration override
    * SJM : Maximum time to diagnosis
    * Summary of sensing, detection and therapy

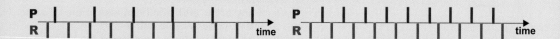

Figure 6.00

ARRHYTHMIA DETECTION AND DISCRIMINATION

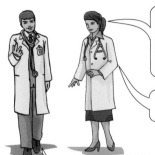

I know that the detection of VF/VT in all ICDs is based upon the mean ventricular rate being higher than a preset value. I learned that such criterion can be obtained sequentially, or better and safer with a sliding window or with a running average.

Now you are talking about discriminators ! Can you tell me what they are and why they are needed ?

Discriminators are intended primarily to avoid inappropriate therapy of SVT by discriminating between VT and SVT.
Let me start with an overview of all excisting discriminators ! In the following pages, I'll give some more details.

DISCRIMINATORS

Single Chamber ICDs	Dual Chamber ICDs
Also called detection enhancements : * Stability (R-R interval regularity) * Sudden onset of ventricular activity * Morphology of ventricular EGM *Not a real discriminator :* * Sustained-duration override	* Atrial and ventricular rate counting (V-rate higher than A-rate ?) * Atrioventricular association * P : R pattern * Chamber of origin * Active or premature stimulation

A. F. Sinnaeve

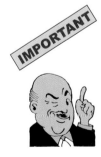

IMPORTANT

Detection : based on cycle length/rate and number of intervals.
VT diagnosis : device has interpreted the detected arrhythmia as ventricular tachycardia.
Therapy can only be initiated by VT diagnosis.
Discriminators : can inhibit the VT diagnosis !
Necessary to avoid inappropriate therapy of SVT.
Programmable to OFF, MONITOR, or ON.
* OFF : not applied, no diagnostics.
* MONITOR : not applied, diagnostics collected.
* ON : applied to diagnosis, diagnostics collected.
If discriminators are not programmed ON, detection = diagnosis.

Abbreviations : EGM = electrogram; SVT = supraventricular tachycardia; VF = ventricular fibrillation; VT = ventricular tachycardia;

Figure 6.01

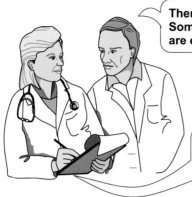

There are many different algorithms for arrhythmia detection ! Some are really sophisticated, but how do we know that they are efficient ? And how can we compare them ?

SENSITIVITY AND SPECIFICITY

We need some statistics ! The foundation of science and all evidence-based medicine ! Let me explain a couple of things...

 POSSIBILITIES WHILE USING AN ALGORITHM FOR VF DETECTION

* TRUE POSITIVES (TP) : The patient has VF and the algorithm has detected it correctly

* FALSE NEGATIVES (FN) : The patient has VF, but the algorithm has not detected it

* TRUE NEGATIVES (TN) : The patient has no VF and the algorithm has detected none

* FALSE POSITIVES (FP) : The patient has no VF, yet the algorithm has detected it

	DETECTION YES	NO
FIBRILLATION YES	TP	FN
FIBRILLATION NO	FP	TN

2
$$\text{SENSITIVITY of the algorithm (\%)} = \frac{TP}{TP + FN} \times 100$$

The sensitivity is a measure of the capability to detect all rhythms that should be treated. It is defined as the percentage of patients with VF that is correctly detected as VF.
The sensitivity should be as high as possible (ideally it should be 100%) i.e. the number of false negatives should be as small as possible.

$$\text{SPECIFICITY of the algorithm (\%)} = \frac{TN}{TN + FP} \times 100$$

The specificity is a measure of the capability to reject all rhythms that should not be treated. It is defined as the percentage of patients without VF correctly interpreted as VF being absent.
The specificity should be as high as possible (ideally it should be 100%) i.e. the number of false positives should be as small as possible.

ABBREVIATIONS : VF = ventricular fibrillation

A. F. Sinnaeve

Figure 6.02

Discriminators in single chamber and dual chamber ICDs are imperfect !
They are helpful in reducing inappropriate shocks but they do not eliminate
them. The terminology and algorithms vary from manufacturer to manufacturer. In some devices the discriminators are available only in the lower
zone VT. The follow-up procedures are complex.

SINGLE CHAMBER DISCRIMINATORS

① **VENTRICULAR STABILITY :** discriminates monomorphic VT from AF based on regularity of the RR interval.

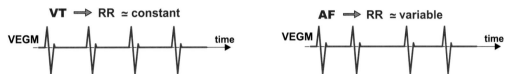

VT ⟹ RR ≃ constant   **AF** ⟹ RR ≃ variable

Weak points : The RR interval in atrial fibrillation tends to become more regular at faster rates. Interval stability cannot reliably differentiate VT vs AF with ventricular rates above 170/min. Unstable polymorphic VT may result in false negatives.

② **SUDDEN ONSET :** discriminates VT from ST by withholding therapy from tachy-cardias in which the rate increases gradually.

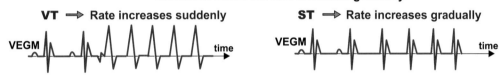

VT ⟹ Rate increases suddenly   **ST** ⟹ Rate increases gradually

Weak points : (1) Will not discriminate sudden onset SVT. (2) May miss VT that starts below the tachycardia detection rate and then accelerates gradually. (3) May miss VT originating during SVT or sinus tachycardia (ST). (4) Before using this discriminator for slow VT, it is important to deter-mine whether inappropriate treatment for SVT is likely (exercise stress test, Holter recordings, etc.). Consider using beta-blockers.

③ **MORPHOLOGY :** discriminates VT from any SVT based on morphologic differences between electrograms in sinus rhythm (template) and tachycardia (using near-field EGM - St Jude).

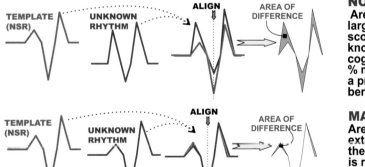

NO MATCH ! ➡ VT Area of difference is large and the % match score is low. The un-known rhythm is re-cognized as VT if the % match is lower than a programmable num-ber (e.g. 70%)

MATCH ! ➡ SVT Area of difference is extremely small and the unknown rhythm is recognized as SVT (% match higher than programmed number)

Weak points : (1) Template recorded with many VPCs or idioventricular rhythm ; (2) Electrogram truncation for very large signals ; (3) Alignment errors ; (4) Oversensing pectoral myopotentials for systems that use the far-field EGM ; (5) Bundle branch block ; (6) Distortion of EGM soon after shock
Note : about 5 - 10% of VTs produce a VEGM similar to that in sinus rhythm.

Abbreviations : AF = atrial fibrillation; EGM = electrogram; NSR = normal sinus rate; ST = sinus tachycardia; SVT = supraventricular tachycardia; VEGM = ventricular electrogram; VF = ventricular fibrillation; VT = ventricular tachycardia;

Figure 6.03

The interval **STABILITY CRITERION** uses the inherent variability of the RR interval in AF to distinguish it from VT which is often regular.
A particular stability algorithm "looks back" at the duration of the preceding cycle. The algorithm works only after the VT counter reaches 3. With a stability of 60 ms (programmable), an interval shorter than the TDI will not be counted (and labeled) as VT if its duration is more than 60 ms longer than the preceding cycle. In such a case, a VT algorithm based on sensing consecutive VT cycles, will reset the counter to zero.

THE STABILITY CRITERION

Remember, the stability as well as the onset enhancement do not function in the VF zone !

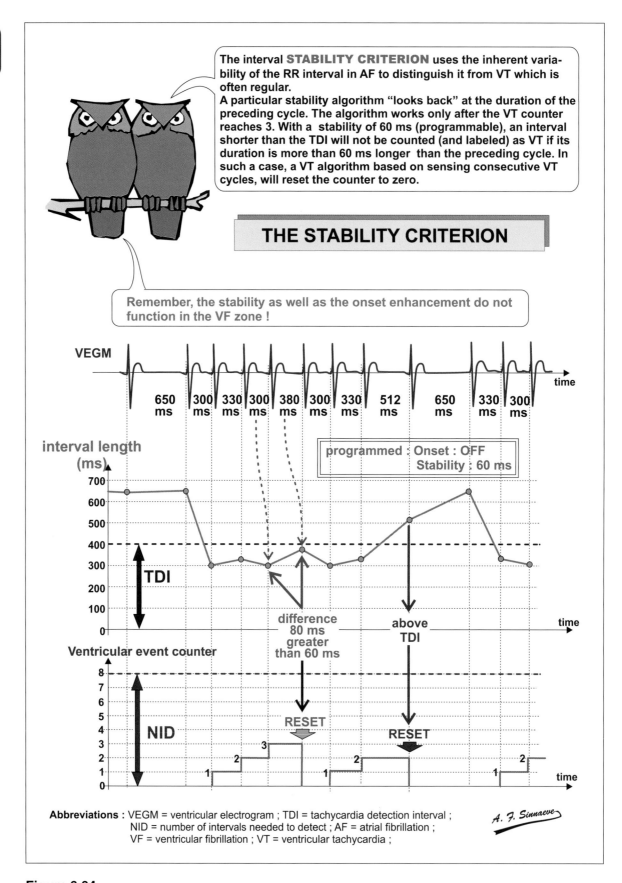

Abbreviations : VEGM = ventricular electrogram ; TDI = tachycardia detection interval ; NID = number of intervals needed to detect ; AF = atrial fibrillation ; VF = ventricular fibrillation ; VT = ventricular tachycardia ;

Figure 6.04

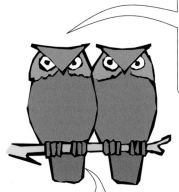

The ONSET criterion is useful to distinguish a relatively slow VT from sinus tachycardia. A sudden reduction in cycle length will be detected as VT, but a gradual rate increase is interpreted as sinus tachycardia and not detected.

Let us consider a relatively simple algorithm that "looks back" at the average of some cycles (e.g. 4) preceding a tachycardia cycle shorter than the TDI. This tachycardia cycle will not be counted when it is longer than a percentage of the average (e.g. 80%).

THE SUDDEN ONSET CRITERION

The algorithm and the terminology vary according ICD models & manufacturers.
Remember, these detection enhancements do not function in the VF zone !

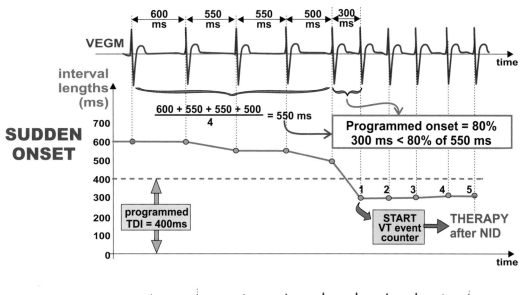

SUDDEN ONSET

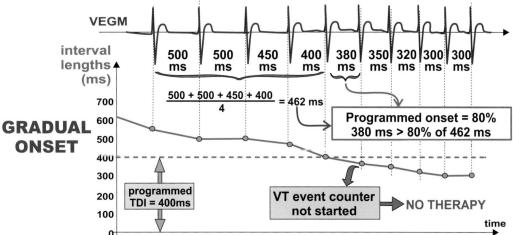

GRADUAL ONSET

Abbreviations : NID = number of intervals needed to detect ; TDI = tachycardia detection interval ; VEGM = ventricular electrogram ; VF = ventricular fibrillation ; VT = ventricular tachycardia ;

Figure 6.05

DETECTION BY ELECTROGRAM MORPHOLOGY - 1

Tell me doctor, why is it so difficult to program an ICD ?
I'm seeing the difference between sinus rhythm and ventricular
fibrillation at a glance. Everybody will notice the difference
between a premature ventricular complex and a regular beat !

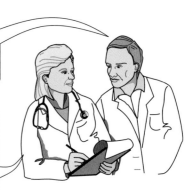

Remember, an ICD cannot "see" the same way we do !
An ICD is a relatively simple device equipped with some computing power and memory. For exploration of the external
world, it can only measure time and voltage ! So, what we call
"form" or "morphology" has to be translated for the ICD in
terms of time and voltage. That's why we need an algorithm.

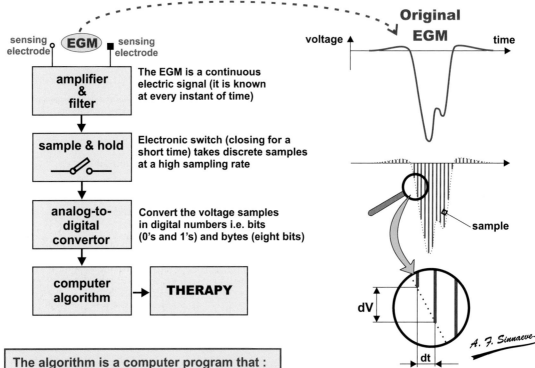

sensing electrode ○ — **EGM** — ■ **sensing electrode**

amplifier & filter — The EGM is a continuous electric signal (it is known at every instant of time)

sample & hold — Electronic switch (closing for a short time) takes discrete samples at a high sampling rate

analog-to-digital convertor — Convert the voltage samples in digital numbers i.e. bits (0's and 1's) and bytes (eight bits)

computer algorithm → **THERAPY**

Original EGM — voltage ↑ — time →

sample

dV

dt

A. F. Sinnaeve

The algorithm is a computer program that :
* determines the maximum (+ or -) of each EGM
* aligns the EGMs (i.e. corresponding peaks)
* takes an average of a number of EGMs during
  sinus rhythm (called a template ; this template
  is stored in device memory for comparison)
* compares every new VEGM with the template
  (i.e. makes some calculations)
* expresses the differences between the VEGM
  and the template as a number
* decides if the new EGM is a VT or a SVT

Contemporary morphology algorithms :
* St Jude : compares the surface areas
  of the peaks
* Medtronic : decomposes the VEGM in
  a number of Haar wavelets
* Guidant : calculates the direction of
  the heart vector

Figure 6.06

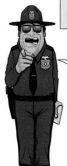

DETECTION BY ELECTROGRAM MORPHOLOGY - 2

Morphology detection is based on comparison of the VEGM of a suspected tachy-arrhythmia with the stored VEGM of a normally conducted sinus beat. Theoretically the VEGM of a SVT should be virtually the same as that of a normal ventricular complex while that of a VT should be substantially different. This distinction works fairly well in practice but there are exceptions (as in patients who develop BBB with a wide QRS complex, only with a rapid sinus rate or SVT). The VEGM pattern used by the device for detection is stored as a template which is the average of a given number "n" of sinus VEGMs.

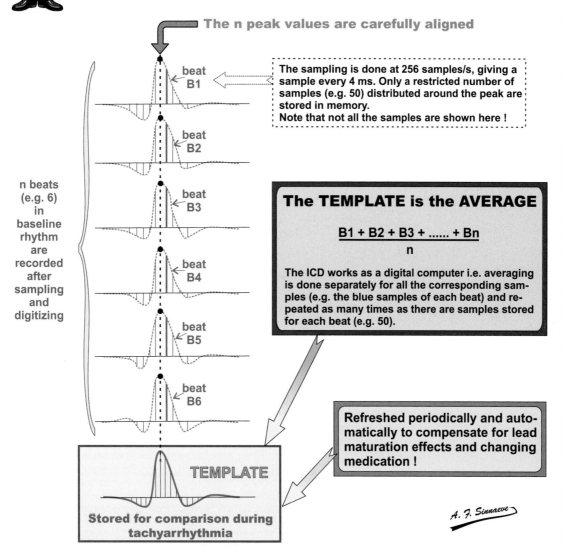

The n peak values are carefully aligned

beat B1

The sampling is done at 256 samples/s, giving a sample every 4 ms. Only a restricted number of samples (e.g. 50) distributed around the peak are stored in memory.
Note that not all the samples are shown here !

beat B2

n beats (e.g. 6) in baseline rhythm are recorded after sampling and digitizing

beat B3

The TEMPLATE is the AVERAGE

$$\frac{B1 + B2 + B3 + ... + Bn}{n}$$

The ICD works as a digital computer i.e. averaging is done separately for all the corresponding samples (e.g. the blue samples of each beat) and repeated as many times as there are samples stored for each beat (e.g. 50).

beat B4

beat B5

beat B6

Refreshed periodically and automatically to compensate for lead maturation effects and changing medication !

A. F. Sinnaeve

TEMPLATE

Stored for comparison during tachyarrhythmia

Contemporary ICDs can acquire a template automatically or manually on demand. (paced beats are ignored as well as those beats immediately following a paced beat, beats too fast for the normal sinus zone are also excluded)

Abbreviations : BBB = Bundle branch block ; SVT = supraventricular tachycardia ; VT = ventricular tachycardia ; VEGM = ventricular electrogram ;

Figure 6.07

DETECTION BY ELECTROGRAM MORPHOLOGY
MEDTRONIC MARQUIS VR - part 1

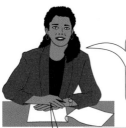

* To minimize the calculations (and hence the power consumption!), the template as well as the VEGMs under investigation, are decomposed into a series of "Haar" wavelets.
* To discriminate between VT and SVT, the wavelet reconstructions of both template and unknown VEGM are compared.

* The more (i.e. smaller) wavelets used, the more closely the reconstruction approximates the original.
* After noise filtering (i.e. omitting very small wavelets) typically between 8 and 20 coefficients are used to describe a template or a VEGM signal.

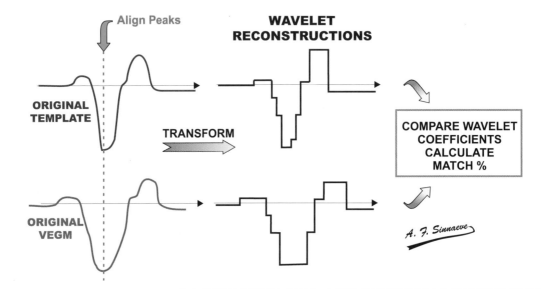

Align Peaks

WAVELET RECONSTRUCTIONS

ORIGINAL TEMPLATE

TRANSFORM

ORIGINAL VEGM

COMPARE WAVELET COEFFICIENTS CALCULATE MATCH %

A. F. Sinnaeve

The matching is done in the ICD by comparing the coefficients of the wavelets of the template to those of the wavelets of tachycardia VEGM. The match is expressed by the ICD as a percentage. If both sets of coefficients are identical the match is 100% and the tachycardia is recognized as SVT. The greater the difference between the two sets of coefficients, the lower the matching percentage. If this percentage is smaller than a preset "%match" (programmable e.g. 70%), the tachycardia is recognized as VT.

* The EGM source and range used for morphology analysis is user programmable and can be near-field or far-field.
* The wavelet algorithm is only activated when a VT episode reaches the NID (number of intervals to detect) and the ICD reviews the QRS complexes in a "look back" window consisting of eight complexes.
* The wavelet algorithm is only applied during initial detection. If the VT detection criterion is met the algorithm will not be applied during redetection.

Abbreviations : NID = number of intervals needed for detection; SVT = supraventricular tachycardia; VEGM = ventricular electrogram; VT = ventricular tachycardia;

Figure 6.08

DETECTION BY ELECTROGRAM MORPHOLOGY
MEDTRONIC   MARQUIS VR - part 2

UNDERSTANDING WAVELETS

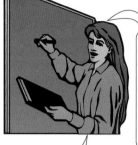

* Each waveform, no matter how jagged or irregular, can be expressed as the sum of a series of simple basic waveforms. These basic waveforms are called wavelets. There many kinds of wavelets.

* "Haar" wavelets are simple rectangular waveforms. They are straightforward mathematical functions which are easily defined by a couple of coefficients (amplitude & position). The duration of each higher Haar wavelet is half of that of the preceding lower one (e.g. the duration of H2 is 50% of the duration of H1).

* I'll spare you the integrals and the higher mathematics of the wavelet decomposition... Let's just show that the algebraic summation of only three Haar wavelets already gives a complicated waveform.

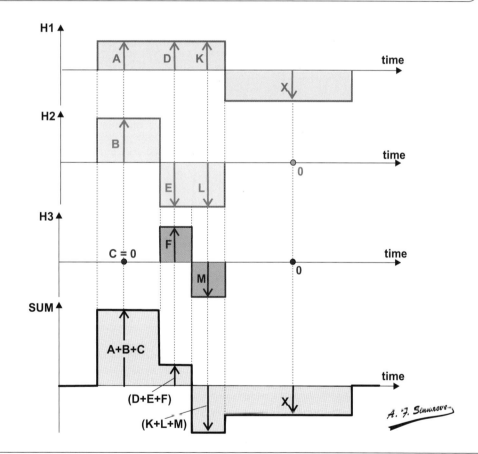

HISTORICAL NOTE :
* Alfred HAAR was a Hungarian mathematician (born in Budapest in 1885 - died in Szeged in 1933). He was the first to describe simple (not sinusoidal) waveforms that are known nowadays as wavelets.
* Wavelet analysis is the contemporary successor of the well known Fourier analysis (which decomposes in a series of sine and cosine functions). The two languages clearly belong to the same family.

Figure 6.09

DETECTION BY ELECTROGRAM MORPHOLOGY
MEDTRONIC MARQUIS VR - part 3

OK ! I understand how the ICD decomposes a QRS complex in a number of simple wavelets and compares it with an equally decomposed template. I also understand how a single VEGM is recognized as VT or SVT. But, how is this information used to classify a rapid rate as SVT or VT and when is ATP therapy started ?

Well, the wavelet algorithm is only activated when a VT episode reaches the NID (initial or combined).
Then, the ICD reviews the QRS complexes in a "look back" window consisting of eight complexes preceding, but not including, the event that fulfilled detection...

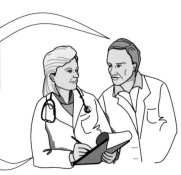

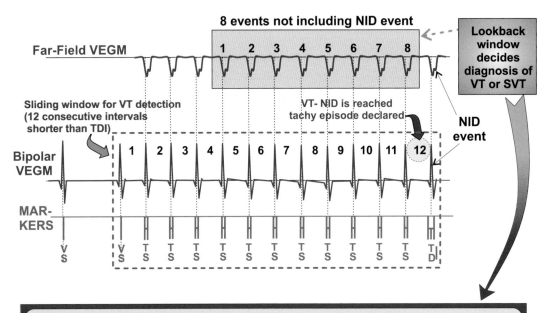

* If six or more of the eight complexes in the "lookback window" are declared as "no-match" to the template, the ICD detects the episode as VT.
* If three or more complexes are a "match" to the template, the ICD detects the episode as SVT and the VT counter (sliding window) is reset to zero.

Note : The wavelet algorithm replaces the former SVT vs. VT enhancement algorithm based on QRS width.

Abbreviations : NID = number of intervals to detect; SVT = supraventricular tachycardia;VT = ventricular tachycardia; VEGM = ventricular electrogram;

Figure 6.10

DETECTION BY ELECTROGRAM MORPHOLOGY
St JUDE MEDICAL

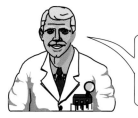

More computational power of contemporary ICDs makes newer dis-
criminators possible, based on more complex electrogram features.
One of these morphology algorithms is the "AREA OF DIFFERENCE
METHOD". Its principle is still relatively simple, but it looks to the
VEGM like an expert cardiologist.

* The "Morphology Discriminator" of St Jude Medical uses the bipolar VEGM of the rate channel.
* The algorithm is based upon several morphologic characteristics : (1) number of peaks (positive
  or negative) (2) sequence of peaks (3) peak polarity (4) amplitude and area of peaks.
* The manufacturer recommends using the system with a "good" template (i.e. if the baseline
  rhythm matches 80% or more with the template).
* The morphology enhancement is inappropriate in patients with rate-related BBB or VT with morphology similar to baseline.
* The morphology template match can be programmed to "monitor only" for storage of data not
  used by the ICD for diagnosis.

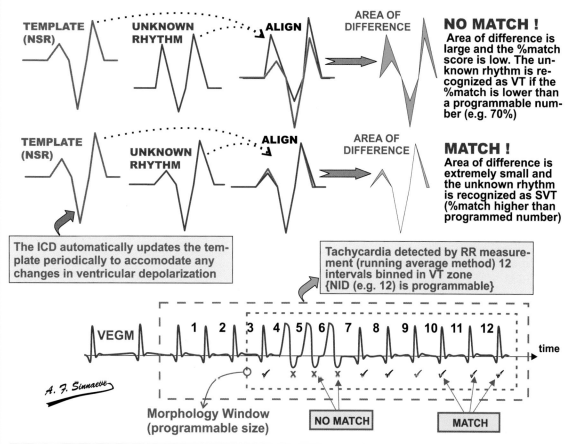

NO MATCH !
Area of difference is large and the %match score is low. The unknown rhythm is recognized as VT if the %match is lower than a programmable number (e.g. 70%)

MATCH !
Area of difference is extremely small and the unknown rhythm is recognized as SVT (%match higher than programmed number)

The ICD automatically updates the template periodically to accomodate any changes in ventricular depolarization

Tachycardia detected by RR measurement (running average method) 12 intervals binned in VT zone {NID (e.g. 12) is programmable}

Morphology Window (programmable size)

NO MATCH

MATCH

The tachycardia is declared as SVT if the number of "matches" in the morphology window equals or exceeds a programmable percentage (e.g. 5 of 8 with 60% match). If the number of matches is less, the device makes the diagnosis of VT.

Abbreviations : BBB= bundle branch block; NID = number of intervals needed for detection; NSR= normal sinus rhythm; SVT = supraventricular tachycardia; VT = ventricular tachycardia; VEGM = ventricular electrogram;

Figure 6.11

DETECTION BY ELECTROGRAM MORPHOLOGY
GUIDANT VITALITY - VECTOR TIMING ALGORITRHM

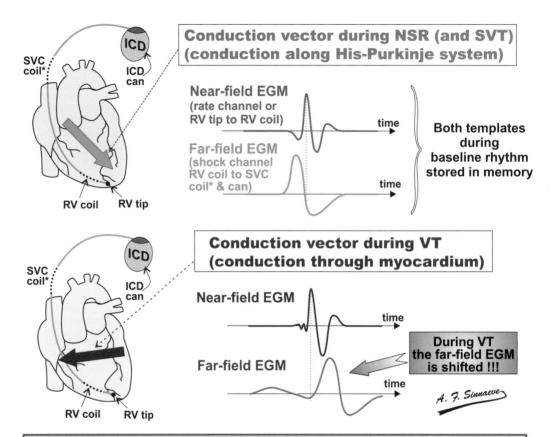

**Conduction vector during NSR (and SVT)
(conduction along His-Purkinje system)**

SVC coil*

ICD
ICD can

RV coil   RV tip

Near-field EGM
(rate channel or
RV tip to RV coil)

time

Far-field EGM
(shock channel
RV coil to SVC
coil* & can)

time

Both templates
during
baseline rhythm
stored in memory

**Conduction vector during VT
(conduction through myocardium)**

SVC coil*

ICD
ICD can

RV coil   RV tip

Near-field EGM

time

Far-field EGM

time

During VT
the far-field EGM
is shifted !!!

A. F. Sinnaeve

The peaks of both near-field EGMs (recorded during NSR and tachycardia) are aligned for
analysis of the timing differences of the far-field signals for the diagnosis of VT vs. SVT.

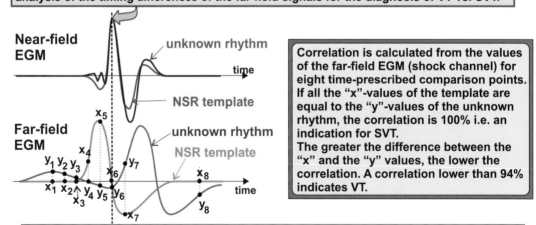

**Near-field
EGM**

unknown rhythm

time

NSR template

**Far-field
EGM**

x_5

x_4

y_1 y_2 y_3

x_6 y_7

x_8

x_1 x_2 y_4 y_5 y_6

time

x_3

y_8

x_7

unknown rhythm
NSR template

Correlation is calculated from the values
of the far-field EGM (shock channel) for
eight time-prescribed comparison points.
If all the "x"-values of the template are
equal to the "y"-values of the unknown
rhythm, the correlation is 100% i.e. an
indication for SVT.
The greater the difference between the
"x" and the "y" values, the lower the
correlation. A correlation lower than 94%
indicates VT.

At the end of the programmable "duration period", the *vector timing algorithm* is looking
back : if 8 of the last 10 beats are uncorrelated (i.e. correlation < 94%) the tachycardia is
classified and treated as VT.

Abbreviations : EGM = electrogram; NSR = normal sinus rhythm; RV = right ventricle; SVC = superior vena
cava; SVT = supraventricular tachycardia; VT = ventricular tachycardia; SVC coil* : if present ;

Figure 6.12

DUAL CHAMBER DISCRIMINATORS
GENERAL PRINCIPLES

This ain't easy, you know !

The design of dual chamber ICDs is based on single chamber experience. Discriminators used in single chamber ICDs (stability, sudden onset and morphology) may or may not be incorporated into dual chamber ICDs according to design and manufacturer. Dual chamber algorithms use both the atrial and the ventricular electrograms for diagnosis.

A. F. Sinnaeve

① ATRIAL & VENTRICULAR RATE COUNTING :

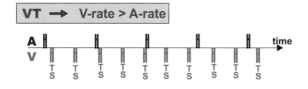

VT ➝ V-rate > A-rate

A dual chamber ICD makes the diagnosis of VT whenever the V rate exceeds the A rate. Fortunately this occurs commonly during VT (in more than 90% of VTs) !

VT with 1:1 AV relationship & constant PR presents the most difficult chalenge in SVT vs VT discrimination.

Weak points :
* undersensing (during AF) & oversensing (during VT, due to VA far-field sensing).
* inability to classify VT with 1:1 AV relationship; false negatives in dual tachycardias such as AF + VT

② ATRIOVENTRICULAR ASSOCIATION :

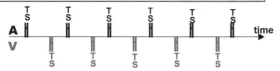

A flut ➝ stable 2:1 AV association

An AV association discriminator monitors the stability of the PR or RP intervals during tachycardia.
Methodology varies according to the manufacturer.

A flut + VT ➝ AV dissociation

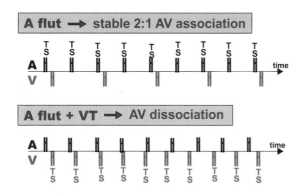

Weak points :
* tachycardias with 1:1 AV or VA conduction;
* undersensing & oversensing; degree of block and hence PR or RP intervals may vary during tachycardia;

③ DETAILED ANALYSIS of P/QRS RELATIONSHIP :

Medtronic's PR Logic algorithm classifies tachycardias with 1:1 AV relationship as sinus or AV junctional according to the location of the AEGM in the VV interval. It looks for atrial fibrillation by counting the number of atrial events in each VV cycle. It can also differentiate far-field R wave sensing from a true atrial event according to the location of the signals in the atrial EGM.

Abbreviations : AEGM = atrial electrogram; A flut = atrial flutter; AF = A fib = atrial fibrillation; AV = atrioventricular; EGM = electrogram; VA = ventriculoatrial; SVT = supraventricular tachycardia; VT = ventricular tachycardia;

Figure 6.13

DISCRIMINATION ALGORITHMS
RHYTHM ID™ (Guidant) - 1

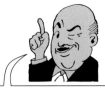

This is an SVT discrimination feature that is straightforward to engage and manage !
And with a minimal programming parameters !

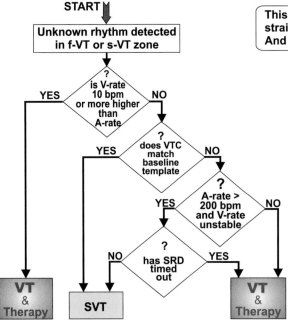

START

Unknown rhythm detected in f-VT or s-VT zone

? is V-rate 10 bpm or more higher than A-rate

YES — NO

? does VTC match baseline template

YES — NO

? A-rate > 200 bpm and V-rate unstable

YES — NO

? has SRD timed out

NO — YES

VT & Therapy

SVT

VT & Therapy

"RHYTHM ID" is a sophisticated algorithm that discriminates SVT from VT for purposes of reducing inappropriate therapy.
* Utilizes a morphology-based method called Vector Timing and Correlation or VTC (automatically adjusts stored template to changing patient rhythm during periodic updates).
* Integrates additional interval based discriminators (i.e. A fib rate threshold and interval stability)

A. F. Sinnaeve

1 V-rate > A-rate

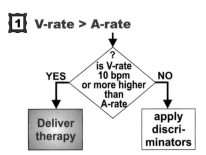

? is V-rate 10 bpm or more higher than A-rate

YES — NO

Deliver therapy

apply discriminators

* Once a fast rhythm is detected, ventricular and atrial rates are analyzed.
* If the ventricular rate is significantly faster than the atrial rate (at least 10 bpm higher), VT is diagnosed and therapy is delivered.
* If the ventricular rate is not faster than the atrial rate, SVT discriminators (enhancement criteria) may be applied.

2 V-rate ≤ A-rate
Morphology based discrimination

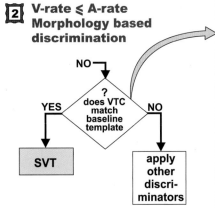

NO

? does VTC match baseline template

YES — NO

SVT

apply other discriminators

timing reference

Near-field EGM (rate channel or RV tip to RV coil)

Far-field EGM (shock channel RV coil to SVC coil* & can)   Actual signal

Template

* Vector Timing and Correlation (VTC) calculates a coefficient of correlation between a template (recorded during baseline rhythm) and the actual signal *(as discussed before)*.

* If there is a good match (correlation coefficient > 94%) between the template and the actual signal, the rhythm is classified as SVT.

* If there is no match (8 of the last 10 beats are uncorrelated), other discriminators may be used.

* The template can be automatically updated every 140 minutes, but manual updating is also possible.

Abbreviations : *SRD = sustained rate duration; SVT = supraventricular tachycardia; VT = ventricular tachycardia;*

Figure 6.14

DISCRIMINATION ALGORITHMS RHYTHM ID™ (Guidant) - 2

Very easy to use and to program ! And yet an excellent specificity without compromising the sensitivity !

3 **V-rate ≤ A-rate**
Interval based discrimination

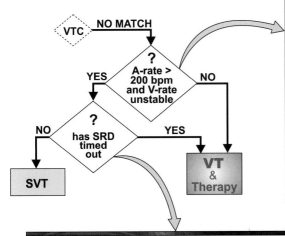

When "VTC" (morphology) does not find a proper match, the rhythm is probably VT and additional enhancement criteria are applied :

* *A fib rate threshold* : the rhythm may be classified as SVT if the atrial rate is above the A fib threshold (fixed at 200 bpm).
* *V rate stabilty* : the stability of the arrhythmia is evaluated by calculating the R-R differences. If the average difference is greater than 20 ms (fixed), the rhythm can be classified as SVT.

Note : *Both "Stability" and "A fib rate" must be met* (**AND** decision) *to declare a rhythm as SVT and to inhibit therapy* !

---

* Sustained Rate Duration (SRD) allows the therapy to be delivered when a tachycardia is sustained for a programmed period of time but SVT inhibit criteria indicates to withhold therapy.
* The SRD timer is programmable (setting : OFF, 10 s, ... 60 min - nominal 3 min)
* The "Rhythm ID" algorithm continues to evaluate the rhythm beat-by-beat throughout SRD while therapy is inhibited until :
  - SRD timer expires
  - Rate increases to higher zone and meets criteria for treatment in that zone
  - Rhythm ID determines that rhythm meets treatment criteria (e.g. if V becomes greater than A, or VTC determines that rhythm is no longer correlated)

---

4 **Post-Shock discrimination**

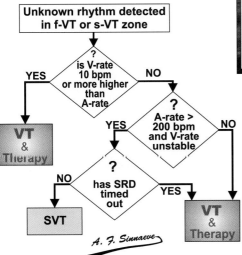

* Since shock delivery may alter rhythm morphology, the "Rhythm ID" algorithm does not use Vector Timing and Correlation (VTC). The rate dependent enhancements (V > A, A fib rate threshold, and stability) are used without VTC.
* Post-shock "Sustained rate duration" (SRD) is independently programmable (nominal value 15 s)

NOTE : VR or single chamber devices

The VR mode may be selected in dual chamber devices in circumstances where atrial information would not be needed or desired, e.g. if atrial port is plugged or if atrial sensing is questionable.
In the VR mode, atrial information (V > A, A fib rate threshold) is not used. In addition Stability is not used.
Only VTC is used for initial detection and only stability (max. difference 30 ms) is used for post-shock operation.

Abbreviations : A fib = atrial fibrillation; SRD = sustained rate duration; SVT = supraventricular tachycardia; VT = ventricular tachycardia; VTC = vector timing and correlation

Figure 6.15

DISCRIMINATION ALGORITHMS
OBDE   (Guidant) - 3

SUDDEN ONSET (SO)

※ The algorithm differentiates between monomorphic ventricular tachy-cardia (MVT) and sinus activity related to exercise.
※ In two stages, the algorithm evaluates how abruptly the cycle length changes from a "normal rhythm" to a rapid rhythm.
※ SO is only available in the lowest zone of multizone devices and may be programmed in ms or in % .
※ SO is measured only once per episode at the time an episode is declared.

STAGE 1 : Find Pivot Interval

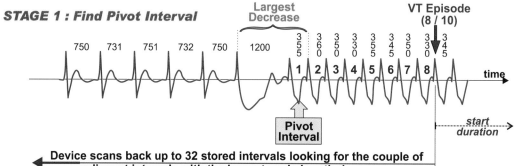

Device scans back up to 32 stored intervals looking for the couple of adjacent intervals with the largest cycle length decrease.

* The shortest of the two adjacent intervals is the pivot interval.
* The pivot delta is the difference between the two adjacent intervals : 1200 - 355 = 845 ms

STAGE 2 : Baseline Average Comparison

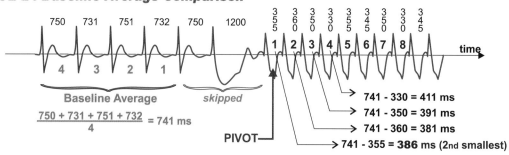

$$\frac{750 + 731 + 751 + 732}{4} = 741\ ms$$

741 - 330 = 411 ms
741 - 350 = 391 ms
741 - 360 = 381 ms
741 - 355 = **386** ms (2nd smallest)

* The device averages 4 intervals prior to the pivot interval to determine baseline average (first two intervals before pivot interval are skipped) : 741 ms
* The difference between baseline average and each of the 4 intervals following the pivot interval is calculated. If 3/4 of the interval differences following the pivot interval are greater than the "Onset Threshold" the onset is declared to be sudden.
* The second smallest difference is identified and used for comparison : 386 ms. (Note that the faster rates - i.e. shorter intervals - give a larger difference with the baseline average).

STAGE 3 : Final Comparison and Decision

* The shorter of pivot delta (stage 1) and the second smallest difference (stage 2) is the measured value reported in episode detail : 845 ms > 386 ms, so 386 ms is used
* This reported value is compared to the programmed "Onset Value" (wich is programmable between 9 and 50 % e.g. 12 %) :

$$\frac{386}{741} \times 100\% = 52\ \% > 12\ \% \longrightarrow \text{SUDDEN onset !!!}$$

Note : **OBDE = One Button Detection Enhancement**

Figure 6.16

DISCRIMINATION ALGORITHMS
RHYTHM ID™ & OBDE (Guidant) - 4

STABILITY

J. F. Cantens MD. PhD.

❖ The Stability Algorithm evaluates the cycle length variability to differentiate stable ventricular rhythms from unstable rhythms.

❖ There are 2 possibilities:
  > "Stability to inhibit" *(RhythmID)* : if a rhythm is declared "unstable" the therapy is withhold (Used to distinguish irregular ventricular response during AF from regular MTV). Available only in the lowest zone of a multizone device.
  > "Shock if unstable" *(OBDE)* (therapy accelerator) : if a rhythm is declared "unstable" initial or remaining ATP therapy is skipped and shock therapy is initiated (Used to differentiate MVT from polymorphic VT/VF). Available in the VT zone (f-VT) of 2 or 3 zone configuration. In a 3 zone device, 'shock if unstable' can be used in the f-VT zone while therapy inhibitors can be used inthe s-VT zone. Applied during 'Initial Detection' and during 'Redetection' (between bursts of ATP).

---

* Stability calculation starts when detection is met (VT declared) and continues throughout "Duration".
* Uses the last 5 consecutive intervals (4 variances) before VT declared to calculate the average variance.
* Adjusts this average variance as new intervals are added during duration
   87.5% of weighted variance + 12.5% of next delta = new weighted average variance
* At the end of Duration the weighted average is compared to the programmed stability threshold
   If measured weighted average is **>** than programmed stability threshold **➜** rhythm is declared UNSTABLE

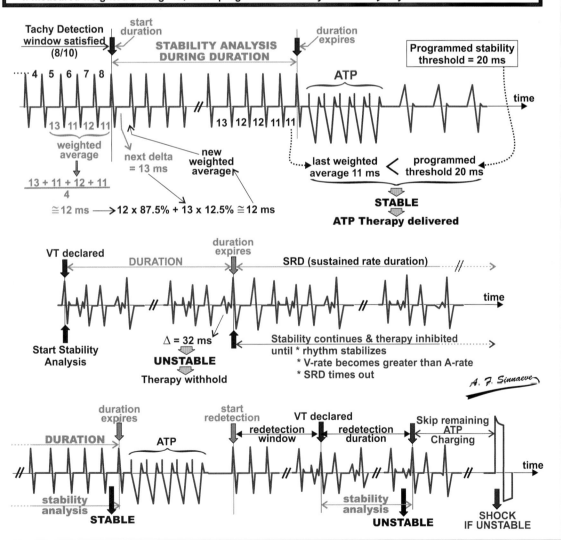

Figure 6.17

DISCRIMINATION ALGORITHMS
The St JUDE system - part 1

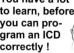

You have a lot to learn, before you can program an ICD correctly !

THE DUAL CHAMBER APPROACH

⭐1 RATE BRANCH ALGORITHM

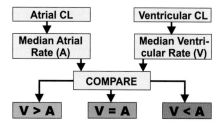

Atrial CL	Ventricular CL
Median Atrial Rate (A)	Median Ventricular Rate (V)

COMPARE

V > A **V = A** **V < A**

> 🌸 The "Rate Branch" algorithm looks at the AA and VV intervals in a window at the time of detection.
>
> 🌸 A and V rates are determined as the median of the AA (or VV) intervals in that window.

⭐2 THE V > A BRANCH

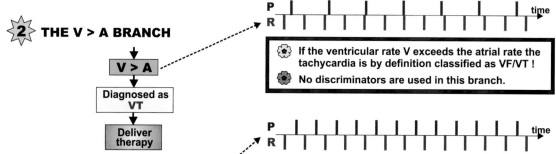

V > A

Diagnosed as **VT**

Deliver therapy

> 🌸 If the ventricular rate V exceeds the atrial rate the tachycardia is by definition classified as VF/VT !
>
> 🌸 No discriminators are used in this branch.

⭐3 THE V = A BRANCH

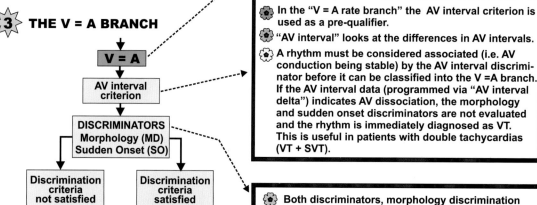

V = A

AV interval criterion

DISCRIMINATORS
Morphology (MD)
Sudden Onset (SO)

Discrimination criteria not satisfied	Discrimination criteria satisfied
Diagnosed as VT with 1:1 retro conduction	Diagnosed as ST, AT, SVT with 1:1 conduction
Deliver therapy	**Inhibit therapy**

> 🌸 In the "V = A rate branch" the AV interval criterion is used as a pre-qualifier.
>
> 🌸 "AV interval" looks at the differences in AV intervals.
>
> 🌸 A rhythm must be considered associated (i.e. AV conduction being stable) by the AV interval discriminator before it can be classified into the V =A branch. If the AV interval data (programmed via "AV interval delta") indicates AV dissociation, the morphology and sudden onset discriminators are not evaluated and the rhythm is immediately diagnosed as VT. This is useful in patients with double tachycardias (VT + SVT).

> 🌸 Both discriminators, morphology discrimination (MD) and sudden onset (SO), may programmed ON or OFF
>
> 🌸 Diagnosis settings can programmed ANY or ALL
>   * setting ANY : one satisfied discriminator (MD or SO) is sufficient to inhibit the therapy
>   * setting ALL : both discriminators (MD and SO) are to be satisfied to inhibit therapy
>
> 🌸 Safest setting : MD = ON, SO = ON, criteria = ANY

A. F. Sinnaeve

Abbreviations : *AT = atrial tachycardia; AV = atrioventricular; CL = cycle length; MD = morphology discrimination; SO = sudden onset discriminator; ST = sinus tachycardia; SVT = supraventricular tachycardia; VF = ventricular fibrillation; VT = ventricular tachycardia;*

Figure 6.18

DISCRIMINATION ALGORITHMS
The St JUDE system - part 2

OK ! Difficult, but so far, I'm able to follow.

THE DUAL CHAMBER APPROACH

4 THE V < A BRANCH

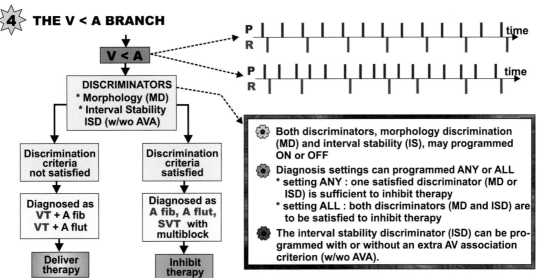

V < A

DISCRIMINATORS
* Morphology (MD)
* Interval Stability ISD (w/wo AVA)

Discrimination criteria **not satisfied**	Discrimination criteria **satisfied**
Diagnosed as **VT + A fib** **VT + A flut**	Diagnosed as **A fib, A flut, SVT** with multiblock
Deliver therapy	**Inhibit therapy**

- Both discriminators, morphology discrimination (MD) and interval stability (IS), may programmed ON or OFF
- Diagnosis settings can programmed ANY or ALL
  * setting ANY : one satisfied discriminator (MD or ISD) is sufficient to inhibit therapy
  * setting ALL : both discriminators (MD and ISD) are to be satisfied to inhibit therapy
- The interval stability discriminator (ISD) can be programmed with or without an extra AV association criterion (w/wo AVA).

SUMMARY :

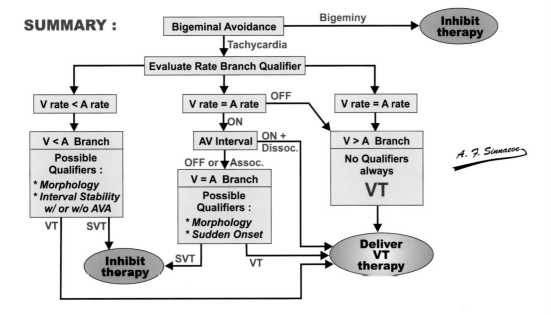

A. F. Sinnaeve

NOTE :
A bigeminal rhythm may have average intervals shorter than the tachycardia detection interval. To prevent against delivering therapy in single Tach configuration or Tachy A configuration (slower tachycardia if 2 tachycardia rates are programmed), the ICD must detect more tachycardia intervals than sinus intervals before it delivers therapy !

Abbreviations : A fib = atrial fibrillation; A flut = atrial flutter; AVA = AV association; SVT = supraventricular tachycardia; VT = ventricular tachycardia;

Figure 6.19

DISCRIMINATION ALGORITHMS
The St JUDE system - part 3

INTERVAL STABILITY DISCRIMINATION (ISD)

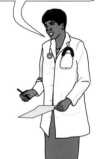

The Interval Stability Discriminator (ISD) was introduced in single chamber ICDs, but is also used in dual chamber devices in the V<A branch.

⭐ "Interval Stability" is designed to discriminate between VT and atrial fibrillation that conducts rapidly to the ventricle.

⭐ This discriminator attempts to differentiate between the rhythms by measuring the beat-to-beat variations in cycle length during the tachycardia. The ventricular rate and cycle length are irregular in atrial fibrillation but VT typically shows little rate variability.

Programming :

Tachy Detect (average interval):	Interval Stability : ON
535 ms / 112 bpm	Interval Stability Delta : 50 ms
NID = 12	Stability window (ISD counter) : 12

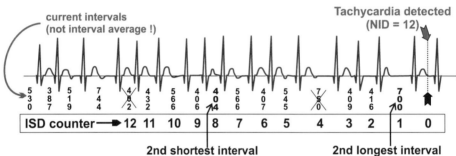

current intervals (not interval average !)

Tachycardia detected (NID = 12)

| ISD counter → | 12 | 11 | 10 | 9 | 8 | 7 | 6 | 5 | 4 | 3 | 2 | 1 | 0 |

2nd shortest interval   2nd longest interval

2nd longest interval - 2nd shortest interval = 700 - 404 = 296
Compare to programmed stability delta : 296 > 50 ms

CONCLUSION : **UNSTABLE** ⟹ (**AF**)

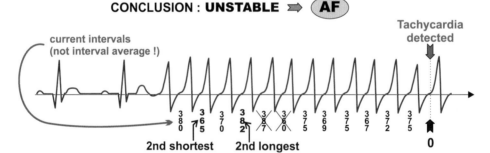

current intervals (not interval average !)

Tachycardia detected

2nd shortest   2nd longest

2nd longest interval - 2nd shortest interval = 382 - 365 = 17
Compare to programmed stability delta : 17 < 50 ms

CONCLUSION : **STABLE** ⟹ (**VT**)

A. F. Sinnaeve

---

* For tachycardia detection, the device looks at the average interval of 4 cycles as defined before (sum of current interval plus 3 previous intervals, divided by 4) as well as the current interval. Both intervals are required for the binning scheme !
* When a tachycardia is detected, the ICD looks back at a programmable number of actual R-R intervals (settings 8, 9, ... 20; nominal 12). The difference between the 2nd longest and the 2nd shortest intervals is calculated and compared to a programmable "Stability Delta" (settings 30, 35, ... 500 ms; nominal 80 ms).
* If the difference is larger than the programmed "Delta", the rhythm is classified as unstable (AF); if the difference is smaller than "Delta", the rhythm is stable and treated as VT.

Abbreviations : AF = atrial fibrillation; Δ = Delta = mathematical symbol for difference; ISD = interval stability discriminator; NID = number of intervals to detect; VT = ventricular tachycardia;

Figure 6.20

DISCRIMINATION ALGORITHMS
The St JUDE system - part 4

AV ASSOCIATION (AVA) in DUAL CHAMBER ICDs

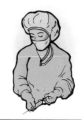

> * The AVA or AV association algorithm looks at the atrial and ventricular electrograms to determine whether they are related or behaving independently. The ICD measures the interval from the R wave to the preceding P wave, searching for variations in the timing.
> * The range of variation is programmable and VT is detected when there is lack of AV association.
> * In St Jude devices this criterion must be used only in combination with the interval stability discrimination algorithm (ISD).
> * This function is most useful when the ventricular rate is lower than the atrial rate and SVT appears regular such as atrial flutter. AV association suggests SVT.

Atrial Flutter + VT

"Interval Stability Discriminator" (ISD) indicates **VT** ; check AVA !

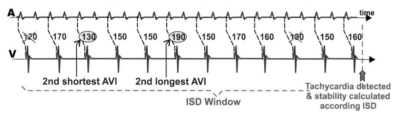

Programmed AVA delta : 40 ms

AVI Difference :
2nd longest - 2nd shortest
= 190 - 130 = 60 ms

AVI Difference > AVA delta :
60 ms > 40 ms
AVA → DISSOCIATED

Final stability indication = VT

Atrial Flutter with 2:1 conduction

"Interval Stability Discriminator" (ISD) indicates **VT** ; check AVA !

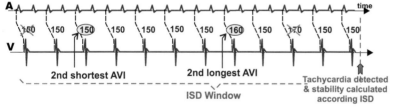

Programmed AVA delta : 40 ms

AVI Difference :
2nd longest - 2nd shortest
= 160 - 150 = 10 ms

AVI Difference > AVA delta :
10 ms < 40 ms
AVA → ASSOCIATED

Final stability indication = SVT

> * If the Interval Stability Discriminator (ISD) is "ON with AVA" and ISD indicates VT, the AV association is examined. A valid AV interval (AVI) is measured from each ventricular sensed event to its preceding atrial event.
> * The difference between the second longest and the second shortest AVI is calculated in a recent group of intervals defined by the progammable ISD window (which was used to verify the stability). This difference is then compared with the programmable AVA-Delta (settings : 30, 40, ..., 150 ms ; nominal : 60 ms).
> * If the measured AVI difference is smaller than the programmed AVA Delta, the AV interval is stable or associated and SVT is indicated. When the AVI difference is larger than AVA-Delta, VT is indicated.
> * NOTE : The smaller the programmed AVA-Delta, the more likely it is that the rhythm will be classified as VT

A. F. Sinnaeve

Abbreviations : AF = A fib = atrial fibrillation; A flut = atrial flutter; AV = atrioventricular; AVA = AV association criterion; AVI = atrioventricular interval; ISD = interval stability discriminator; SVT = supraventricular tachycardia; VT = ventricular tachycardia;

Figure 6.21

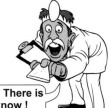

DISCRIMINATION ALGORITHMS
The St JUDE system - part 5

SUDDEN ONSET (SO) :

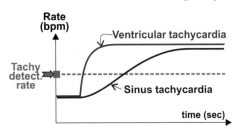

It's not easy ! Not at all ! There is a lot to remember, you know !

★ This discriminator attempts to differentiate rhythms by determining the rate of onset of the tachycardias. Theoretically, VT starts abruptly while ST has a more gradual onset.

★ Feature designed to discriminate ST from VT in patients whose maximum sinus rate can exceed the rate of their slowest VT.

★ Used in single chamber ICDs and in dual chamber ICDs (as part of the V = A branch).

---

* The *"Sudden Onset"* criterion uses a programmable *"Sudden Onset Delta"* to evaluate the rate of onset of the tachycardia (settings : 30, 35, ... 500 ms - nominal 100 ms - or 4, 6, ... 86%).
* For tachycardia detection (performed by counting the number of <u>binned</u> tachycardia events), the St Jude system uses both a <u>running average</u> and a <u>current interval</u>. Binning is done by comparing the running average with the current interval according to previously described methodology.
* As soon as a tachycardia event is binned and therefore detected as tachycardia, the device looks at the previous 8 average intervals, using every other average interval for comparison with the tachycardia average interval (in the following case 428 ms is the first binned interval as VT) in order to determine whether the difference is large enough to satisfy the sudden onset criterion.
* If any of the interval averages minus the tachy average interval is larger than the programmed SO-Delta, the sudden onset is satisfied and the discriminator indicates SVT. Comparison continues with each new interval until detection is satisfied.

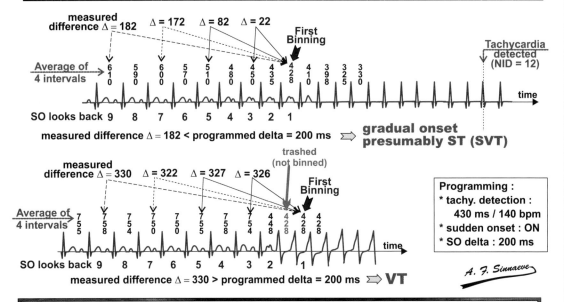

* Since average intervals are used for comparison, a single long interval during a gradual increase in rate may (appropriately) result in failure to satisfy the SO criterion.
* Alternatively, after an abrupt change in cycle length greater than the selected SO-Delta, a single long interval amid several short intervals will probably still allow the SO criterion to be satisfied.
* The smaller the programmed SO-Delta, the more likely a rhythm will be classified as VT.
* An exercise stress test may occasionally be very helpful in selecting an appropriate SO-Delta.

Abbreviations : *NID = number of intervals needed to detect; SO = sudden onset; ST = sinus tachycardia; SVT = supraventricular tachycardia; VT = ventricular tachycardia;* **NOTE** : *Δ = Delta = mathematic symbol for difference;*

Figure 6.22

DISCRIMINATION ALGORITHMS
The St JUDE system - part 6

This is a single chamber discriminator ! It is only used with Ventricular Only Arrhythmia Sensing.

SINUS INTERVAL HISTORY (SIH)

★ SIH gives an additional evaluation of interval irregularity over time.
★ SIH recognizes long intervals that have occurred during "Tachycardia Detection".
★ SIH may be used to identify AF that may have regularized.
★ SIH is only examined if "Interval Stability Discriminator" identifies the rhythm as VT-like

---

* SIH defines the number of sinus intervals or average intervals that can occur during detection of a rhythm considered to be VT.

* If the number of sinus intervals or average intervals is greater than or equal to this threshold, the rhythm may be regularized AF.

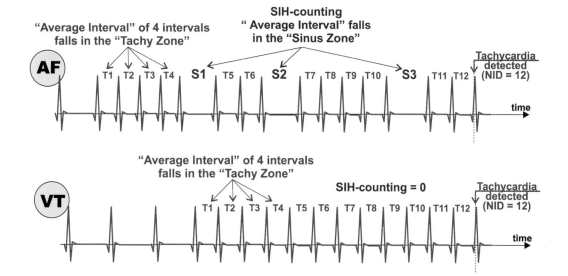

---

* If "Interval Stability" is "ON with SIH" and Interval Stability indicates VT, the number of sinus intervals or average intervals during detection of the arrhythmia is examined. The maximum SIH-count can be programmed. SIH count is increased once for every interval where either :
> The interval's "Current Interval" value is in the sinus zone
> The interval's "Average Interval" value is in the sinus zone
> Both "Current Interval" and "Average Interval" values are in the sinus zone

* If the counted number of sinus intervals is less than the programmed SIH-count, the combination Stability/SIH-count indicates VT.

* When Interval Stability is "ON with SIH" and Interval Stability indicates SVT, the SIH-count is not checked.

* The larger the programmed SIH-count, the more likely it is that a rhythm will be classified as VT

Abbreviations : AF = atrial fibrillation; SIH = sinus interval history; SVT = supraventricular tachycardia; VT = ventricular tachycardia; NID = number of intervals to detect;

Figure 6.23

DISCRIMINATION ALGORITHMS
PR LOGIC™ (Medtronic) - 1

The PR Logic® analyzes the 2 previous RR intervals for the number and location of atrial signals relative to the R wave, i.e. it uses VV, AA, AV and VA intervals to discriminate VT from SVT. Atrial activity is classified as antegrade, retrograde, or junctional based on the position of the atrial signal within the RR interval. The algorithm assigns 19 codes to the number of atrial events relative to the R wave. The codes are compared with sequences known to occur in specific rhythms and patterns of SVT. The code includes variations of P/R patterns and takes into account the presence of VPCs. The information from the coding is used together with other parts of the complex algorithm.

1 ventricular sense, atrial sense, ventricular sense

an atrial sense in these parts of VV is junctional
50%
50 ms / 80 ms
Vs
an atrial sense in this part is retrograde
an atrial sense in this part is antegrade
Vs

The 1:1 VT-ST boundary separates the antegrade and retrograde zones. The nominal value of the antegrade zone is 50% of the V-V cycle (minus 80 ms), but it can be programmed to different values, changing the relative size of the antegrade and retrograde zones. This may be useful if slow retrograde or antegrade events occur in the incorrect zone.
* If a long PR interval pushes the P wave into the retrograde zone : expand the anterograde zone (for example from 50% to 66%), thereby reducing the retrograde zone to 34%.
* If a long retrograde RP interval falls into the anterograde zone : reduce the anterograde zone (for example from 50% to 25%) thereby expanding the retrograde zone to 75%.

2 start of 1st VV interval, 50% of VV interval, end of 1st VV interval, 50%, end of 2nd VV interval. ventricular sense, ventricular sense, ventricular sense.
2 consecutive Vs - Vs intervals form a **pattern code**

3 19 different pattern codes can be recognized. They are identified by a letter and are ordered in a look-up table.

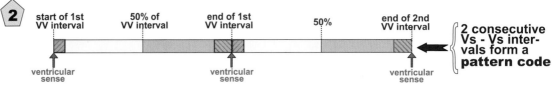
examples → A
→ B
→ C etc.
19 letters for 19 pattern codes

4 Any cardiac rhythm generates a series of code letters. The device interprets the string of code letters to determine if there is a match with a stored pattern consistent with known sequences of SVT or VT or VF or double arrhythmia (SVT & VT)

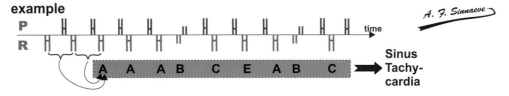
example
A A A B C E A B C → Sinus Tachycardia

A. F. Sinnaeve

Abbreviations : As = atrial sense; ST = sinus tachycardia; SVT = supraventricular tachycardia; VF= ventricular fibrillation; VPC = ventricular premature contraction; Vs = ventricular sense; VT = ventricular tachycardia;

Figure 6.24

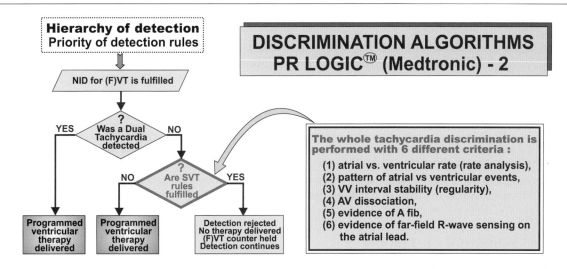

Hierarchy of detection
Priority of detection rules

NID for (F)VT is fulfilled

? Was a Dual Tachycardia detected

YES / NO

? Are SVT rules fulfilled

NO / YES

Programmed ventricular therapy delivered

Programmed ventricular therapy delivered

Detection rejected
No therapy delivered
(F)VT counter held
Detection continues

DISCRIMINATION ALGORITHMS PR LOGIC™ (Medtronic) - 2

137

The whole tachycardia discrimination is performed with 6 different criteria :
(1) atrial vs. ventricular rate (rate analysis),
(2) pattern of atrial vs ventricular events,
(3) VV interval stability (regularity),
(4) AV dissociation,
(5) evidence of A fib,
(6) evidence of far-field R-wave sensing on the atrial lead.

SVT limit : Defines the minimum ventricular interval in which the device applies the PR logic criteria (nominal 320 ms - it is usually programmed at the same value as the VF interval). The device will deliver therapy when the median ventricular interval is less than the programmed SVT limit, provided VT, VF or fast VT detection criteria are satisfied.

1 RATE ANALYSIS

The *VV median* is used to determine whether a rhythm falls within the SVT limit. If the VV median is less than the SVT limit, the rhythm is treated as VF/FVT/VT.

The most recent 12 ventricular intervals are stored in a buffer (fifo) :
350 370 390 390 350 350 380 400 390 350 360 400
The VV median is the larger of the middle two sorted intervals :
350 350 350 350 360 370 380 390 390 390 400 400

The *AA median* is calculated and compared to the median VV median. This information is one of the criteria used for classifying arrhythmias.

The most recent 12 atrial intervals are stored in a buffer (fifo) :
280 270 290 300 270 260 280 290 290 270 250 300
The AA median is the larger of the middle two sorted intervals :
250 260 270 270 270 280 280 290 290 290 300 300

VV median > AA median ⟹ SVT

A. F. Sinnaeve

2 PATTERN : see previous page

3 REGULARITY or VV-INTERVAL STABILITY

Regularity is one of the criteria used to define A fib or A flut and to detect double tachycardias (VT & SVT). The regularity is determined by comparing how often the two most common intervals occur during the most recent 18 ventricular events (all VV intervals ≥ 240 ms are included). The intervals do not need to be next to each other. The value must be ≥ 75% to classify a rhythm as regular.

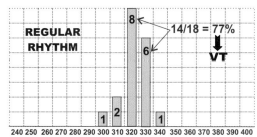

A result of 75% or greater is used for VT recognition during "Dual Tachycardias"

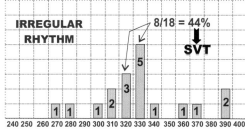

A result of 50% or less will reject VT detection (based on the A fib rule)

Abbreviations : AV = atrioventricular; A fib = atrial fibrillation; A flut = atrial flutter; VF = ventricular fibrillation; VT = ventricular tachycardia; (F)VT = fast ventricular tachycardia; SVT = supraventricular tachycardia; fifo = first in first out buffer memory;

Figure 6.25

DISCRIMINATION ALGORITHMS
PR LOGIC™ (Medtronic) - 3

It is hard to remember all this stuff. I'm lucky to have the book !

4 AV DISSOCIATION

The device looks at each VV interval and determines whether the AV intervals are consistent (AV association) or inconsistent (AV dissociation). This part of the algorithm aims (along with other detection criteria) to determine the presence of dual tachycardias (VT & SVT).

A rhythm is considered dissociated if 4 of the most recent 8 VV intervals exhibit either :
* No atrial events in the ventricular interval
* An AV interval that differs from the average of the previous 8 AV intervals by more than 40 ms

5 AF EVIDENCE CRITERION

The AF evidence criterion recognizes atrial tachyarrhythmias that may not have repeating couple code patterns. A counter is incremented or decremented according to the number of atrial events within each VV interval. The criterion is initially satisfied when the counter is ≥ 6 and remains satisfied as long as the counter remains ≥ 5.

* The counter is incremented (+1) when 2 or more atrial events occur within 1 VV interval.
* If none or one atrial event occurs in the VV interval, the count remains unchanged.
* If the present and the previous VV intervals both show 0 or 1 atrial events, the count is decreased by 1.

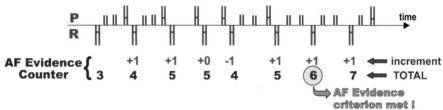

6 FAR-FIELD R-WAVE CRITERION

The Far-Field R-wave criterion analyzes the AA pattern anytime there are 2 atrial events within a VV interval. Consistency of the pattern and placement of the atrial events suggests that one of the atrial events is actually a far-field R-wave.

The Far-Field R-wave criterion is fulfilled under the following circumstances :
* A short-long pattern of AA (PP) intervals and ...
* A short PR interval (< 60 ms) or ...
* A short RP interval (<160 ms).
* A far-field R-wave is identified in at least 10 of the most recent 12 VV intervals

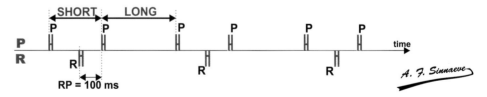

NOTE : There are always several criteria involved for the identification of a tachyarrhythmia. *e.g. Atrial Fibrillation* is recognized if : (1) the RR median is within the SVT limit; (2) the far-field R-wave criterion is not satisfied; (3) AF Evidence counter is satisfied; (4) the regularity criterion shows an irregular rhythm; (5) the PP median is less than the RR median.

Abbreviations : AF = atrial fibrillation; AV = atrioventricular; SVT = supraventricular tachycardia; VT = ventricular tachycardia;

Figure 6.26

DISCRIMINATION ALGORITHMS
PR LOGIC™ (Medtronic) - 4

The PR Logic is easy to program :
* One-touch programming for 3 discrimination criteria (ST, A fib/A flut , Other 1:1 SVTs)
* No testing or reprogramming necessary.

1:1 VT-SVT BOUNDARY %

The VT-SVT boundary may be programmed fo 35, 50, 66, 75, 85%. In the case of slow conduction (retrograde or antegrade), events may occur in the wrong zone. Thus a 1:1 SVT with a long AV delay would have its atrial event falling in the retrograde zone and be classified as VT. Similarly VT with delayed 1:1 VA conduction could be classified as SVT if the atrial event falls within the antegrade zone. The electrophysiology of the patient must be known to avoid such misclassifications.

1:1 VT-SVT boundary can be programmed to increase the size of the appropriate zone. For example, if a patient exhibits long VA conduction during VT, select 35%. If SVT has long AV intervals, select a value that exceeds the AV/VV ratio observed during the tachycardia.

OTHER 1:1 SVTs

This identifies 1:1 SVTs where the atrial and the ventricular activation are approximately simultaneous so that the atrial events fall within the "junctional" segment of the ventricular interval. It is designed to discriminate against common SVTs such as AVNRT and AVRT.

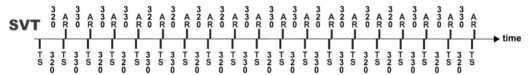

This criterion could inappropriately withhold therapy if atrial sensing is disturbed as with a dislodged atrial lead. This function should not be programmed until the atrial lead has matured. Therefore it is advised to wait a month before this function is programmed. Use caution when programming this function in patients exhibiting slow 1:1 VA conduction during VT/VF. In some cases therapy may not be withheld and ATP may be intentionally programmed to treat AVNRT and AVRT that terminate frequently with ventricular ATP.

ATRIAL FIBRILLATION

In addition to satisfying the AF evidence counter (and far-field R wave sensing has been ruled out), the A fib rule requires that the AA median < 94% of the VV median (or 6% shorter) and the ventricular cycle length regularity < 50%.

ATRIAL FLUTTER

Diagnosis of A flut requires AV association. Device diagnosis of A flut does not require the regularity count. VT during 2:1 atrial flutter is identified by AV dissociation.

SINUS TACHYCARDIA

A typical pattern is recognized by the ICD : one atrial event for each ventricular event, typically in the antegrade segment of the ventricular interval.

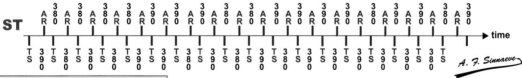

FAR-FIELD R WAVE SENSING

This is common because there is no atrial blanking period after ventricular sensing (PVAB) and only 30 ms after ventricular pacing. Far-field sensing is easily recognized and discarded by the PR Logic algorithm.

REDETECTION

Dual chamber discriminators do not apply during redetection. Thus redetection cannot reject ST or SVT.

Abbreviations : AF = A fib = atrial fibrillation ; A flut = atrial flutter ; AV = atrioventricular ; AVNRT = AV nodal reentry tachycardia ; AVRT = atrioventricular tachycardia with participation of an accessory pathway ; PVAB = postventricular atrial blanking period ; ST = sinus tachycardia ; SVT = supraventricular tachycardia ; VA = ventriculoatrial ; VF = ventricular fibrillation ; VT = ventricular tachycardia ;

Figure 6.27

UPGRADED PR LOGIC ALGORITHM IN MEDTRONIC ICDs
THE ST RULE

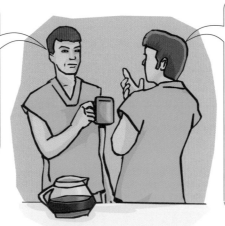

The PR Logic algorithm of Medtronic ICDs is difficult to understand. I have found like others that the most common cause of inappropriate therapy with the PR Logic algorithm is sinus tachycardia (ST) or atrial tachycardia with long PR intervals.

The withholding algorithm for ST is the most "utilized" component of PR Logic, and it needed improvement. PR Logic is primarily changed with the addition of a new ST detection rule. The new PR Logic was implemented starting with Entrust DR. The new ST detection rule eliminates the need to adjust the VT/ST boundary so that there is no longer a programmable anterograde/retrograde zone. This new ST rule appears to reduce the number of inappropriate shocks for ST.

The new ST detection rule provides discrimination of ST from VT based on :

⚙ **1:1 conducton. Only beats with 1:1 AV conduction are used in subsequent calculations.**

✸ **Recent history of heart rate (R-R intervals) and intrinsic P-R intervals. In other words, the device determines on the basis of memorized data whether these measurements fall inside the expected range for the patient or outside where they are labeled "unexpected".**

✸ **The combination of results being sent to the cumulative ST evidence counter.**

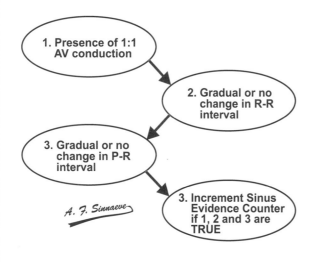

1. Presence of 1:1 AV conduction

2. Gradual or no change in R-R interval

3. Gradual or no change in P-R interval

3. Increment Sinus Evidence Counter if 1, 2 and 3 are TRUE

A. F. Sinnaeve

One-to-One AV Conduction

R-R interval classified as 1:1 if

✸ **1 atrial event OR**

✸ **2 atrial events with FFRW oversensing in at least 4 of the last 12 beats**

AND

Recent history consistent with 1:1 if

✸ **Majority of recent beats classified as 1:1 AV OR**

✸ **Most recent 4 beats classified as 1:1 AV**

Sinus Tach is present when ST Evidence Counter >= 6. At that point the PR Logic will withhold therapy on the basis of Sinus Tach assuming NID is met.
The rule considers the presence of :
* atrial oversensing or FFRW sensing
* intermittent ectopy (PVC, PAC)
* pacing

Abbreviations : AV = atrioventricular; FFRW = far-field R wave; NID = number of intervals needed for detection; PAC = premature atrial complex; PVC = premature ventricular complex; ST = sinus tachycardia; VT = ventricular tachycardia.

Figure 6.28

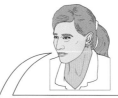

DURATION-BASED FEATURES TO OVERRIDE DISCRIMINATORS - 1

SVT-VT discriminators can prevent or delay therapy if they misclassify VT or VF as SVT. These programmable features prevent the sustained inhibition of therapy if an arrhythmia satisfies the ventricular criterion (VF or VT) for a sufficiently long duration even if discriminators indicate SVT. Overriding the discriminators and inhibition of ICD therapy is an option that can be programmed in terms of maximum duration of detected tachycardia before the ICD delivers therapy. This constitutes a "safety net". Using this duration-based feature implies that one does not have full confidence in the capability of an ICD to make a certain diagnosis of SVT and one fears VT might be missed and continue for a long time without proper therapy.

Remember "Tiered Therapy" and the actions that may be programmed :

blan-king	VF	f-VT	s-VT	normal sinus	bradycardia
	Hi shock	ATP2 Lo shock Hi shock	ATP1 & 2 Lo shock Hi shock	none	brady pacing

* The "safety net" function cannot be used for VF or when only VF is programmed for detection.
* It is important to remember that this function can deliver inappropriate therapy for SVT or sinus tachycardia though SVT can occasionally be terminated by ventricular therapy. Therefore the safety net function must be used judiciously.

GUIDANT : Sustained-Duration Override (EXAMPLE)

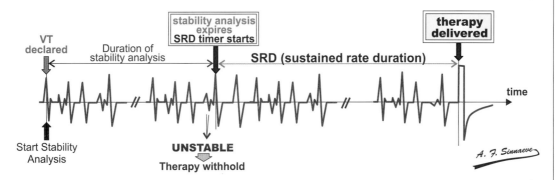

When a decision is made to inhibit therapy, the SRD timer begins at the end of "Duration". If the detection criterion in the lowest zone is maintained for the programmed SRD period, the programmed therapy will be delivered at the end of the SRD period. If arrhythmia drops out during SRD, the episode ends.

SRD is programmable from 10 s to 60 min. It is not available in the VF zone.

Therapy delivery is inhibited until one of the following occurs :
1. The rate increases to a higher zone and "Duration" for that zone is met (all zones are active simultaneously).
2. Stability is inhibiting therapy and the rhythm becomes reclassified as stable.
3. AFib Rate Threshold is inhibiting therapy delivery and the atrial rate falls below the threshold.
4. V-rate > A-rate is programmed ON and becomes "True" (VF or VT is detected).
5. The SRD timer expires.

Abbreviations : ATP = antitachycardia pacing ; f-VT = fast ventricular tachycardia ; s-VT = slow ventricular tachycardia ; SVT = supraventricular tachycardia ; VF = ventricular fibrillation ;

Figure 6.29

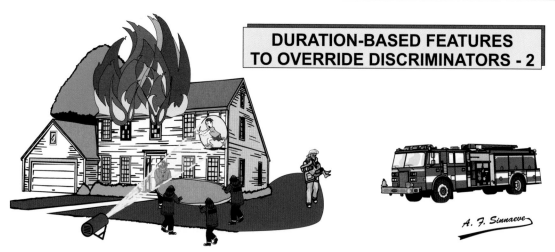

DURATION-BASED FEATURES TO OVERRIDE DISCRIMINATORS - 2

A. F. Sinnaeve

St JUDE : Maximum Time to Diagnosis (MTD)

* If an arrhythmia satisfying the slowest tachyarrhythmia detection interval exists longer than a programmed duration (the MTD detection time, programmable from 20 s to 60 min), the ICD abandons use of all SVT discriminators (including Rate Branch) and initiates the programmed MTD therapy.
* If MTD therapy is programmed to "Fib Therapy", the device begins charging to the first programmed fibrillation therapy when the MTD timer expires.
* If MTD therapy is programmed to "Tach Therapy" and the MTD timer expires, the ICD initiates the first programmed therapy for the s-VT or f-VT zone (ATP or charging for cardioversion)

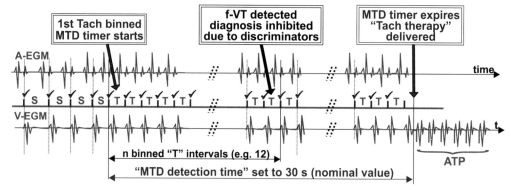

* The "Maximum Time to Fib Therapies" (MTF) is useful for patients who tolerate their arrhythmias for only a limited time during delivery of less agressive therapies. When the MTF timer expires, the ICD abandons tachycardia therapies and delivers fibrillation therapies.

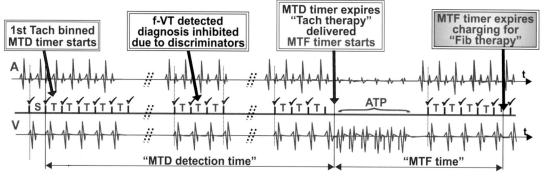

* MTD is not available if the SVT Discriminators are not turned on ! In this case MTF starts when the first "Tach interval" is binned. The MTF is programmable from 10 s to 5 min (nominal 20 s)

Abbreviations : ATP = antitachycardia pacing ; f-VT = fast ventricular tachycardia ; s-VT = slow ventricular tachycardia ; SVT = supraventricular tachycardia ; T = tachy interval ; S = sinus interval ;

Figure 6.30

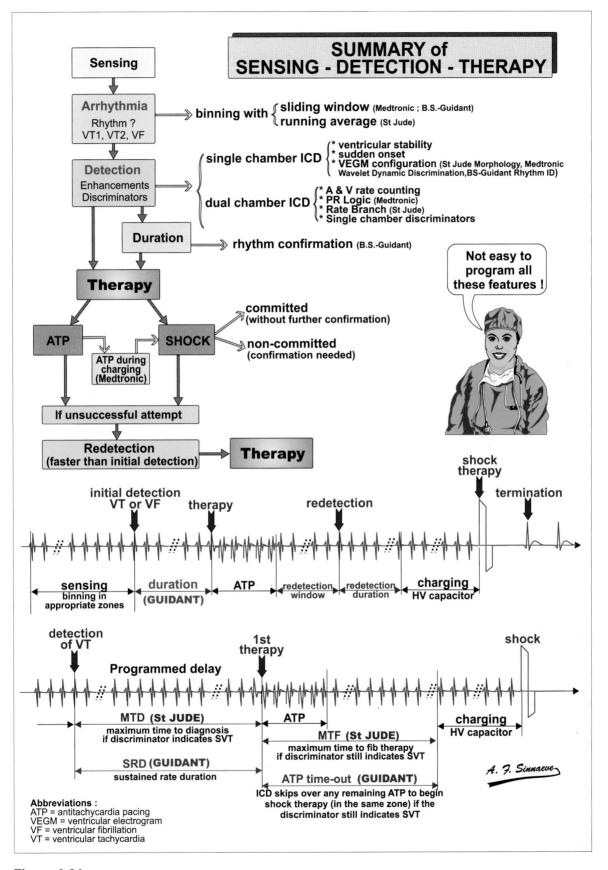

Figure 6.31

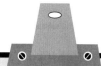

⑦ ICD THERAPIES

✿ HIGH-ENERGY SHOCK THERAPY

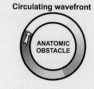

* Tachycardia detection & shock therapy
* Committed shock therapy
* Non-committed shock therapy
* Redetection - parts 1& 2

✿ ANTITACHYCARDIA PACING (ATP)

* Termination of reentrant tachycardias by ATP - parts 1 & 2
* Tiered therapy
* Antitachycardia pacing - part 1 : BURST
* Antitachycardia pacing - part 2 : RAMP
* Secrets of ATP - parts 1 & 2
* Decrementing in ATP therapy
* Programmability of ATP sequences - parts 1 & 2
* Simplified ICD programming : rule of 8 for fast VT
* Simplified programming of Medtronic ICDs for the treatment of fast VT
* Capacitor charging during ATP - parts 1 & 2

✿ BRADYCARDIA PACING BY THE ICD

* Differences between pacing parameters
* Minimizing RV pacing

✿ ATRIAL THERAPIES

* Special ICD functions
* Atrial therapies

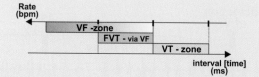

Figure 7.00

COMMITTED OR NONCOMMITTED ? Part 1

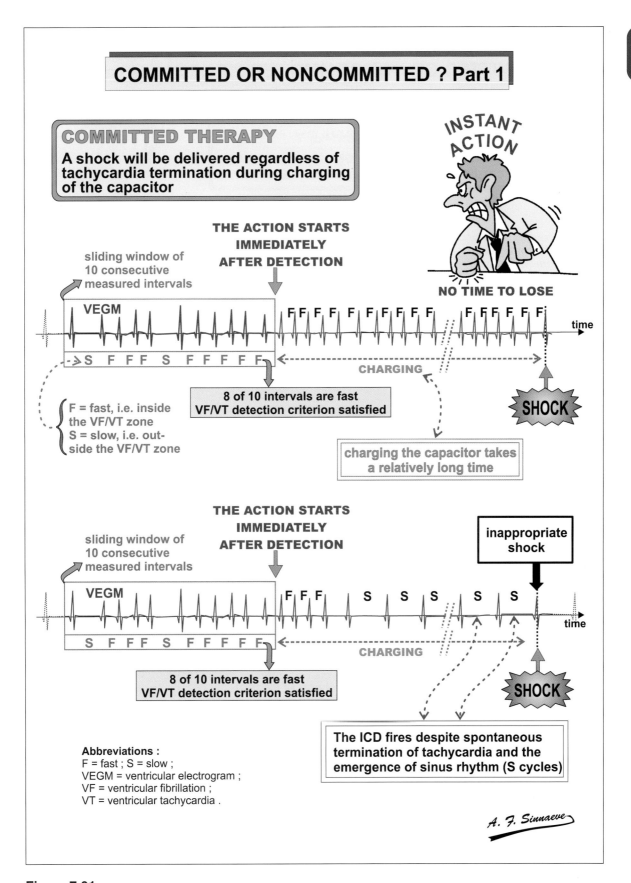

COMMITTED THERAPY

A shock will be delivered regardless of tachycardia termination during charging of the capacitor

INSTANT ACTION

NO TIME TO LOSE

THE ACTION STARTS IMMEDIATELY AFTER DETECTION

sliding window of 10 consecutive measured intervals

VEGM

F F F F F F F F F   F F F F F F

time

- S F F F S F F F F F   CHARGING

F = fast, i.e. inside the VF/VT zone
S = slow, i.e. outside the VF/VT zone

8 of 10 intervals are fast
VF/VT detection criterion satisfied

SHOCK

charging the capacitor takes a relatively long time

THE ACTION STARTS IMMEDIATELY AFTER DETECTION

sliding window of 10 consecutive measured intervals

VEGM

F F F   S   S   S   S   S

time

S F F S F F F F F   CHARGING

inappropriate shock

8 of 10 intervals are fast
VF/VT detection criterion satisfied

SHOCK

The ICD fires despite spontaneous termination of tachycardia and the emergence of sinus rhythm (S cycles)

Abbreviations :
F = fast ; S = slow ;
VEGM = ventricular electrogram ;
VF = ventricular fibrillation ;
VT = ventricular tachycardia .

A. F. Sinnaeve

Figure 7.01

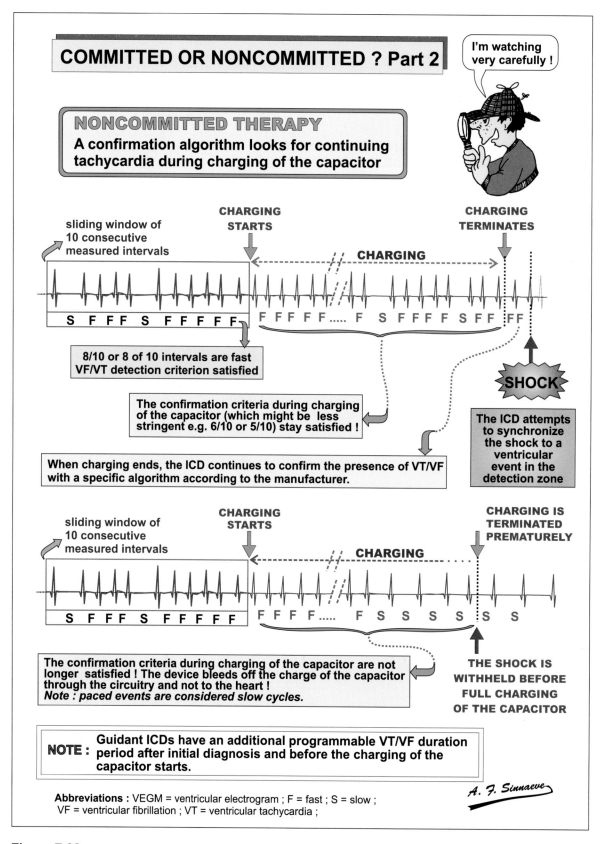

Figure 7.02

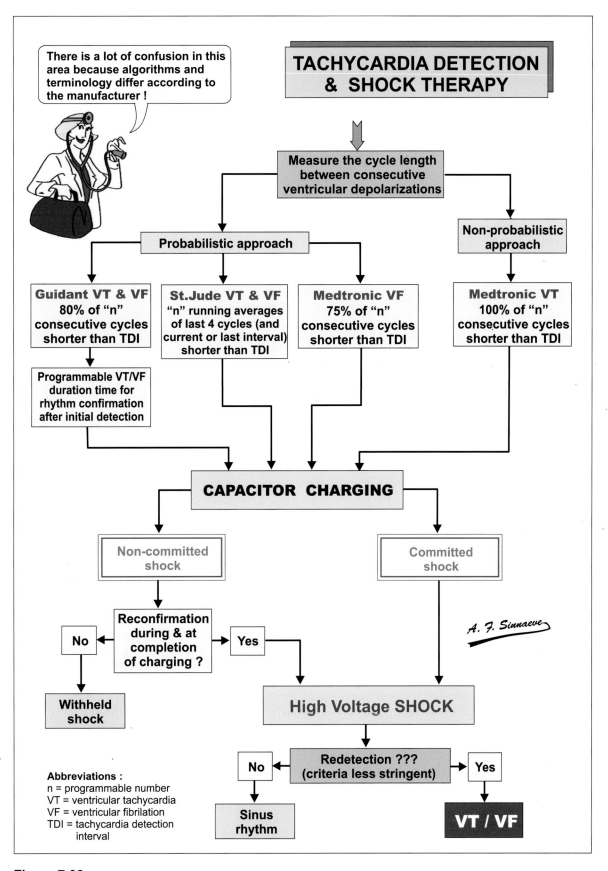

Figure 7.03

148

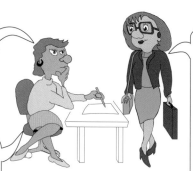

What do you mean, redetection? Is one detection not sufficient ?

REDETECTION - 1

So, after therapy we have three possibilities : the heart can return to sinus rhythm, the tachycardia can continue unchanged or it can accelerate into a faster (organized or polymorphic) VT or degenerate into VF !

Unfortunately, the delivered therapy of the ICD is not always successful ! Attempts of antitachycardia pacing (ATP) or shocks may fail or, worse, aggravate the tachy-arrhythmia.
It is essential that the ICD reassess the heart rhythm immediately after therapy is delivered.

EXAMPLE

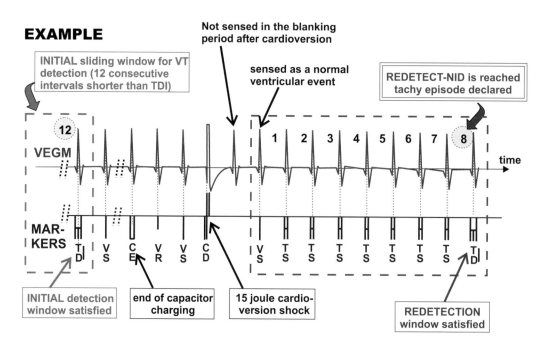

* **Post-therapy detection algorithms** are similar to the ones used for initial detection.
* Most algorithms simplify the initial detection criteria by disabling detection enhancements following delivery of therapy.
* Allowing reduction of the number of intervals for redetection or programming the duration timer for a shorter time, the overall duration of episodes is minimized.
* Since a persistent arrhythmia indicates failed therapy, redetection of an arrhythmia normally provokes more aggressive treatment measures (tiered therapy!)

A. F. Sinnaeve

Abbreviations : ATP = antitachycardia pacing ; NID = number of intervals needed to detect ; TDI = tachycardia detection interval ; VT = ventricular tachycardia ; VEGM = ventricular electrogram ; The markers are depicted in the Medtronic format ;

Figure 7.04

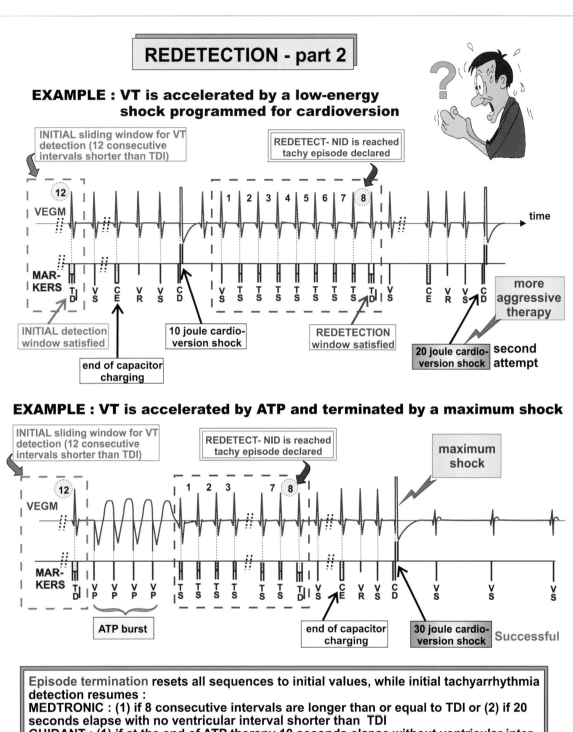

REDETECTION - part 2

EXAMPLE : VT is accelerated by a low-energy shock programmed for cardioversion

EXAMPLE : VT is accelerated by ATP and terminated by a maximum shock

Episode termination resets all sequences to initial values, while initial tachyarrhythmia detection resumes :
MEDTRONIC : (1) if 8 consecutive intervals are longer than or equal to TDI or (2) if 20 seconds elapse with no ventricular interval shorter than TDI
GUIDANT : (1) if at the end of ATP therapy 10 seconds elapse without ventricular intervals shorter than TDI or (2) 30 seconds after shock therapy
St JUDE : the ICD considers the episode as over, if a programmed number of intervals (3, 5 or 7) is binned in the sinus zone (according to the averaging algorithm used for detection)

A. F. Sinnaeve

Abbreviations : ATP = antitachycardia pacing ; NID = number of intervals needed to detect ; TDI tachycardia detection interval ; VT = ventricular tachycardia ; VEGM = ventricular electrogram;
The markers are depicted in the Medtronic format

Figure 7.05

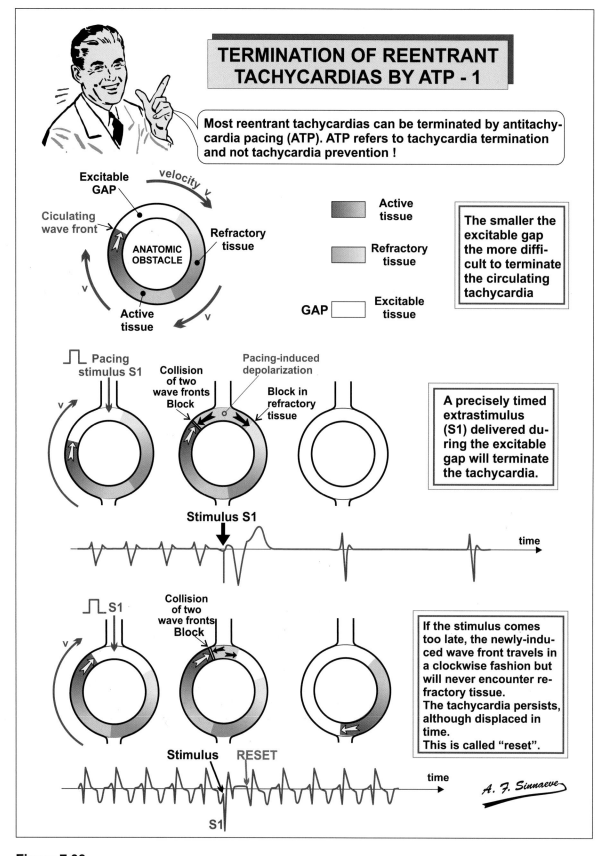

TERMINATION OF REENTRANT TACHYCARDIAS BY ATP - 1

Most reentrant tachycardias can be terminated by antitachycardia pacing (ATP). ATP refers to tachycardia termination and not tachycardia prevention !

Excitable GAP

velocity v

Ciculating wave front

ANATOMIC OBSTACLE

Refractory tissue

Active tissue

v

v

Active tissue

Refractory tissue

GAP — Excitable tissue

The smaller the excitable gap the more difficult to terminate the circulating tachycardia

Pacing stimulus S1

Collision of two wave fronts Block

Pacing-induced depolarization

Block in refractory tissue

A precisely timed extrastimulus (S1) delivered during the excitable gap will terminate the tachycardia.

Stimulus S1

time

S1

Collision of two wave fronts Block

If the stimulus comes too late, the newly-induced wave front travels in a clockwise fashion but will never encounter refractory tissue.
The tachycardia persists, although displaced in time.
This is called "reset".

Stimulus   RESET

time

S1

A. F. Sinnaeve

Figure 7.06

TERMINATION OF REENTRANT TACHYCARDIAS BY ATP - 2

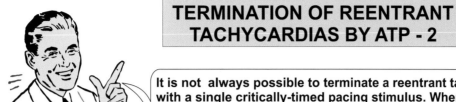

It is not always possible to terminate a reentrant tachycardia with a single critically-timed pacing stimulus. When the pacing site is too far from the reentrant loop, the pacemaker-induced depolarization cannot reach the excitable gap.

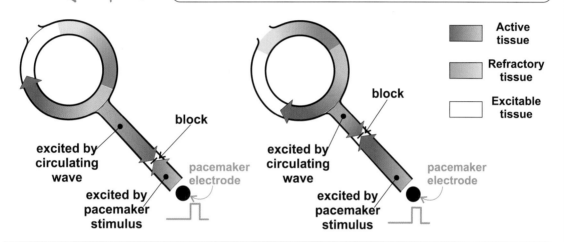

If two closely coupled stimuli are applied, the first one will "clear the way" from refractoriness in order for the second one to penetrate the loop at the right moment ! (Myocardial refractory period is rate-dependent and gradual decreases in duration with an increase in the rate. Increase in the pacing rate thus decreases the duration of myocardial refractoriness).

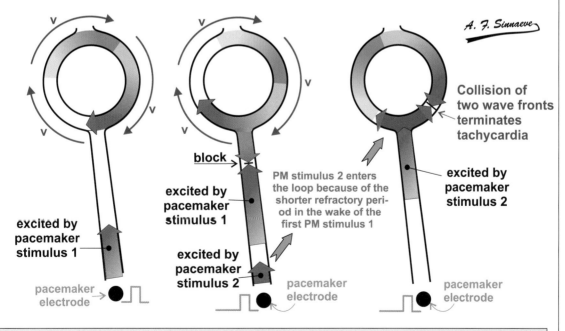

This process is known as "peeling-back" of the refractory period and may require more than two PM stimuli to allow a critically-timed PM stimulus to enter the loop to extinguish the reentrant process

Figure 7.07

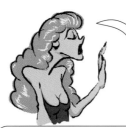
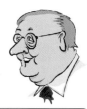

TIERED THERAPY

> Tiered therapy ? Isn't that something about the rows and the ranks in the theater, that are placed one above the other ?

Actually, it is simply the hierarchical approach to the treatment of ventricular tachyarrhythmias ! Different ventricular tachyarrhythmias are best treated according to their mechanism and rate. Tiered therapy consists of 2 or 3 zones which are generally not overlapping. It aims at treating less serious ventricular tachyarrhythmias (such as relatively slow VT) with less aggressive therapy (such as ATP or low-energy cardioversion) to avoid delivery of a maximum shock usually reserved for VF. Thus less aggressive therapy with a more extensive ATP sequence (with longer detection times) could be programmed in the lowest of the 3 zones (i.e. slow VT zone) where the VT is better tolerated hemodynamically. More aggressive therapy is programmed for faster VTs that may still be terminated with ATP. In other words, tiered therapy attempts to delay the delivery of a shock in the two VT zones (slow and fast VT zones).

DECREASING TOLERANCE ← **OK** → **DECREASING TOLERANCE**

overlapping possible of FVT & VF zones

ZONE	BRADY-CARDIA	NORMAL SINUS	SLOW VT	FAST VT	VF
RATE (bpm)	below 50	50 - 140*	140 - 200	with overlapping 200 - 250 / without overlapping 200 - 230	with overlapping > 200 even if FVT is 200 to 230 / without overlapping > 230
THERAPY	Brady-pacing	NONE	ATP Lo shock Hi shock	ATP Hi shock	Hi shock

A. F. Sinnaeve

* Use <140 cautiously for very slow VT

SVT detection enhancements may be used.

No SVT detection enhancements can be used ! Therapy consists only of a medium or high energy shock

WARNING !

After initial therapy the ICD never allows a lesser sequence to follow so that therapy becomes progressively more aggressive

Advantage of tiered therapy :
* ATP is a more gentle way of terminating VT than the delivery of a high-energy shock (treating a slow and well-tolerated VT with a 20 or 30 J shock is similar to shooting a mouse with an elephant gun).
* The VT zones can be monitored for diagnosis while therapy is turned off.

Disadvantages of tiered therapy :
* Potentially long delays may be introduced before essential high-energy therapy is delivered. This limitation can now be overcome by delivering one ATP sequence for fast VT during capacitor charging. If ATP terminates the fast VT, the shock is aborted.
* May precipitate a faster ventricular tachyarrhythmia (proarrhythmia) but this is uncommon in slower VTs.
* Adds complexity in programming and follow-up.
* Programming lower rate zones increases the chance of inappropriate therapy for SVT

> Programming a faster rate for FVT than for VF is confusing ! I look forward to some explanation as to how this is possible in ICDs with overlapping FVT and VF zones. Also, I'd like to know about ICDs that can deliver ATP during charging.

Abbreviations : ATP = antitachycardia pacing; FVT = fast ventricular tachycardia; SVT = supraventrivular tachycardia; VF = ventricular fibrillation; VT = ventricular tachycardia

Figure 7.08

152

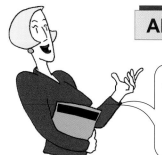

ANTITACHYCARDIA PACING - 1 - BURST

In "Burst Pacing" a programmable number of stimuli are delivered at fixed cycle length, faster than the rate of the VT.
The number of pacing stimuli and the stimulation rate should not be excessive to minimize the risk of VT acceleration or degeneration into VF. Regardless of the programmed sequence, the pacing rate can never be delivered at a cycle length less than the programmed minimum pacing interval (e.g. 200 ms) for safety considerations.

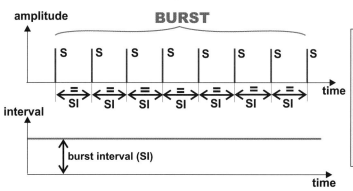

The burst interval (SI) is shorter than the tachycardia interval (TI). SI can be a fixed percentage of the tachycardia cycle length or a programmable percentage of the average of the last four intervals (the % is often adaptive).
The number of pulses in each burst is always programmable.

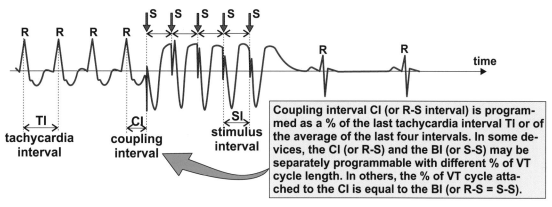

Coupling interval CI (or R-S interval) is programmed as a % of the last tachycardia interval TI or of the average of the last four intervals. In some devices, the CI (or R-S) and the BI (or S-S) may be separately programmable with different % of VT cycle length. In others, the % of VT cycle attached to the CI is equal to the BI (or R-S = S-S).

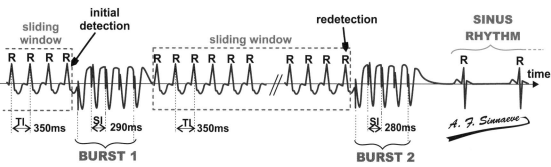

The number of burst sequences is programmable (1 to n) in case of unsuccessful VT termination. Upon redetection of VT, the device delivers another burst if n > 1. The pacing interval (SI) may be decreased in the next burst by a programmable decrement (e.g. 10 ms). This is called "interval decrement".
The number of stimuli per burst can be increased (usually by one) for each successive burst in the scheme.

Figure 7.09

What do you mean with ramp pacing ? I cannot see any ramp ! How should it be programmed ?

ANTITACHYCARDIA PACING - 2 - RAMP

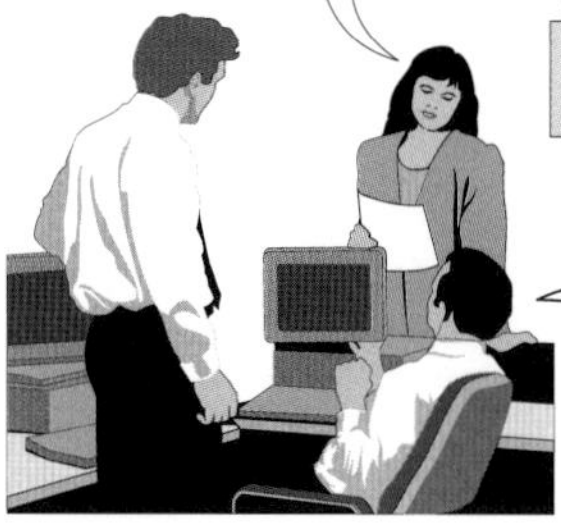

In "Ramp Pacing", the pacing rate is continually altered from slower to faster. It can be defined as a burst in which each successive stimulus-to-stimulus interval is shortened or decremented.

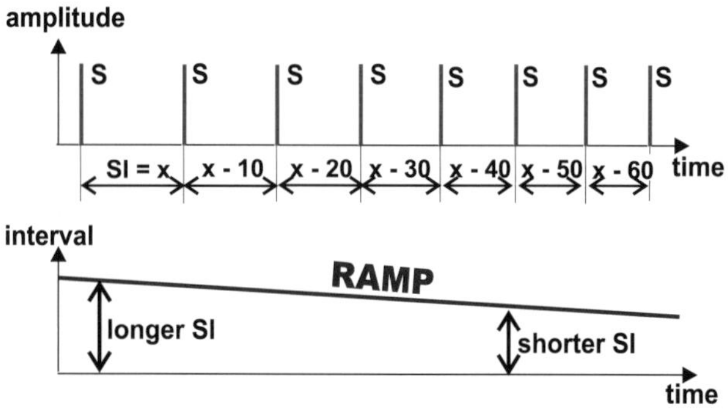

amplitude

S S S S S S S S

SI = x | x - 10 | x - 20 | x - 30 | x - 40 | x - 50 | x - 60   time

interval

RAMP

longer SI   shorter SI

time

1. The first stimulus interval (SI) of each ramp sequence is usually a fixed percentage of the tachycardia cycle length (TI) or a programmable percentage of the average of the last four intervals.
2. The interstimulus interval (SI) is progressively shortened by a programmable interval decrement (e.g. 10 ms).
3. The number of pulses in the ramp is always programmable.
4. The pulse increment parameter allows the number of stimuli in the burst to be increased for each successive burst in the scheme (e.g. Burst 1 = 4 pulses, burst 2 = 5 pulses, etc.)
5. The number of bursts in each therapy is programmable
6. The burst cycle length (SI) cannot be shorter than the programmed minimum cycle length

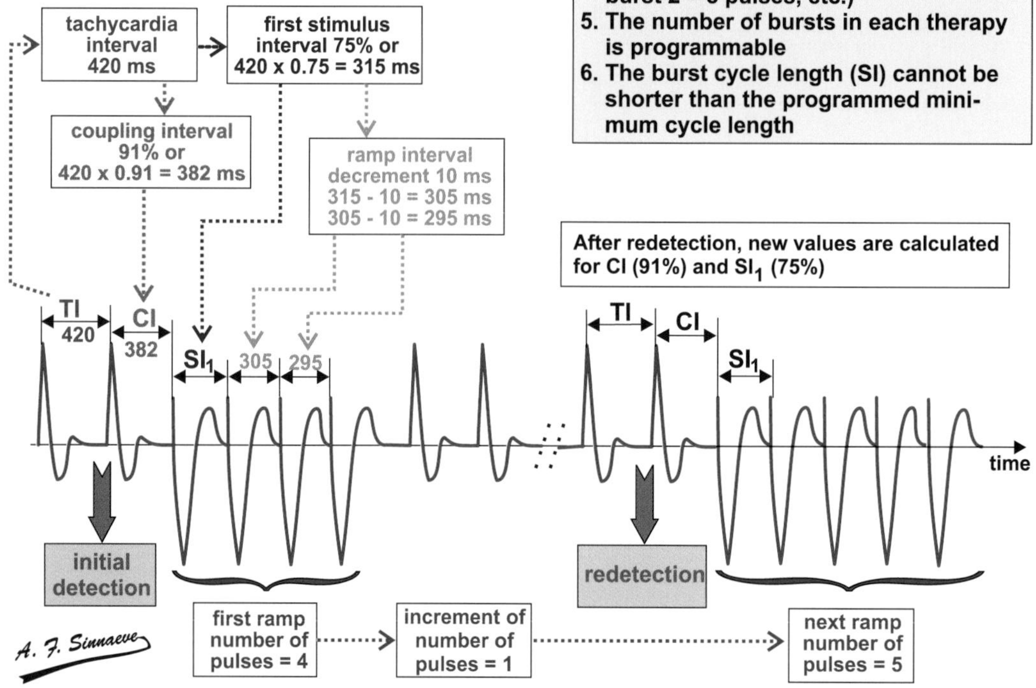

tachycardia interval 420 ms → first stimulus interval 75% or 420 x 0.75 = 315 ms

coupling interval 91% or 420 x 0.91 = 382 ms

ramp interval decrement 10 ms
315 - 10 = 305 ms
305 - 10 = 295 ms

After redetection, new values are calculated for CI (91%) and SI$_1$ (75%)

TI 420 | CI 382 | SI$_1$ | 305 | 295

TI | CI | SI$_1$

initial detection

redetection

first ramp number of pulses = 4 ·····> increment of number of pulses = 1 ·····················> next ramp number of pulses = 5

A. F. Sinnaeve

time

Adaptive rather than fixed values (absolute timing in ms) are usually applied to calculate and program the CI and the SI. In this example CI is adaptive with timing as a % of computed ventricular rate. The SI is also adaptive with a % value different from that used for the CI.

Abbreviations : ATP = antitachycardia pacing; CI = coupling interval; TI = tachycardia interval; SI = stimulus interval or burst cycle length.

Figure 7.10

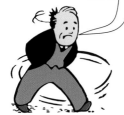

What do they mean by acceleration induced by ATP ?

There is no formal definition but many consider acceleration present when there is more than 10 - 25% change in CL, development of polymorphic VT or degeneration into VF.

SECRETS OF ATP - part 1

What predisposes to acceleration ?

The risk of acceleration increases as the CL decreases (i.e. fast VT)

What do you mean by slow and fast VT ?

In terms of ATP therapy slow VT has a CL > 320 - 300 ms (corresponding with a rate lower than 188 - 200 bpm), while fast VT has a CL of 320 - 240 ms (i.e. a rate of 188 - 250 bpm). The distinction is important because ATP can reliably terminate 85 - 90% of slow VT with a low risk of acceleration (1 - 5%). Recently it has been shown that fast VT can also be terminated by ATP in about 75% of cases with a low acceleration rate.

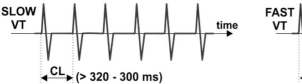
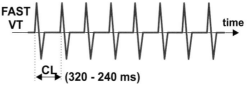

SLOW VT ... time CL (> 320 - 300 ms)

FAST VT ... time CL (320 - 240 ms)

Does this mean that ATP should be programmed for fast VT in virtually all patients ?

Yes, because slow and fast VT are common. Fast VT that could destabilize into VF can therefore be treated by ATP early without a shock. Thus in a patient with only a past history of VF, programming of ATP should be seriously considered.

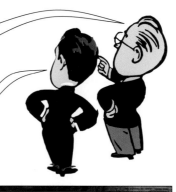

I used to get terrible shocks from time to time and that was very unpleasant. Then my doctor changed my ICD to ATP and that goes really painlessly !

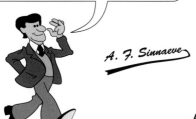

A. F. Sinnaeve

ATP can terminate VT painlessly in 70 - 90% of cases.
ATP improves the quality-of-life.
ATP may extend the longevity of an ICD.
ATP used for fast VT may reduce the number of shocks by more than 70% without increasing the time to termination or a major increase in acceleration. In the past fast VT was detected as VF for which a shock was delivered.

Abbreviations : ATP = antitachycardia pacing; CL = cycle length; VF = ventricular fibrillation; VT = ventricular tachycardia;

Figure 7.11

There are so many variations of ATP ! How does one know how to program ATP ? Do we have to induce VT to test the efficacy of ATP ?

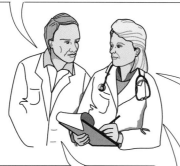

SECRETS OF ATP - part 2

It's simpler than you think.
* First you have to realize that there is little clinical advantage to the various ATP schemes.
* Second, for slow VT burst pacing and ramp pacing are equally effective. Ramp pacing is more likely to induce acceleration in fast VT than burst pacing.
* Third, there is no need to test the ATP scheme on induced VT before discharge from the hospital.

Are you saying that you can program ATP without VT induction ? How do you do that ?

Remember that about 50% of the tachyarrhythmias detected in the traditional VF zone (< 300-320 ms) consist of monomorphic VT. Programming ATP depends on the clinical scenario.

In a patient with a history of only VF (no VT), you program 3 zones : fast VT (CL : 300-240 ms) detection 12/16, 2 sequences of 8 pulses, burst pacing at 88% of CL of VT works very well. The coupling interval of the second burst decreases by 10 ms (10 ms decrement). The VF zone is programmed at 240 ms and slow VT at 340 ms.

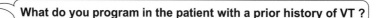

What do you program in the patient with a prior history of VT ?

The same as I told you for VF and fast VT. Program the VTDI according to the documented VT rate.

How do you program the ATP sequence for slow VT ?

A good scheme consists of 3-5 bursts at 88% CL (8 pulses) and 10 ms decrement followed by 2-3 attempts at ramp pacing at 91%

In the Medtronic devices fast VT is programmed via VF with overlapping zones. What about devices from other manufacturers ?

You program ATP for fast VT with 1-2 bursts and then a shock (at DFT level, then maximum). VF is programmed at < 220-240 ms thereby allowing ATP for VT from 220-240 ms CL to 300-320 ms CL according to programming.

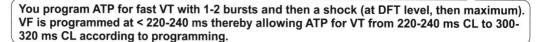

In most cases you don't have to tailor the ATP sequence for a patient's inducible VT. That simplifies programming as well as follow-up !!!

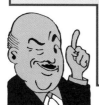

It seems that an ICD has become an ATP device with defibrillation back-up as needed ! There are now ICDs that can charge their capacitor during ATP so that a shock can be delivered, if necessary, without undue delay.

A. F. Sinnaeve

Factors influencing the success of ATP
1. VT cycle length
2. Presence and duration of excitable gap
3. Conduction time from stimulation site to VT site
4. Refractoriness at the stimulation site and the VT site
THE CL IS THE MOST IMPORTANT FACTOR !
A SHORTER CL CREATES A SHORTER EXCITABLE GAP

Abbreviations : ATP = antitachycardia pacing; CL = cycle length; DFT = defibrillation threshold; VF = ventricular fibrillation; VT = ventricular tachycardia; VTDI = ventricular tachycardia detection interval;

Figure 7.12

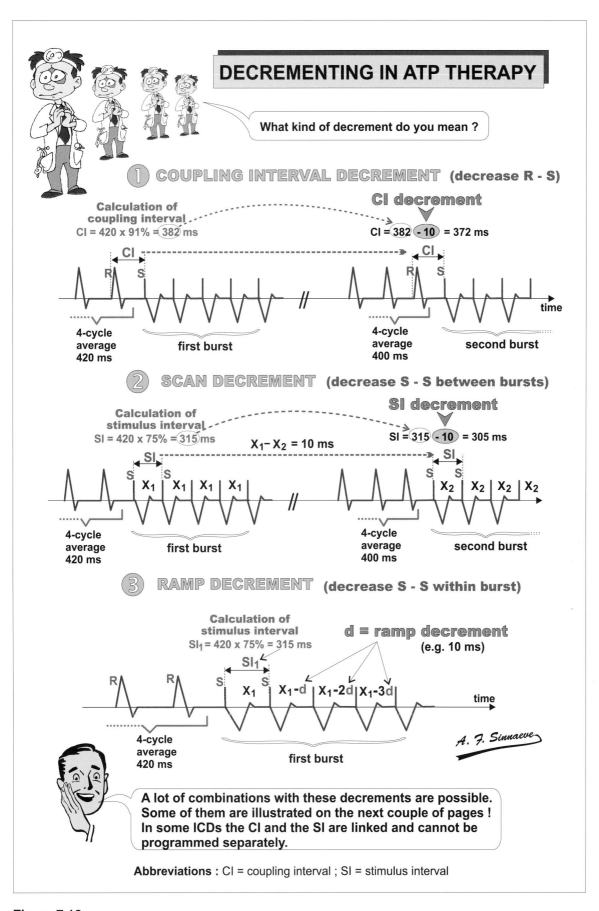

Figure 7.13

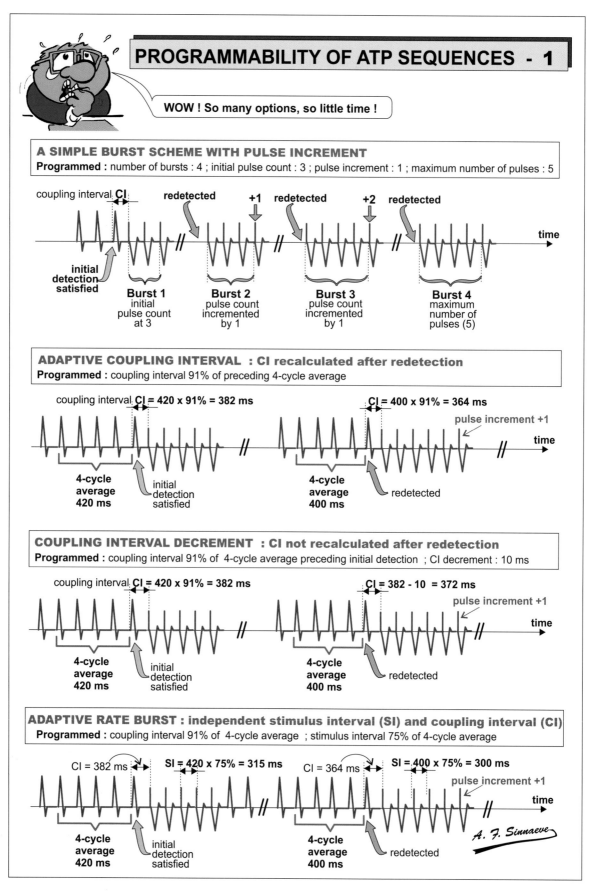

PROGRAMMABILITY OF ATP SEQUENCES - 1

WOW ! So many options, so little time !

A SIMPLE BURST SCHEME WITH PULSE INCREMENT

Programmed : number of bursts : 4 ; initial pulse count : 3 ; pulse increment : 1 ; maximum number of pulses : 5

coupling interval **CI**   **redetected**   **+1**   **redetected**   **+2**   **redetected**

time

initial detection satisfied

Burst 1
initial pulse count at 3

Burst 2
pulse count incremented by 1

Burst 3
pulse count incremented by 1

Burst 4
maximum number of pulses (5)

ADAPTIVE COUPLING INTERVAL : CI recalculated after redetection

Programmed : coupling interval 91% of preceding 4-cycle average

coupling interval **CI = 420 x 91% = 382 ms**   **CI = 400 x 91% = 364 ms**

pulse increment +1

time

4-cycle average 420 ms   initial detection satisfied

4-cycle average 400 ms   redetected

COUPLING INTERVAL DECREMENT : CI not recalculated after redetection

Programmed : coupling interval 91% of 4-cycle average preceding initial detection ; CI decrement : 10 ms

coupling interval **CI = 420 x 91% = 382 ms**   **CI = 382 - 10 = 372 ms**

pulse increment +1

time

4-cycle average 420 ms   initial detection satisfied

4-cycle average 400 ms   redetected

ADAPTIVE RATE BURST : independent stimulus interval (SI) and coupling interval (CI)

Programmed : coupling interval 91% of 4-cycle average ; stimulus interval 75% of 4-cycle average

CI = 382 ms   **SI = 420 x 75% = 315 ms**   **CI = 364 ms**   **SI = 400 x 75% = 300 ms**

pulse increment +1

time

4-cycle average 420 ms   initial detection satisfied

4-cycle average 400 ms   redetected

A. F. Sinnaeve

Figure 7.14

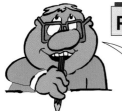

PROGRAMMABILITY OF ATP SEQUENCES - 2

Unbelievable ! Still more parameters for ATP therapy !?

ADAPTIVE RAMP SCHEME : ramp decrement (decrease of R-R within burst)
Programmed : coupling interval 91% of 4-cycle average ; stimulus interval 75% of 4-cycle average ; ramp decrement = 10 ms ; minimum interval = 270 ms

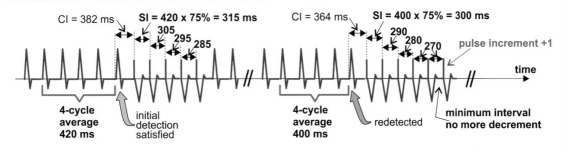

BURST-SCAN SCHEME : bursts with nonadaptive stimulus interval (SI)
with scan decrement (decrease of R-R between bursts)
Programmed : coupling interval 91% of 4-cycle average ; stimulus interval 75% of 4-cycle average ; scan decrement = 10 ms ; minimum interval = 270 ms

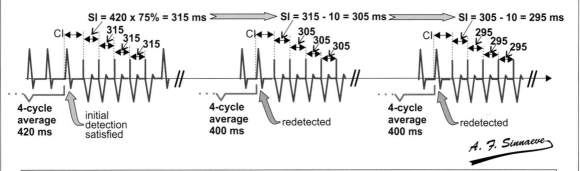

RAMP-SCAN SCHEME : ramp decrement (stimulus interval (SI within ramp)
versus scan decrement (decrease of R-R between ramps)
Programmed : initial stimulus interval 75% of 4-cycle average ; initial number of pulses per burst = 3 ; pulse increment = 1; maximum pulses per burst = 6 ; ramp decrement = 10 ms ; scan decrement = 20 ms ; minimum interval =235 ms ;

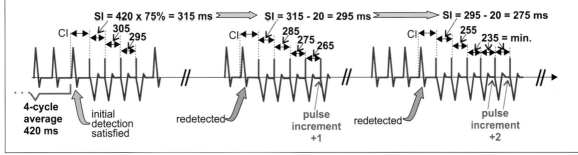

Figure 7.15

SIMPLIFIED ICD PROGRAMMING

1. Rule of 8 for fast VT

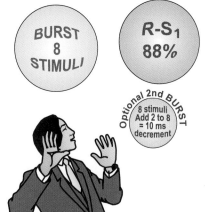

BURST 8 STIMULI

$R-S_1$ 88%

Optional 2nd BURST
8 stimuli
Add 2 to 8
= 10 ms decrement

The rule of 8 extends to the letter B in BURST because a B looks like an 8.

$R - S_1$ = coupling or adaptive interval
If VT cycle length is x, the cycle length of the first burst will be 88% of x or 0.88x. The cycle length of the optional second burst will be 10 ms shorter.

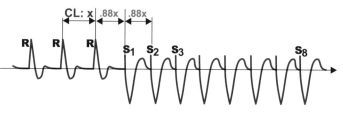

CL: x | .88x | .88x

R R R S_1 S_2 S_3 ... S_8

A. F. Sinnaeve

2. Empiric ICD programming

A recent study demonstrated that (empiric) simplified pre-specified programming of Medtronic ICDs was just as effective as physician-tailored programming in terms of clinical parameters and shock-related morbidity.

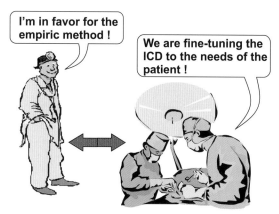

I'm in favor for the empiric method !

We are fine-tuning the ICD to the needs of the patient !

EMPIRIC SETTINGS OF MEDTRONIC ICDs FOR VT/VF

Ventricular Tachyarrhytmia	Cutoff	Detection	Therapies
VF on	250 beats/min	18 of 24	30 J x 6
FVT via VF	200 beats/min	(18 of 24)	Burst (1sequence), 30 J x 5
VT on	150 beats/min	16	Burst (2), ramp (1), 20 J, 30 J x3

Supraventricular tachycardia criteria on : atrial fibrillation / atrial flutter, sinus tachy (1:1 VT-ST boundary = 66%), SVT limit = 200 beats/min. Burst ATP : 8 intervals, R-S1 = 88%, 20 ms decrement. Ramp ATP : 8 intervals, R-S1 = 81%, 10 ms decrement.
A decrement in cycle length from burst to burst (inter-burst decrement) is called decremental scanning but the cycle length of a given burst remains constant. In ramp pacing the change in cycle length occurs from stimulus to stimulus (intra-burst step size). Inter- and intra-decrement functions can be combined.

Abbreviations : ATP = antitachycardia pacing ; VF = Ventricular fibrillation ; VT = ventricular tachycardia ; FVT = fast ventricular tachycardia ; SVT = supraventricular tachycardia ; ST = sinus tachycardia ;

Figure 7.16

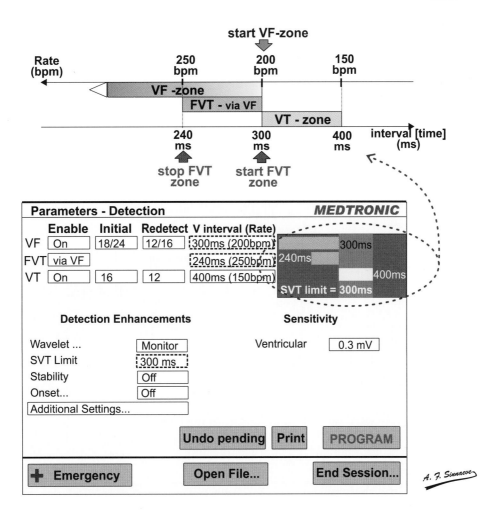

"Empiric" ICD programming ? OK ! OK ! ...
But I am not an engineer and it is all very confusing to me. Programming a VT that is faster than VF is not an obvious choice to me !

SIMPLIFIED PROGRAMMING of MEDTRONIC ICDs FOR THE TREATMENT OF FAST VT

When programming fast VT via VF a "last eight intervals look-back" is applied. If 18/24 intervals are < 300 ms (FDI), then a separate running counter determines whether the last 8 intervals are < 300 ms but > 240 ms. When the last 8 intervals are all within this FVT zone, the rhythm is classified as FVT and is treated with ATP. If 1 or more of these last 8 intervals is shorter than 240 ms the rhythm is classified as VF and treated with a shock.

Abbreviations : ATP = antitachycardia pacing ; FDI = ventricular fibrillation interval ; FVT or fVT = fast ventricular tachycardia ; VF = ventricular fibrillation ; VT = ventricular tachycardia ;

Figure 7.17

CAPACITOR CHARGING DURING ATP - part 1

**ATP during charging allows ATP events to occur
without delaying shock therapy if required**

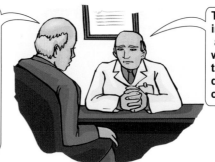

I know that one ATP sequence is painless and can terminate a lot of fast tachycardias (especially monomorphic VTs).
However, if ATP fails to stop the rapid VT (or even accelerates it) a lot of time is wasted by redetection and capacitor charging before a shock can be delivered. Such a delay may increase the incidence of syncope and reduce shock efficacy.

To prevent delay in shock therapy, a new feature was designed to deliver ATP during capacitor charging.

The Medtronic Solution

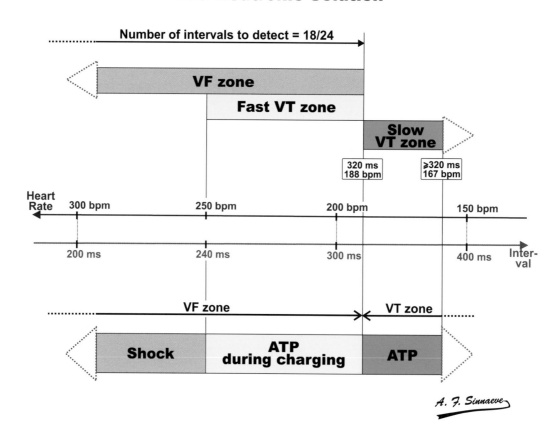

Number of intervals to detect = 18/24

VF zone

Fast VT zone

Slow VT zone

320 ms
188 bpm

≥320 ms
167 bpm

Heart Rate

300 bpm   250 bpm   200 bpm   150 bpm

200 ms   240 ms   300 ms   400 ms   Interval

VF zone   VT zone

Shock   ATP during charging   ATP

A. F. Sinnaeve

Abbreviations: ATP = antitachycardia pacing ; VF = ventricular fibrillation ; VT = ventricular tachycardia ;

Figure 7.18

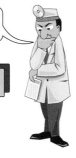

I 'm convinced that ATP during charging is very useful !
But, can you explain how it works ?

CAPACITOR CHARGING DURING ATP - part 2

ATP during charging allows ATP events to occur without delaying shock therapy if required

Successful ATP during charging

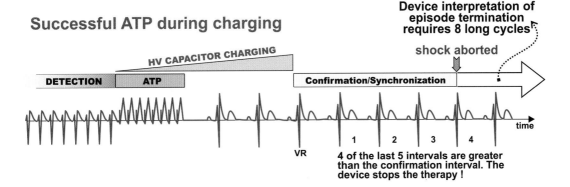

Device interpretation of episode termination requires 8 long cycles

shock aborted

HV CAPACITOR CHARGING

DETECTION | ATP | Confirmation/Synchronization

time

VR

4 of the last 5 intervals are greater than the confirmation interval. The device stops the therapy !

Unsuccessful ATP during charging

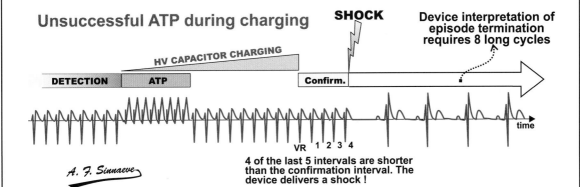

SHOCK

Device interpretation of episode termination requires 8 long cycles

HV CAPACITOR CHARGING

DETECTION | ATP | Confirm.

time

VR 1 2 3 4

4 of the last 5 intervals are shorter than the confirmation interval. The device delivers a shock !

A. F. Sinnaeve

* ATP during charging must be programmed "ON".
* Confirmation interval : programmed VT interval + 60 ms.
* If ATP during charging is enabled, the device applies VF (fast VT) confirmation after charging ends. In contrast, if ATP during charging is disabled, the ICD applies VF (fast VT) confirmation as soon as capacitor charging starts.
* If ATP during charging is enabled, counting of confirmation intervals begins after the first interval beyond completion of charging.The device cancels therapy if 4 of 5 cycles are longer than the confirmation interval. This means that 2 long cycles abort the shock. On the other hand 2 short cycles will trigger a shock ! Therefore, despite successful VT termination, VPCs may create 2 short cycles and trigger shock delivery.

Abbreviations: ATP = antitachycardia pacing ; HV = high voltage ; VPC = ventricular premature complex ; VS = sensed ventricular event ; VT = ventricular tachycardia ;

Figure 7.19

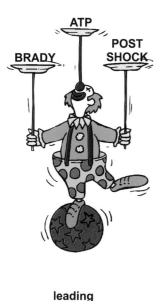

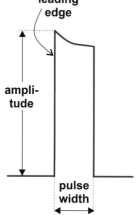

leading
edge

ampli-
tude

pulse
width

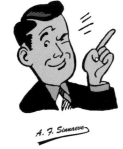

A. F. Sinnaeve

Abbreviations :
HV = high voltage

DIFFERENCES BETWEEN PACING PARAMETERS

REGULAR ANTIBRADYCARDIA PACING

Normal settings of the voltage output according the strength - duration curve, pacing threshold and safety margin.

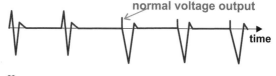

normal voltage output

time

ATP PACING

The ATP voltage output (amplitude and pulse width) is program-mable separately from the "brady pacing" and the "post-shock" parameters. However, ATP pulse width and ATP amplitude are common for all ATP schemes, regardless of zone and position in a prescription.

A high ATP voltage output (to near maximum values) is program-med because the pacing threshold is elevated at very fast pacing rates. To ensure capture manufactures use nominal settings of 7.5 or 8 V and 1 or 1.6 ms.

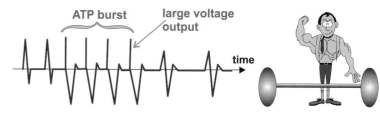

ATP burst   large voltage output

time

POSTSHOCK PACING

After delivery of an HV shock, the pacing threshold is temporarily elevated usually for less than a minute. Post-shock bradycardia pacing is programmed at a high voltage output and pulse width for a relatively short duration which may be programmable. Because bradycardia pacing may be proarrhythmic, some ICDs permit programming of a post-shock pause before pacing begins. In some ICDs the post-shock pacing mode and the pacing rate may also be programmable in the immediate post-shock period. The ICD eventually reverts to its usual programmed antibrady-cardia parameters.

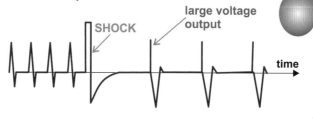

large voltage output

SHOCK

time

Figure 7.20

MINIMIZING RV PACING

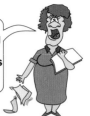

I'm stunned...
The professor just said that RV pacing might be harmful ! RV pacing impairs the LV function, he said, and increases the risk for AF and for hospitalization due to CHF !?

RV pacing mimics LBBB

LBBB
→ altered ventricular contraction
→ delayed LV contraction
→ LV & RV asynchrony → decreased LV diastolic time
→ abnormal septal motion
→ *abnormal LVEF*

How to minimize RV pacing ?

① **Do not pace if not necessary**
* Use DDD(R) with a long AV delay
  (caveat ! several drawbacks !)
* Program a slow lower rate
  (according to the behavior of the spontaneous rhythm)
* Use an AV search algorithm
  (overcomes some drawbacks of fixed long AV delay)

② **Use AAI and AAIR modes**   * Used in Europe in carefully screened patients with SSS without bundle branch block and without delayed AV conduction

③ **Use biventricular (BiV) or single-chamber LV pacing**
* For selected patients with LVEF ≤ 35% (even in the absence of CHF)
* Especially patients with mitral regurgitation and those with cumulative % VP expected to be high (e.g. complete AV block)

④ **Use an algorithm that maintains AAI or AAIR pacing**
* *Managed Ventricular Pacing*[R] (**MVP**) : this algorithm of Medtronic provides AAIR pacing (or AAI) with ventricular monitoring and backup DDDR pacing (or DDD) during AV block

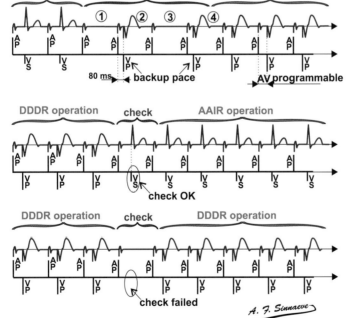

Switching from AAI(R) to DDD(R)

For transient loss of AV conduction, the device remains in AAIR mode and provides backup pacing (80 ms after the A-A escape interval).

If two of the four most recent A-A intervals are missing a ventricular event, the device identifies a persistent loss of AV conduction and switches to DDDR.

Switching from DDD(R) to AAI(R)

The device performs periodic one-cycle checks for AV conduction. The first check occurs after 1 minute. Consequent checks occur after progressively longer intervals (2, 4, 8... min) up to 16 hours and then occur every 16 hours thereafter.
If a ventricular event is sensed during the check, the device returns to the AAI(R) mode.

A. F. Sinnaeve

Abbreviations : AF = atrial fibrillation ; AP = atrial pace ; AV = atrioventricular ; CHF = congestive heart failure ; LBBB = left bundle branch block ; LV = left ventricle ; LVEF = left ventricular ejection fraction ; RV = right ventricle ; VP = ventricular pace ; VS = ventricular sense ;

Figure 7.21

SPECIAL ICD FUNCTIONS

Some ICDs provide both ventricular and atrial defibrillation using the standard leads for ventricular defibrillation. However, detection and therapy of atrial fibrillation are independent of the ventricular detection and defibrillation system.
Other ICDs also provide ventricular resynchronization by pacing in the left as well as in the right ventricle in patients with left ventricular dyssynchrony.

ATRIAL & VENTRICULAR ICD PROVIDING ATP AND DEFIBRILLATION TO BOTH ATRIUM AND VENTRICLE

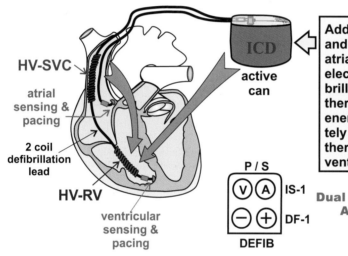

HV-SVC

atrial sensing & pacing

2 coil defibrillation lead

HV-RV

ventricular sensing & pacing

ICD
active can

P / S
V A   IS-1
– +   DF-1
DEFIB

Additional capability for atrial ATP and defibrillation. The shock for atrial defibrillation uses the same electrodes as for ventricular defibrillation. Atrial sensing and atrial therapy sequence (ATP and shock energy) are programmable separately from ventricular detection and therapy (ATP, shock energy) for ventricular tachyarrhythmias.

Dual chamber ICD Active can

BIVENTRICULAR ICD

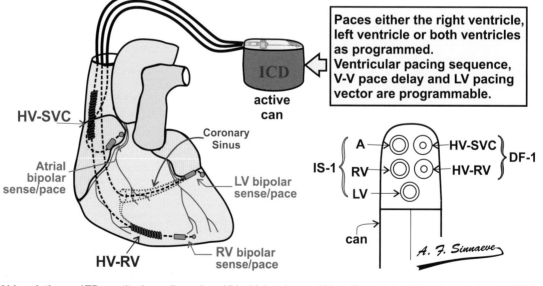

HV-SVC

Atrial bipolar sense/pace

Coronary Sinus

LV bipolar sense/pace

HV-RV

RV bipolar sense/pace

ICD
active can

Paces either the right ventricle, left ventricle or both ventricles as programmed.
Ventricular pacing sequence, V-V pace delay and LV pacing vector are programmable.

A   HV-SVC
IS-1 RV   HV-RV   DF-1
LV

can

A. F. Sinnaeve

Abbreviations : ATP = antitachycardia pacing ; HV = high voltage ; LV = left ventricle ; RV = right ventricle ; SVC = superior vena cava ; V-V delay = time interval between the pacing pulse in the RV and the one in the LV ;

Figure 7.22

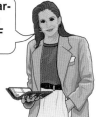

Atrial fibrillation (AF) is a common clinical arrhythmia, particularly in patients with organic heart disease and in the elderly ! About 25% of ICD recipients have a history of AF at the time of implantation.

ATRIAL THERAPIES

The technology is amazing ! Some ICDs provide both ventricular and atrial defibrillation with a standard ICD lead system.
These devices function as implanted coronary care units capable of treating virtually all slow and fast arrhythmias.

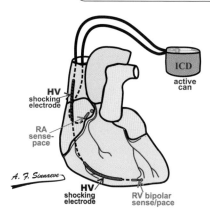

HV shocking electrode

RA sense-pace

A. F. Sinnaeve

HV shocking electrode

RV bipolar sense/pace

ICD active can

Dual-chamber Atrial Defibrillator

* Able to deliver shocks with a programmable energy using conventional ventricular electrode configurations.

* Tiered atrial therapy is possible : ATP (ramp or burst), HF burst pacing (50 Hz) and shock.

* AF occurs more frequently than VF and may terminate spontaneously

* There is less urgency for therapy with AF

* Two operating modes: patient activated or automatic. In the automatic mode, shocks can be delivered at a prespecified time e.g. early morning while the patient is asleep.

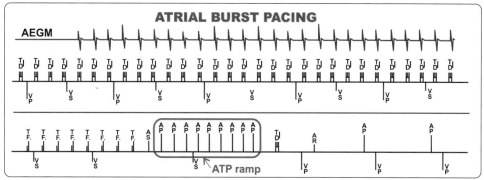

ATRIAL BURST PACING

AEGM

ATP ramp

MARKERS : AP = atrial pace; AS = atrial sense; TD = AT/AF detection; TF. = FAT detection via AT; VS = ventricular sense; VP = ventricular pace; CE = charge end; CD = cardioversion/defibrillation pulse

(The TF marker was used by Medtronic prior to the release of the EnRhythm/EnTrust devices. It represents an AT/AF event that occurs in the AT/AF overlap zone. This marker is no longer used in Medtronic devices with atrial therapies)

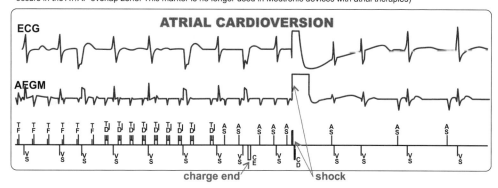

ATRIAL CARDIOVERSION

ECG

AEGM

charge end   shock

Abbreviations : AEGM = atrial electrogram; AF = atrial fibrillation; AT = atrial tachycardia; ATP = antitachycardia pacing; FAT = fast atrial tachycardia; HF = high frequency; HV = high voltage; RA = right atrium; RV = right ventricle;

Figure 7.23

168

ICD TIMING CYCLES

* Refractory & blanking periods

* Basic timing cycles of Medtronic ICDs - parts 1 & 2

* Basic timing cycles of Boston Scientific (Guidant) ICDs

* Basic timing cycles of Guidant (BS) Vitality - parts 1 & 2

* Basic timing cycles of St Jude Medical ICDs

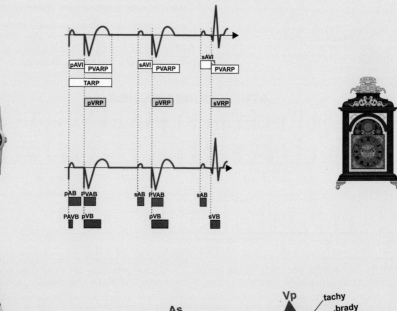

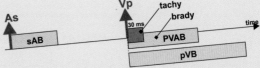

Figure 8.00

TIMING in ICDs
REFRACTORY and BLANKING PERIODS

It is important to understand the function of blanking and refractory periods as well as their relationships and differences !

 REFRACTORY PERIODS :

✷ **BIOLOGICAL :**

The length of time during which the myocardium is incapable of responding to a stimulus (an electrical stimulus cannot evoke any response because repolarization of the cells is still incomplete for the sodium channels to operate properly).

✷ **FOR DEVICES :**

The length of time, following certain events, during which the sensing amplifier is not responsive to events such as the evoked response, T waves, retrograde P waves, etc.
During a refractory period some events can be detected and shown on the marker channel. They may be stored in the device memory for retrieval and analysis by the operator.
Events detected during a refractory period cannot start an AV delay or lower rate interval. However events detected during a refractory period may be used for a variety of functions such as automatic mode switching (AMS).

 BLANKING PERIODS :

✷ A short preset or programmable interval during which the sense amplifier is temporarily disabled or blinded for all incoming signals.
Blanking periods start with the delivery of an output pulse or when the device senses intrinsic activity.
Cross chamber blanking periods in dual chamber devices are intended to prevent inappropriate detection of signals from the opposite chamber (i.e. to eliminate crosstalk).

NOTE 1 : The first part of a refractory period is blanked.
NOTE 2 : In some devices pAB may extend through the entire AV delay (pAVI)

pAVI | PVARP   **sAVI** | PVARP   sAVI | PVARP
TARP
pVRP   pVRP   sVRP

0 ms   500 ms   1000 ms   1500 ms

pAB PVAB   sAB PVAB   sAB
PAVB pVB   pVB   sVB

A. F. Sinnaeve

Abbreviations : AVI = atrioventricular interval (pAVI = AV delay after atrial pacing ; sAVI = AV delay after atrial sensing)
PVARP = postventricular atrial refractory period
TARP = total atrial refractory period = AVI + PVARP
VRP = ventricular refractory period (pVRP = after ventricular pacing ; sVRP = after ventricular sensing)
AB = atrial blanking (pAB = after atrial pacing ; sAB = after atrial sensing)
PVAB = postventricular atrial blanking
PAVB = postatrial ventricular blanking
VB = ventricular blanking (pVB = after ventricular pacing ; sVB = after ventricular sensing)

Figure 8.01

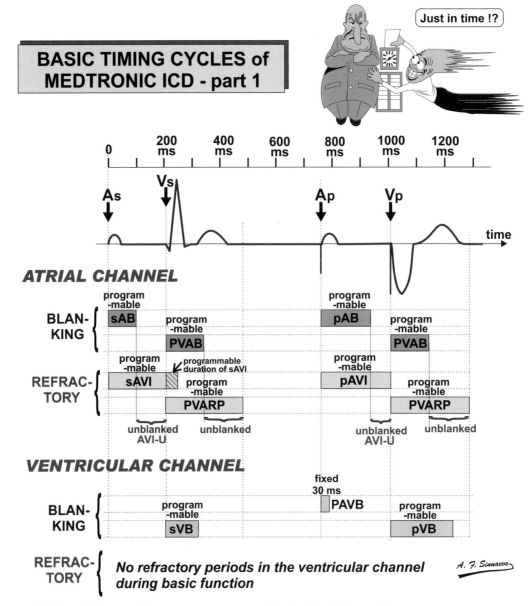

BASIC TIMING CYCLES of MEDTRONIC ICD - part 1

Just in time !?

NOTE : sAB and sVB were non-programmable in older ICD models.

! *PVAB in this diagram refers to the bradycardia function only. For the ICD to detect atrial tachyarrhythmias or activity for the discriminator algorithms, the PVAB is only 30 ms as shown in the next page.*

The duration of sVB is important to prevent double counting of the QRS by the ventricular channel.
The duration of pVB is important to prevent T wave oversensing by the ventricular channel.

Abbreviations :
pAVI = atrioventricular interval after atrial pace ; AVI-U = unblanked part of the AV delay
AB = atrial blanking period (pAB : after pacing; sAB : after sensing)
PVAB = postventricular atrial blanking ; PAVB = postatrial ventricular blanking (to prevent crosstalk)
PVARP = postventricular atrial refractory period
VB = ventricular blanking period (pVB : after pacing; sVB : after sensing)

Figure 8.02

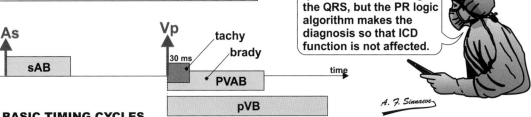

BASIC TIMING CYCLES of MEDTRONIC ICDs - part 2

The very short PVAB for tachycardia causes frequent far-field sensing of the QRS, but the PR logic algorithm makes the diagnosis so that ICD function is not affected.

A. F. Sinnaeve

BASIC TIMING CYCLES (Medtronic - ENTRUST)

ATRIAL BLANKING :

pAB = programmable 150 - 250 ms
    (nominal = 200 ms)
sAB = programmable 100 - 170 ms
    (nominal = 100 ms)
brady PVAB = programmable 10 - 300 ms
    (nominal = 150 ms)
tachy PVAB = 30 ms (fixed)

ATRIAL REFRACTORY :

PVARP = programmable: Varied or 150 - 500 ms
    (minimun PVARP = PVAB)
    (nominal 310 ms)
    PVARP extension after a PVC : 400 ms
    (if programmed less than that value)
pAVI = programmable 30 - 350 ms
    (rate-adaptive)
sAVI = programmable 30 - 350 ms
    (rate-adaptive)
Unblanked AVI (AVI-U) starts after completion of pAB or sAB provided pAVI > pAB or sAVI > sAB

VENTRICULAR BLANKING :

pVB = programmable 150 - 450 ms
    (nominal 200 ms)

sVB = programmable 120 - 170 ms
    (nominal 120 ms)

PAVB = 30 ms (fixed)

VENTRICULAR SAFETY PACING :

VSP = 110 ms. A shorter value (70 ms) takes effect when the pacing rate exceeds the VSP switch rate calculated according to :
$$\frac{60\,000}{2 \times (pVB + 110\ ms)} \text{ per minute.}$$

Postventricular atrial blanking (PVAB)

Three forms of PVAB are programmable :

Partial PVAB

There is a 30 ms non-programmable atrial blanking interval after a ventricular paced beat and none (0 ms) after a ventricular sensed beat. No markers can be seen in this hardware blanking interval (i.e. first 30 ms). Atrial events falling in the progammable PVAB for bradycardia ("software blanking" period) are used only by the PR Logic and are labeled AR in the models before Entrust. Ab markers are new, starting with the Entrust ICD, and depict atrial sensing in the PVAB. If the programmed PVAB is 150 ms, atrial signals detected between 30 ms and 150 ms from the onset of the PVARP will now be labeled Ab. Events depicted as Ab are ignored by the mode switch, PVC response, non-competitive atrial pacing (NCAP) and PMT intervention algorithms.

Absolute PVAB

All of the 150 ms (assumed value of PVAB) is blanked for tachy and brady functions. No events are used for the PR Logic. Nevertheless Ab markers will be seen.

Partial PVAB+

This interval is similar to the Partial PVAB but the atrial sensitivity is decreased (higher numerical value) for a brief period following a paced or sensed *ventricular* event to provide amplitude-based discrimination between far-field R waves and intrinsic atrial events.

Although the differences between the successive models are small, it is better to have a good look in the manual !

I have some more ICD technical manuals from all manufacturers and their various device models ! Where shall I put them ?

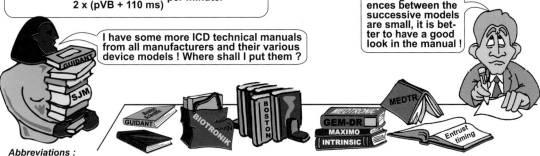

Abbreviations :
AB = atrial blanking period (pAB : after pacing ; sAB : after sensing) ; PAVB = postatrial ventricular blanking (to prevent crosstalk) ; PVC = premature ventricular complex ; PVAB = postventricular atrial blanking ; AVI = atrioventricular interval or AV delay (pAVI : after atrial pace ; sAVI = after atrial sense) ; PVARP = postventricular atrial refractory period ; VB = ventricular blanking period (pVB : after pacing ; sVB : after sensing) ; VSP = ventricular safety pacing ; PMT = pacemaker mediated tachycardia ;

Figure 8.03

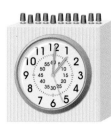

BASIC TIMING CYCLES of
BOSTON SCIENTIFIC (GUIDANT) ICDs

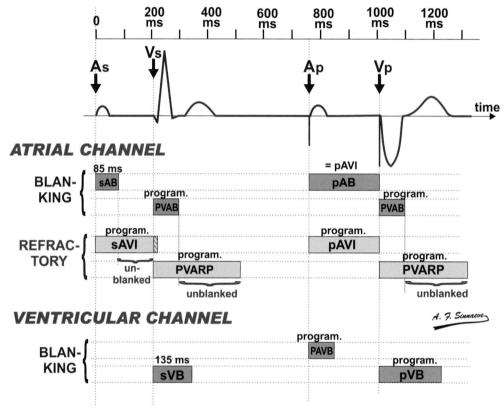

A. F. Sinnaeve

sAB = atrial blanking period after atrial sense : fixed 85 ms

pAB = atrial blanking period after atrial pace : always same as pAVI

pAVI = programmed AV delay after atrial pace : dynamic OFF or dynamic ON
    dynamic OFF : programmable constant value 10, 20, ... 300 ms
    dynamic ON : maximum value programmable 20, 30, ... 300 ms
        minimum value programmable 10, 20, ... 290 ms

sAVI = programmed AV delay after atrial sense : same as pAVI but may be shortened
    by a "Sensed AV Offset" (to compensate for hemodynamic difference between
    sensed and paced atrial events) : programmable OFF, -10, -20, ... -100 ms

PVARP = postventricular atrial refractory period : dynamic OFF or dynamic ON
    dynamic OFF : programmable constant value 150, 160, ... 500 ms
    dynamic ON : maximum value programmable 160, 170, ... 500 ms
        minimum value programmable 150, 160, ... 490 ms

PVAB = postventricular atrial blanking period : programmable 45, 65 or 85 ms

PAVB = postatrial ventricular blanking period : programmable 45, 65 or 85 ms

sVB = ventricular blanking after ventricular sense : fixed 135 ms

pVB = ventricular blanking after ventricular pace : dynamic OFF or dynamic ON
    dynamic OFF : programmable constant value 150, 160, ... 500 ms
    dynamic ON : maximum value programmable 160, 170, ... 500 ms
        minimum value programmable 150, 160, ... 490 ms

Figure 8.04

TIMING CYCLES - Guidant (Vitality) - 1

A good timing is everything !

ATRIAL CHANNEL - DUAL CHAMBER MODE

A sensed V sensed

A sensed V paced

A paced V sensed

A paced V paced

time

A. F. Sinnaeve

sAVI

sAB

PVARP

Programmable AV delay after sensed atrial event (includes 85 ms absolute refractory, i.e. blanked)

AV delay after paced atrial event (entire delay is absolute refractory = blanked)

Programmable atrial refractory PVARP (includes programmable atrial cross chamber blanking)

PVAB A-blank after V-pace (programmable values 45, 65, 85 ms)

PVAB A-blank after V-sense (programmable values 45, 65, 85, and SMART sensing™)

sAB atrial blanking after A-sense (fixed on 85 ms)

1 AV-INTERVAL (AVI) The AV-delay can be programmed to one of two operations :

✦ *AV Delay* : a fixed interval (programmable values 10, 20, ..., 300 ms - nominal setting 180 ms)

✦ *Dynamic AV Delay* : can be programmed Off or On.
The dynamic AV delay is based on the previous A-A interval and shortens automatically the AVI during an increase of rate.

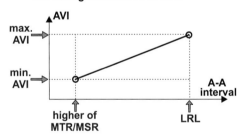

max. AVI : programmable values 20, 30, ..., 300 ms
nominal setting : 180 ms
min. AVI : programmable values 10, 20, ..., 290 ms
nominal setting : 80 ms

longer

shorter

longer

shorter

2 POSTVENTRICULAR ATRIAL REFRACTORY PERIOD (PVARP)

✦ *Fixed PVARP* : programmable values 150, 160, ..., 500 ms - nominal setting 250 ms

✦ *Dynamic PVARP* : can be programmed Off or On.
This feature shortens automatically the PVARP when the rate increases.
Max. PVARP : programmable values 160, 170, ..., 500 ms - nominal setting 250 ms
Min. PVARP : programmable values 150, 160, ..., 490 ms - nominal setting 240 ms

✦ *PVARP after PVC* : helps preventing pacemaker-mediated tachycardia due to retrograde conduction, which is typically associated with PVCs. This feature can be programmed Off or On.
Programmable values 150, 200, ..., 500 ms - nominal setting 400 ms

Abbreviations : AB = atrial blanking; AVI = atrioventricular interval; LRL = lower rate limit; MSR = max. sensor-driven rate; MTR = max. tracking rate; PVAB = postventricular atrial blanking; PVARP = postventricular atrial refractory period; PVC = premature ventricular contraction;
s... = after sensing (e.g. sAB); p... = after pacing (e.g. pAVI);

Figure 8.05

TIMING CYCLES - Guidant (Vitality) - 2

Timing is essential for under-standing PMs and ICDs !

3 SMARTSensing™ : A-blank after V-sense only

Improves the devices ability to sense P waves and to reject FFRW sensing (by auto-matically adjusting the amplifier gain), especially during atrial and/or ventricular tachyarrhythmias.

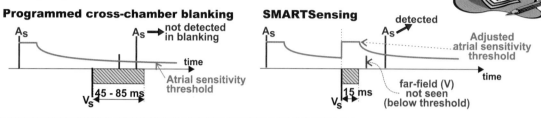

Programmed cross-chamber blanking

SMARTSensing

VENTRICULAR CHANNEL - DUAL CHAMBER MODE

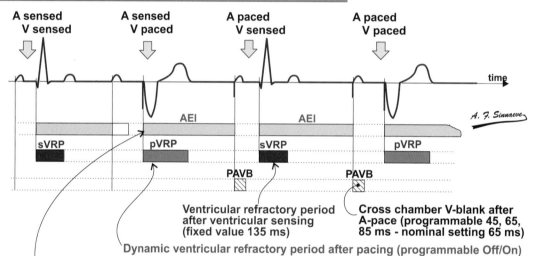

The manufacturer uses the term "ventricular refractory period" for what is really a "ventricular blanking period" in an ICD !

VENTRICULAR REFRACTORY PERIOD (pVRP)

✦ **pVRP** : a fixed interval (programmable values 150, 160, ..., 500 ms - nominal setting 250 ms)

✦ **Dynamic VRP** : can be programmed Off or On.
The dynamic VRP is based on the previous V-V interval and shortens automatically the VRP during an increase of rate.

max. VRP : programmable values 160, 170, ..., 500 ms nominal setting : 250 ms
min. VRP : programmable values 150, 160, ..., 490 ms nominal setting : 240 ms

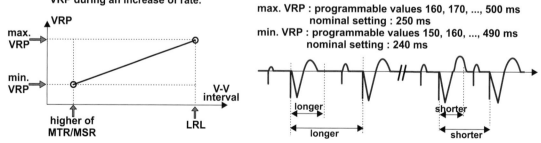

Abbreviations : AEI = atrial escape interval ; PAVB = postatrial ventricular blanking ; pVRP = ventricular refractory period after ventricular pacing ; sVRP = ventricular refractory period after ventricular sensing ;

Figure 8.06

BASIC TIMING CYCLES of St JUDE MEDICAL

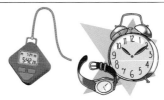

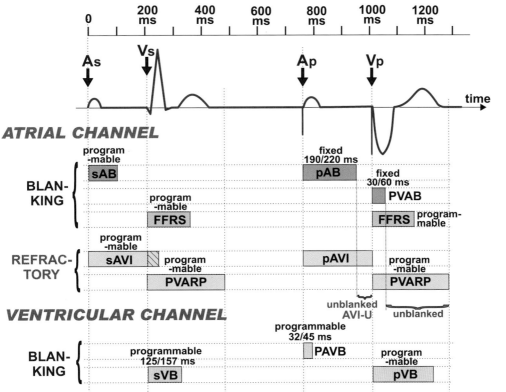

ATRIAL CHANNEL

VENTRICULAR CHANNEL

NOTE : The fixed PVAB and the programmable FFRS in previous models have been replaced by a single programmable PVAB interval

---

pAVI = program. 35 - 350 ms (nominal 170 ms) - max. pAVI limited by programmed "Base Rate"

sAVI = program. 25 - 325 ms (nominal 150 ms) - shorter or equal to pAVI and within 100 ms of pAVI
both pAVI & sAVI may be rate responsive (programmable Off, Low, Medium, High)
if rate responsive : minimum pAVI & sAVI programmable 35 - 120 ms (nominal 50 ms)

pAB = fixed 190 or 220 ms; automatically adapted by device depending on atrial pacing amplitude

sAB = programmable 93, 125 or 157 ms (nominal 93 ms)

pVB = programmable 125 - 470 ms (nominal 250 ms) (= absolute refractory)
must be programmed shorter than PVARP
pVB may be rate responsive (Off, low, medium, high - nominal : medium)
if rate responsive a minimum pVB must be programmed : 125 - 470 ms (nominal 220 ms)

sVB = programmable 125 or 157 ms (nominal 125 ms)

PVARP = programmable 125 - 470 ms (nominal 280 ms) (= relative refractory)

PAVB = choice by clinician : 32 or 45 ms (default 32 ms)
there is no PAVB after a sensed P wave

A. F. Sinnaeve

PVAB = fixed at between 30 and 60 ms, automatically adapted by the device depending on programmed amplitude, pulse width and maximum pacing rate ; there is no PVAB after ventricular sensing.

FFRS = far-field R wave suppression interval is programmable OFF, 20 - 200/250 ms (nominal OFF)
and is only available when arrhythmia sensing is "dual chamber". Unlike PVARP, the FFRS is a true blanking period because atrial events falling in the FFRS do not affect any of the ICD functions, and are not counted for the purpose of automatic mode switching.
FFRS begins with a ventricular paced or sensed beat. After a ventricular stimulus, the first part of the FFRS is the PVAB.

  Use the Far-Field R Suppression with caution as it may have adverse effects on atrial sensing, and indirectly, on SVT discrimination and automatic mode switching !

Figure 8.07

⑨ COMPLICATIONS of ICD THERAPY

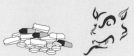

* Summary of complications of ICD therapy - parts 1 - 3

* Reversal of coil or lead connections

* Absent or delayed ICD therapy

* Continuation of tachycardia after therapy

* Misclassification of shock efficacy

* Important interactions between medications and ICDs

* ICD and antiarrhythmic drug therapy
  1. Potential benefits of AA drugs
  2. Classification of AA drugs - interactions with ICDs
  3. Potential adverse effects of AA drugs on ICDs
  4. Proarrhythmia caused by AA drugs

* ICDs and proarrhythmia

* ICD-induced proarrhythmia

* Electrical storm

* Psychological problems and stress

* Patient instructions at hospital discharge - parts 1 & 2

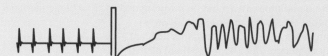

Figure 9.00

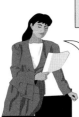

COMPLICATIONS of ICD THERAPY

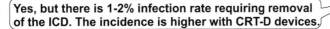

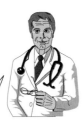

You know, perioperative mortality is less than 0.5% !

Yes, but there is 1-2% infection rate requiring removal of the ICD. The incidence is higher with CRT-D devices.

Complications due to venous access

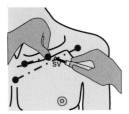

Complications related to blind subclavian venous puncture depend on :
(1) the operator's skill
(2) patient's anatomy

* Pneumothorax
* Hemoptysis
* Hemothorax or hemopneumothorax
* Air embolism
* Venous thrombosis
* Pulmonary embolism
* Brachial plexus injury

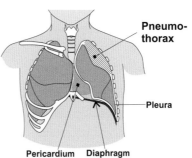

Pocket-related complications

* Pocket seroma
* Pocket hematoma
* Pocket erosion
* Pocket infection either localized or associated with systemic infection.
  (The latter may be associated with septic thrombus on the lead identifiable by echocardiography)

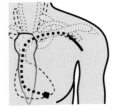

A. F. Sinnaeve

Lead-related complications

* Lead malposition
* Lead dislodgement
* Lead perforation of RV (may cause loss of pacing/sensing, diaphragmatic stimulation and cardiac tamponade)
* Lead fracture
* Insulation break
* Loose set screw
* Defective insulation cap
* Misconnection
* Twidler's syndrome

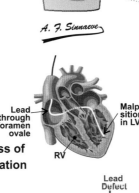

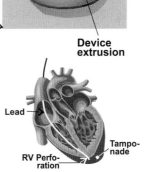

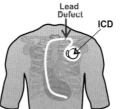

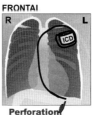

Abbreviations : LV = left ventricle ; RV = right ventricle ; CRT = cardiac resynchronization therapy

Figure 9.01

COMPLICATIONS of ICD THERAPY - cont'd

> ICDs are extremely complicated high-tech devices and their implantation as well as their programming have to be performed with expert skill !

ICD generator - Acute complications

* Malfunction during testing
* Inadequate DFT
* Undersensing of VT/VF

Other complications

* ICD migration into axilla
* Perioperative cerebral ischemia (rare)
* Extracardiac stimulation
  {right phrenic nerve stimulation with atrial lead and with RV lead : diaphragm (with or without perforation) and chest wall intercostal muscle stimulation (with perforation)}
* Significant site pain requiring reoperation
* Postoperative thrombosis of deep femoral vein
* Frozen shoulder

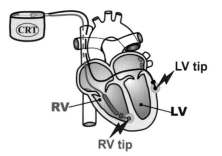

A. F. Sinnaeve

Complications with CRT

* Coronary sinus dissection
* Coronary sinus perforation
* Left phrenic nerve stimulation
* AV block in the setting of LBBB during RV lead manipulation
* Inability to implant LV lead transvenously

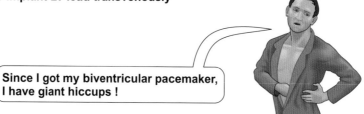

> Since I got my biventricular pacemaker, I have giant hiccups !

Abbreviations : AV = atrioventricular ; CRT = cardiac resynchronization therapy ; DFT = defibrillation threshold ; LBBB = left bundle branch block ; LV = left ventricle ; RV = right ventricle ; VF = ventricular fibrillation ; VT = ventricular tachycardia ;

Figure 9.02

COMPLICATIONS of ICD THERAPY - cont'd

Complications are uncommon, but nevertheless possible !
Acute complications occur at implantation (such as pneumothorax, hematoma, etc.). *Delayed complications* may turn up
after days or even after months (such as lead failure, excessive fibrosis at the electrode tip, etc.).

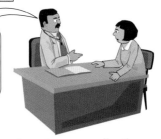

LONG-TERM COMPLICATIONS
Lead malfunction (fracture and/or insulation break) is the most common long-term complication

Interactions between medications and ICD
* drug-induced proarrhythmia
* increase of DFT (transient)
* prolongation of VT cycle length
* conversion of atrial fibrillation to atrial flutter

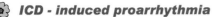

ATP   ACCELERATION OF VT

ICD - induced proarrhythmia
* delivery of a shock in sinus rhythm may rarely be fatal
* tachyarrhythmias with appropriate therapy
  (acceleration of VT by ATP or shock)
* tachyarrhythmias with inappropriate therapy
  (VF induction by low-energy shock)
* bradyarrhythmias

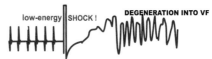

low-energy SHOCK !   DEGENERATION INTO VF

Oversensing causing inappropriate shocks
* intracardiac signals (T wave and P wave sensing
  double counting of R waves)
* myopotentials
* Electromagnetic interference (EMI at home, at work, at the hospital)

Each time when I touch
the coffee machine, my
ICD gives me a shock !?
Is that EMI ?

Programming related problems
* inappropriate rate cutoff for tachycardia detection
* intentional or erroneous device deactivation with
  failure to reactivate the ICD

Patient related problems
* psychological problems and stress
* phantom shocks
* twiddler's syndrome
* pacemaker syndrome and LV dyssynchrony
* increase of DFT (by electrode tissue interface or
  adverse change in the myocardial substrate)

ICD

A. F. Sinnaeve

Miscellaneous problems
* delayed or absent conversion of VT/VF
* gradual reduction of VEGM amplitude (local reaction)
  during basic rhythm causing undersensing of VT/VF
* electrical storm
* pacemaker-mediated tachycardia

SENSING
ATRIAL
DEPOLARIZATION

A

AV Delay

VA con-
duction

ICD

PACING
IN
VENTRICLE

V

Underdetection of tachyarrhythmia
* specificity and sensitivity of algorithm is less than100%
  (inappropriate shocks for SVT and ST)

ICD related problems
* early battery depletion and/or prolonged charge time
* random ICD component failure
* adverse effects from ICD design and not due to malfunction

Abbreviations : ATP = antitachycardia pacing ; DFT = defibrillation threshold ; EMI = electromagnetic interference ;
LV = left ventricle ; ST = sinus tachycardia ; SVT = supraventricular tachycardia ; VEGM = ventricular electrogram ;
VF = ventricular fibrillation ; VT = ventricular tachycardia ;

Figure 9.03

REVERSAL OF COIL OR LEAD CONNECTIONS

Reversal of coils in a dual coil integrated lead

In an integrated lead, the distal defibrillation coil forms part of pacing and sensing function !

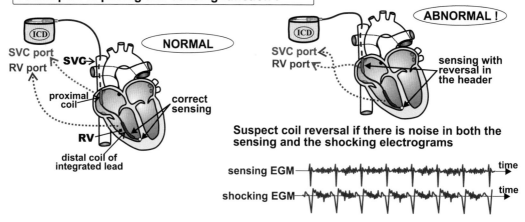

SVC port
RV port
SVC
proximal coil
correct sensing
RV
distal coil of integrated lead
NORMAL

SVC port
RV port
ABNORMAL !
sensing with reversal in the header

Suspect coil reversal if there is noise in both the sensing and the shocking electrograms

sensing EGM ————— time
shocking EGM ————— time

This problem may cause sensing of thoracic myopotentials and atrial activity with resultant ICD inhibition and/or inappropraite therapy (shocks)

Reversal of the two ventricular leads (CRT)

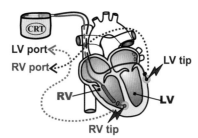

LV port
RV port
RV
LV tip
LV
RV tip

Reversal of the left and the right ventricular lead connections may be inapparent during biventricular pacing if the interventricular interval (V-V) is zero. Programming LV pacing alone will show an RV pacing configuration without a dominant positive QRS complex in V1. Programming RV pacing alone will show a RBBB pacing configuration in lead V1 provided the lead pacing the LV is correctly positoned in the coronary venous system.

Reversal of atrial and right ventricular leads

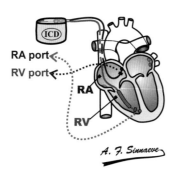

RA port
RV port
RA
RV

A. F. Sinnaeve

* Pacing abnormalities

* VT and VF will be missed because the device interprets them as supraventricular in origin. SVT above the cutoff rate will be interpreted as VT/VF with the delivery of therapy.

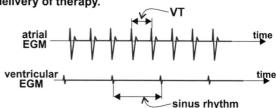

VT
atrial EGM ————— time
ventricular EGM ————— time
sinus rhythm

Abbreviations : CRT = Cardiac resynchronization therapy ; EGM = electrogram ; LV = left ventricle ; RA = right atrium ; RV = right ventricle ; SVC = superior vena cava ; SVT = supraventricular tachycardia ; VF = ventricular fibrillation ; VT = ventricular tachycardia ; RBBB = right bundle branch block ;

Figure 9.04

ABSENT OR DELAYED ICD THERAPY

① INACTIVATED ICD

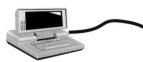

> Don't forget to reprogram the device after general surgery during which the device was deactivated !

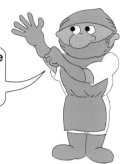

② UNDERSENSING OF VEGM

- Low amplitude of sensed VEGM (uncommon)
- Low amplitude of VEGM after unsuccessful shock
- Amplitude fluctuations of VEGM : spontaneous changes in VEGM may cause signal dropout in ICDs with automatic gain or automatic threshold control

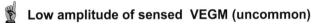

- Lead malfunction (fracture, insulation defect, ...) and displacement
- Device malfunction (battery, capacitor, electronic component, ...)

③ UNDERDETECTION OF TACHYARRHYTHMIA

- VT/VF rate-cutoff programmed too high

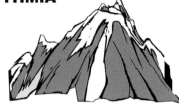

> This is really too high ! I'll never reach the top...

- One or more programmed discriminators not being satisfied
- Multiple programmable tachycardia zones : tachycardias with rates near the VT/VF intervals

④ INAPPROPRIATE PROGRAMMED VT THERAPY :
ATP sequence or low energy shock

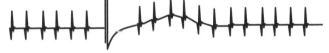

A. F. Sinnaeve

⑤ INTERFERENCE :
Noise or signals from a separate pacemaker (no longer seen with contemporary ICDs)

ABBREVIATIONS : VEGM = ventricular electrogram; VF = ventricular fibrillation; VT = ventricular tachycardia

Figure 9.05

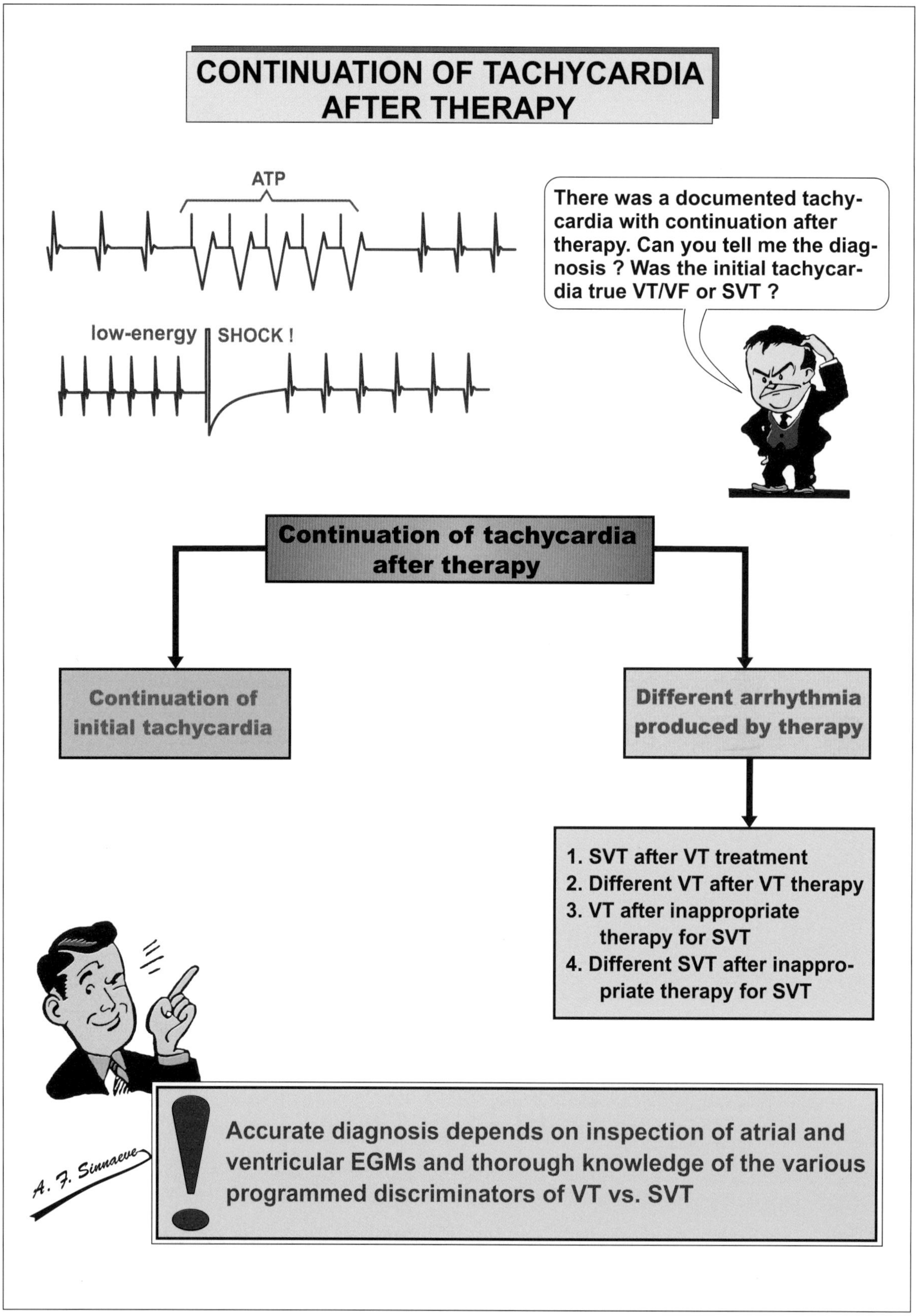
CONTINUATION OF TACHYCARDIA AFTER THERAPY
ATP
low-energy
SHOCK !
There was a documented tachycardia with continuation after therapy. Can you tell me the diagnosis ? Was the initial tachycardia true VT/VF or SVT ?
Continuation of tachycardia after therapy
Continuation of initial tachycardia
Different arrhythmia produced by therapy
1. SVT after VT treatment
2. Different VT after VT therapy
3. VT after inappropriate therapy for SVT
4. Different SVT after inappropriate therapy for SVT
Accurate diagnosis depends on inspection of atrial and ventricular EGMs and thorough knowledge of the various programmed discriminators of VT vs. SVT
A. F. Sinnaeve

Figure 9.06

MISCLASSIFICATION OF SHOCK EFFICACY

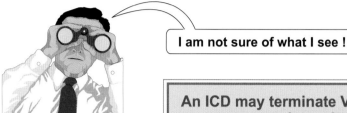

I am not sure of what I see !

An ICD may terminate VT, but all the same, may not detect its termination !

 1 VT recurs before the ICD can detect the return to sinus rhythm after the shock. There is immediate recurrence because of new sustained or unsustained VT.

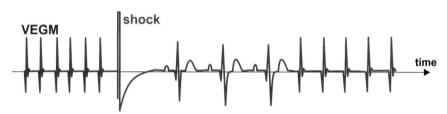

TREATMENT : Reduce the number of beats for redetection of sinus rhythm. For unsustained VT, increase the number of beats required for redetection.

 2 The shock produces SVT in the VT zone

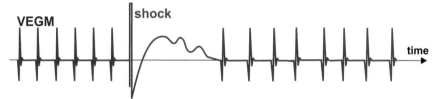

TREATMENT : As with inappropriate SVT detection

A. F. Sinnaeve

ABBREVIATIONS : VEGM = ventricular electrogram; VF = ventricular fibrillation; VT = ventricular tachycardia
SVT = supraventricular tachycardia

Figure 9.07

IMPORTANT INTERACTIONS BETWEEN MEDICATIONS AND ICDs

☹ **ARRHYTHMIA DETECTION can be affected by :**

* Slowing of VT rate below cut-off rate for detection

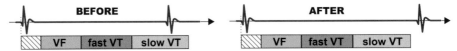

BEFORE — VF | fast VT | slow VT

AFTER — VF | fast VT | slow VT

* Slowing of fast VT may allow termination with ATP rather than a shock
* Diminished slew rate (rate of change of voltage of the EGM)
* QRS widening, altering the criteria for ventricular arrhythmia recognition (e.g. see morphology)

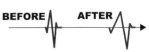

BEFORE   AFTER

👽 **PACING :**

* Increase in capture threshold for antibradycardia pacing

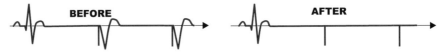

BEFORE   AFTER

* Increase in capture threshold at rapid pacing rates ("use dependency")
* Induction of sinus bradycardia and/or AV block, necessitating antibradycardia pacing

💣 **DEFIBRILLATION :**

* Development of proarrhythmia characterized by aggravation of pre-existing tachyarrhythmia (increased occurrence and/or faster rate) and/or development of new, different and faster ventricular arrhythmias requiring more shocks and occasionally easier inducibility of ventricular fibrillation by ATP or low-shock cardioversion.

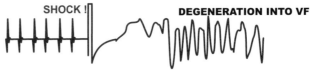

SHOCK !   DEGENERATION INTO VF

* Decrease in defibrillation threshold : Class III drugs (but not amiodarone) may lower the defibrillation threshold and may be helpful in high threshold situations
* Increase in defibrillation threshold

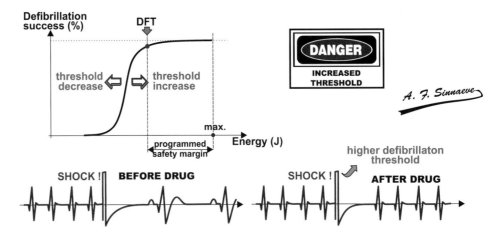

Defibrillation success (%)
DFT
threshold decrease ⇐ ⇒ threshold increase
max.
programmed safety margin
Energy (J)

DANGER
INCREASED THRESHOLD

A. F. Sinnaeve

higher defibrillaton threshold

SHOCK !   BEFORE DRUG

SHOCK !   AFTER DRUG

☺ **ELIMINATION OR REDUCED OCCURENCE OF VT AND SVT**

Figure 9.08

ICD and ANTIARRHYTHMIC DRUG THERAPY - 1

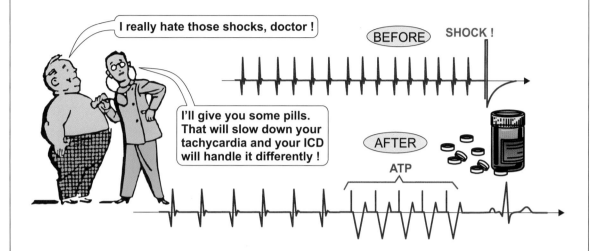

About 50% or more of patients with ICDs require antiarrhythmic (AA) drugs !

POTENTIAL BENEFITS OF AA DRUGS

1. Reduction of the number of sustained (and non-sustained) symptomatic VT/VF episodes thereby limiting the number of painful high-energy shocks and conserving battery longevity.
2. Suppression of coexisting supraventricular tachyarrhythmias limiting the number of inappropriate shocks. Drugs can also reduce the rate of supraventricular tachyarrhythmias and thus reduce inappropriate shocks by this mechanism.
3. Slowing of the VT rate and possibly better organization of irregular VTs. Slower VT is better tolerated hemodynamically and more amenable to painless termination by ATP obviating painful shocks. In other words, the efficacy of painless ATP for VT termination is enhanced. Slowing of VT makes it more amenable to ablative therapy.
4. Slowing of the sinus rate may also reduce inappropriate shocks.
5. Class III drugs (sotalol, dofetilide and azimilide) appear to decrease the energy requirements for defibrillation. This may be potentially beneficial in patients with a marginal defibrillation threshold (DFT).

A. F. Sinnaeve

Abbreviations : AA drug = antiarrhythmic drug ; ATP = antitachycardia pacing ; DFT = defibrillation threshold; VF = ventricular fibrillation ; VT = ventricular tachycardia ;

Figure 9.09

ICD and ANTIARRHYTHMIC DRUG THERAPY - 2

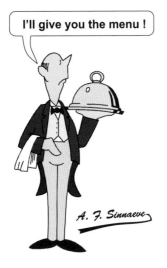

I'll give you the menu !

A. F. Sinnaeve

ANTIARRHYTHMIC DRUGS CLASSIFICATION

Class I : Sodium Channel Blockers
IA : Quinidine, Procainamide, Disopyramide
IB : Lidocaine, Mexiletine
IC : Flecainide, Propafenone

Class II : Beta-Blockers
Propanolol, Metoprolol

Class III : Potassium Channel Blockers
Sotalol, Dofetilide, Amiodarone*, Azimilide

Class IV : Calcium Channel Blockers
Verapamil, Diltiazem

* Amiodarone contains activities of all four classes, yet it is classified as a Class III agent .

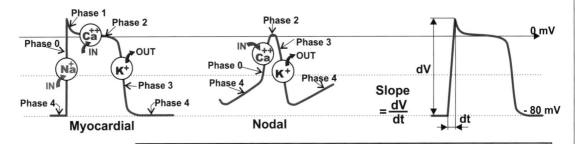

Myocardial   Nodal   Slope $= \dfrac{dV}{dt}$

Everybody has to know these facts !

ICD AND ANTIARRHYTHMIC DRUG INTERACTIONS

* Sodium channel blockers increase the DFT or the energy for successful defibrillation.

* Potassium channel blockers decrease DFTs.

* Antiarrhythmic drugs may affect pacing threshold, making it more difficult to capture.

* Antiarrhythmic drugs substantially slow the conduction i.e. they slow the dV/dt of the action potential, thereby prolonging the QRS in the electrogram with the possibility of double counting and inappropriate shocks.

Important

A change in antiarrhythmic drug therapy, dose or new drug, requires retesting of the DFT (defibrillation threshold) to establish the continuing efficacy of the ICD system.

Figure 9.10

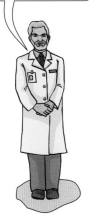

Be very careful with AA drugs for an ICD patient !

A. F. Sinnaeve

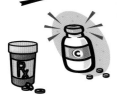

POTENTIAL ADVERSE EFFECTS OF ANTIARRHYTHMIC DRUGS IN PATIENTS WITH ICDs

- Increase in the DFT which may cause device failure to defibrillate. Na-channel blocking drugs (especially class IC) may increase the duration of the ventricular electrogram causing inappropriate shocks from double counting.

- Prolongation of VT cycle length below the programmed tachycardia detection rate. Patients may be unaware of the slower VT and may present in heart failure after several days of persistent slow VT.

- Conversion of atrial fibrillation into atrial flutter with 1:1 AV conduction and rapid ventricular rate leading to hemodynamic impairment and inappropriate shock.

- Bradycardia : Ventricular pacing may cause pacemaker syndrome, LV dyssynchrony with the risk of precipitating heart failure. Pacing also causes faster depletion of the device battery.

- Proarrhythmia.

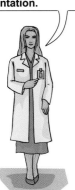

Beware! A change in AA agent (drug and/or dose) is an important event in ICD patients as it often requires retesting of the DFT especially if it was high at the time of implantation.

EFFECT OF AA DRUG THERAPY ON DFTs

INCREASE	DECREASE	VARIABLE
Quinidine* Disopyramide* Procainamide* Lidocaine Mexiletine Flecainide Propranolol Amiodarone** Verapamil Diltiazem	Sotalol Dofetilide	Propafenone Bretylium

* Class IA drugs have shown inconsistent results but Quinidine has increased the DFT in some studies.

** Oral amiodarone can increase the DFT in selected patients with potentially life threatening consequences. IV amiodarone has no important effect on the DFT.

Abbreviations : *AA drug = antiarrhythmic drug ; AV = atrioventricular ; DFT = defibrillation threshold ; LV = left ventricle ; VT = ventricular tachycardia ;*

Figure 9.11

ICD and ANTIARRHYTHMIC DRUG THERAPY - 4

PROARRHYTHMIA

Antiarrhythmic drugs can aggravate the clinical arrhythmia, increase its frequency or cause new arrhythmias. This is called proarrhythmia !

Drug-induced proarrhythmia occurs in patients with or without an ICD. It is more likely to occur in patients with ICDs because they often have ischemic heart disease and decreased left ventricular function and with increasing age. As a rule such patients should not receive antiarrhythmic drugs other than sotalol and amiodarone.

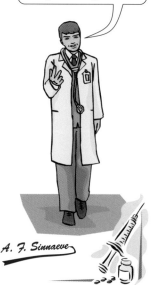

Attention ! For some patients AA drugs may be dangerous !

 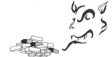

A. F. Sinnaeve

PROARRHYTHMIA CLASSIFICATION	
Antiarrhythmic drug	**Proarrhythmia**
Class IA	Torsades de pointes : Twisting of the points (long QT) magnified by hypokalemia
Class IC Flecainide Propafenone	Sustained or incessant VT, polymorphic VT/VF (rare). VT difficult to defibrillate. VT may be provoked by increased heart rate. Slowing of atrial flutter rate causing 1:1 conduction to the ventricle with fast ventricular rate and wide QRS resembling VT.
Class II Beta-blockers	Severe sinus bradycardia
Class III Sotalol Dofetilide	Torsades de pointes (long QT) magnified by hypokalemia
Class IV Verapamil Diltiazem	Severe sinus bradycardia

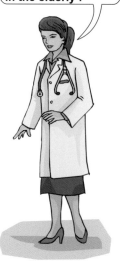

I'm always mindful of the proarrhythmia risk in patients with poor LV function and in the elderly !

Abbreviations : *AA drug = antiarrhythmic drug ; AV = atrioventricular ; LV = left ventricle ; VF = ventricular fibrillation ; VT = ventricular tachycardia ; long QT = long QT-interval ;*

Figure 9.12

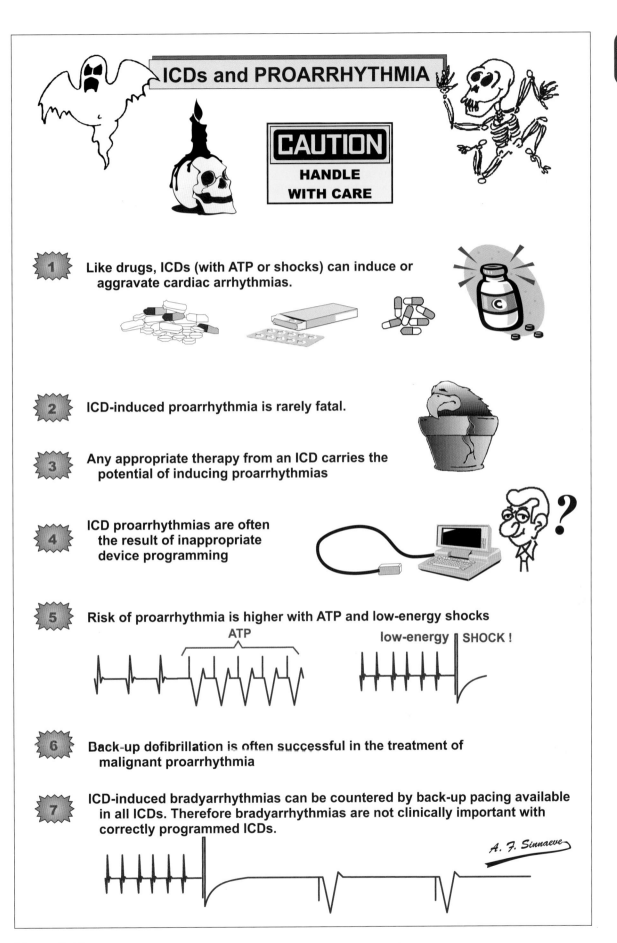

189

ICDs and PROARRHYTHMIA

CAUTION
HANDLE
WITH CARE

1. Like drugs, ICDs (with ATP or shocks) can induce or aggravate cardiac arrhythmias.

2. ICD-induced proarrhythmia is rarely fatal.

3. Any appropriate therapy from an ICD carries the potential of inducing proarrhythmias

4. ICD proarrhythmias are often the result of inappropriate device programming

5. Risk of proarrhythmia is higher with ATP and low-energy shocks

ATP

low-energy ∥ SHOCK !

6. Back-up defibrillation is often successful in the treatment of malignant proarrhythmia

7. ICD-induced bradyarrhythmias can be countered by back-up pacing available in all ICDs. Therefore bradyarrhythmias are not clinically important with correctly programmed ICDs.

A. F. Sinnaeve

Figure 9.13

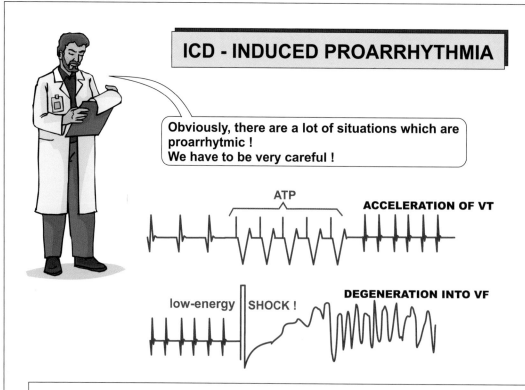

ICD - INDUCED PROARRHYTHMIA

Obviously, there are a lot of situations which are proarrhytmic !
We have to be very careful !

ATP — ACCELERATION OF VT

low-energy SHOCK ! — DEGENERATION INTO VF

1. TACHYARRHYTHMIAS

A. APPROPRIATE TACHYCARDIA THERAPY

i) Acceleration or degeneration of VT into faster VT or VF
ii) Deceleration of VT; slowing VT below the detection rate
iii) SVT (often transient)

B. INAPPROPRIATE TACHYCARDIA THERAPY

i) SVT ; this may induce VT/VF and/or a different SVT
ii) Committed shock for nonsustained VT
iii) Any form of oversensing : VT/VF and/or SVT may be produced by therapy

2. BRADYARRHYTHMIAS

i) Undersensing by pacing system
ii) Postshock bradycardia and conduction blocks
iii) Postshock increase in pacing threshold with loss of capture

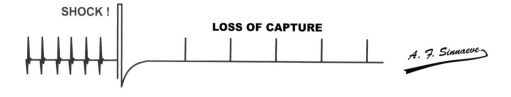

SHOCK ! LOSS OF CAPTURE

A. F. Sinnaeve

Figure 9.14

ELECTRICAL STORM

Repetitive VT in the first week after ICD implantation is not part of the definition of electrical storm ! The definition of electrical storm in the literature is confusing. Electrical storm in ICD patients is now often defined as the occurrence of 3 or more *separate* ventricular tachyarrhythmias in 24 hours regardless of therapy. Untreated VT memorized in the VT zone must be sustained (i.e. >30 sec).

No ! 3 episodes treated with ATP would be considered as an electrical storm. Obviously, the number of shocks for VT will depend on how the ICD is programmed for VT therapy and on the number of VF episodes. Shocks for VT were more common in the past because we have now learned to use ATP more effectively.

I always thought that 3 separate shocks in 24 hrs were required for the diagnosis ?

What about incessant VT ?

Incessant VT restarting soon (after ≥ 1 sinus cycle and within 5 minutes) after a technically successful therapy, forms part of the definition because it represents the most serious manifestation of this entity

CLINICAL MANIFESTATIONS :

* Obvious causes (ischemia, heart failure, hypokalemia) are evident in less than 20% of cases.
* Sympathetic activity plays an important role in the genesis of electrical storm.
* Most patients present with monomorphic VT.
* The prevalence of VF is low.

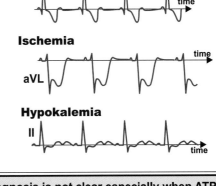

Heart Failure

V6   time

Ischemia

          time
aVL

Hypokalemia

II
          time

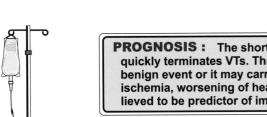

ATP
time

PROGNOSIS : The short-term prognosis is not clear especially when ATP quickly terminates VTs. Thus, ATP may render electrical storm a relatively benign event or it may carry a substantial risk if the underlying cause (e.g. ischemia, worsening of heart failure) is not treated. Electrical storm is believed to be predictor of impaired long-term prognosis.

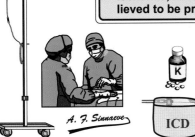

A. F. Sinnaeve

ICD

K

THERAPY :

* Beta-blockers and intravenous amiodarone.
* Radiofrequency ablation.
* Magnesium and potassium may be helpful particularly in patients with prolonged QT intervals or hypokalemia.
* ICD : the number of VT cycles for detection can be increased to allow spontaneous termination.
* ICD : overdrive pacing by increasing the lower rate may terminate electrical storm.

Abbreviations : ATP = antitachycardia pacing ICD = implantable cardioverter defibrillator ; VF = ventricular fibrillation ; VT = ventricular tachycardia .

Figure 9.15

PSYCHOLOGICAL PROBLEMS AND STRESS

WHAT THE DOCTOR SAYS TO THE PATIENT :

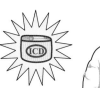

The ICD is a wonderfull piece of electronics : it prevents your heart from beating too slow or too fast. You will feel like you have a new lease on life. It will protect you against syncope or loss of conciousness and sudden death ! Your ICD may safe your life !

WHAT THE PATIENT THINKS :

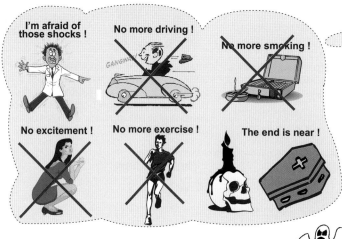

I'm afraid of those shocks !

No more driving !

No more smoking !

No excitement !

No more exercise !

The end is near !

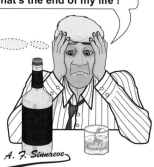

Syncope ? Sudden death !? That's the end of my life !

ICD therapy may have adverse physical, social and psychological consequenses. Panic reactions, negative effect on body image, imaginary shocks, confrontation with death and uncertainty about the future, loss of independency by driving restrictions, etc.

All in all, about half the ICD patients experience depression or anxiety, and a psychiatric consultation is often necessary !

The number of shocks is only one reason for depression and anxiety. Unexpected shock delivery is a stressful event, especially when it is repeated after a short time. This "near-death experience" may trigger a severe anxiety state. In the subset of patients receiving shocks, quality of life is worse especially in those receiving five or more shocks. Therefore, activation of ATP for fast VTs should be performed in every ICD patient to minimize painful shocks that contribute to the detorioration of quality of life.

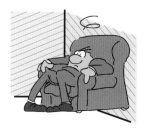

WHAT CAN BE DONE :

* Early incorporation of the patient in a cardiac rehabilitation program
* Assess the concerns of the patient and his/her family and educate them
* Organize and supervise support group meetings for patients with ICDs; stimulate social contacts
* For some patients a cognitive behavior therapy may be very helpful

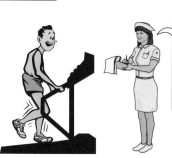

I'm a cardiac nurse and I will help you with your rehabilitation. We will try to find an answer for all your questions !

Figure 9.16

PATIENT INSTRUCTIONS AT HOPITAL DISCHARGE - 1

Before the patient can go home, some tests have to be done and some instructions are to be given :
 * Ensure that the device is activated !
 * Perform final device programming.
 * Document lead position by chest X-ray and measure R wave amplitude to rule out early lead dislodgment.
 * *Provide patient and family education.*
 * *Plan outpatient follow-up.*

General instructions :

* Have always your ICD identification card with you. (or medicalert bracelet or necklace)

* Keep the incision dry for 7 days. (pay attention while showering or bathing)

* Avoid touching or rubbing the incision.

* Steri-strips (or tapes) are to be removed by a nurse. at first office visit (7-10 days after surgery)

* Notify the doctor's office for any observation of redness, heat, swelling, soreness around the ICD. Contact the doctor's office if you have chills or fever.

Activity precautions :

* Resume gradually your daily activities (as well your sexual activities).

* Avoid rough contact with ICD site, heavy lifting and reaching above the head or across the shoulder.

Special precautions :

* Do not drive before clearance from your physician.

* Avoid strong static magnetic fields (large transformers, stereo speakers, unshielded magnetrons, jewellery or toys with neodymium magnets, etc.).

* Avoid strong electromagnetic fields (radio transmitters, radar, leaning over running car engine).

* Inform security agents at the airport and show your ICD identification card. Do not linger at the gates In warehouses, libraries, etc.

* Always notify medical personel about your ICD ! (MRI scans, radiation therapy, diathermy, TENS units, electrocautery).

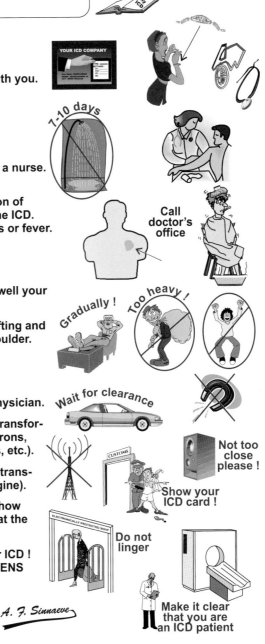

A. F. Sinnaeve

Figure 9.17

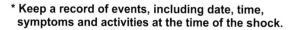

PATIENT INSTRUCTIONS AT HOSPITAL DISCHARGE - 2

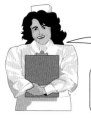

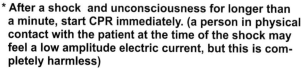

Don't hesitate to call !
I will be glad to answer your questions or
to make an appointment with the doctor.

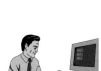

I 'm feeling dizzy and
my heart is pounding

What to do after a shock

* When you have any symptoms that your heart is
going out of rhythm lie down.

Yes, I had a shock.
But now I feel fine !?

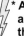 * After receiving a shock and you feel fine afterwards
and your pulse is regular, there is no need to go to
the emergency room.

* Keep a record of events, including date, time,
symptoms and activities at the time of the shock.

Record keeping
(on paper or PC)

* After a shock and unconsciousness for longer than
a minute, start CPR immediately. (a person in physical
contact with the patient at the time of the shock may
feel a low amplitude electric current, but this is completely harmless)

Start CPR
immediately !

 * If two or more shocks are delivered in quick succession, let someone call an ambulance. Under no circumstances the patient should drive a car to go to
the hospital.

Hurry up !
I had three shocks !

Follow-up and device checks

* Chronic follow-up every 3 to 6 months is advisable
for a largely asymptomatic patient (assess and document routine device operation and clinical progress).
For some present-day ICDs chronic follow-up may be
done remotely in conjunction with outpatient visits.
Patients who live far away from the testing center
could be largely followed by remote monitoring.

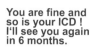

You are fine and
so is your ICD !
I'll see you again
in 6 months.

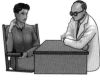

* Unexpected evaluations may be prompted by symptoms,
delivery of ICD therapy, unsuccessful therapy, presumed
failure of the device, patient alerts, patient concerns.
(this often results in changes in therapy, device reprogramming, alteration of patients medical regime).

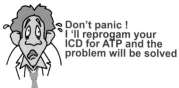

Don't panic !
I 'll reprogam your
ICD for ATP and the
problem will be solved

* The frequency of follow-up visits will be increased
when the battery shows signs of depletion.

* Notify your physician at once when alarms are
observed (sound or vibration).

Doctor, on several
occasions I heard
some ringing and
it was not my GSM
and I was not drunk !

A. F. Sinnaeve

Figure 9.18

FOLLOW-UP of ICDs

* General principles
* Significance of symptoms before a shock
* Analysis of delivered ICD therapy from stored data - Strategy
* Oversensing of intracardiac signals
* Oversensing of extracardiac signals
* VT versus SVT : analysis of single chamber EGMs
* VT versus SVT : analysis of dual chamber EGMs
* VT versus SVT : diagnostic data ancillary to stored EGMs
* Follow-up of ICDs from "A" to "Z" (parts 1 to 5)
* Medtronic Cardiac Compass
* Wireless programming
* Internet-based remote monitoring of ICDs (parts 1 to 3)
* Management of ICD patients undergoing electrosurgery
* Management of ICD patients in the emergery room
* Magnet application over ICDs
* Deactivating a Guidant ICD using a magnet

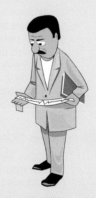

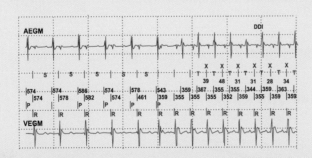

Figure 10.00

FOLLOW-UP : GENERAL PRINCIPLES

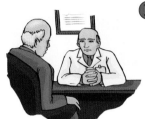

① History & Physical examination

* Occurence of shocks or syncope ?
* Delivered therapy ? What body positions have triggered therapy ?
* ICD infection or erosion ?
* Changes in drug hystory ? New medications ?
* Factors precipitating VT ? (check if CHF, infection, ischemia)
* Factors precipitating SVT ? (check if obstructive pulmonary disease, infection, anemia, dehydration)
* Is it possible to reduce the conditions for sudden cardiac death ? (beta blockers, statins, ACE inhibitors ?)

② System Component Testing

* Sensing : amplitude of EGM in A & V (eventual left and right) ?
    * Check for arm movements, deep breathing, coughing, ...
    * Myopotentials ? T-wave sensing ? Far-field sensing ?
    * Double counting ?
* Lead impedances ?
* Battery voltage ?
    * ERI ?
* HV capacitor charging time ?
    * ERI ?
    * Last reformation of HV capacitor ?
* Pacing thresholds in A & V (left as well as right) ?
    * Can the amplitude (or the duration) of the stimuli be lowered ? (safe the battery)
* Print data

③ ICD programming

BRADY pacing	NORMAL sinus	SLOW VT	FAST VT	VF

* Ventricular tachyarrhythmia detection
    * Oversensing ?
    * SVT or VT criteria ? Discriminators ? Enhancements ?
    * Morphology template ?
* Ventricular tachyarrhythmia therapy
    * Tiered therapy zones ?
    * ATP parameters ? (burst, ramp, scan, increments, ...)
    * Shock parameters ? (energy, duration, ...)
* Brady therapy parameters
    * Mode ?
    * Amplitude & duration of pulses ?
    * Base rate (LRL) ?

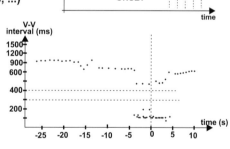

④ Stored EGMs, episodes, trends, ...

* Episodes before shock ? Appropriate shocks ?
* Trends normal ?
* Print strips !

A. F. Sinnaeve

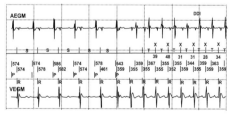

Abbreviations : ATP = antitachycardia pacing ; CHF = congestive heart failure ; EGM = electrogram (endocardial) ; ERI = elective replacement indicator ; HV = high voltage ; LRL = lower rate limit ; SVT = supraventricular tachycardia ; VF = ventricular fibrillation ; VT = ventricular tachycaedia ;

Figure 10.01

SIGNIFICANCE OF SYMPTOMS BEFORE A SHOCK

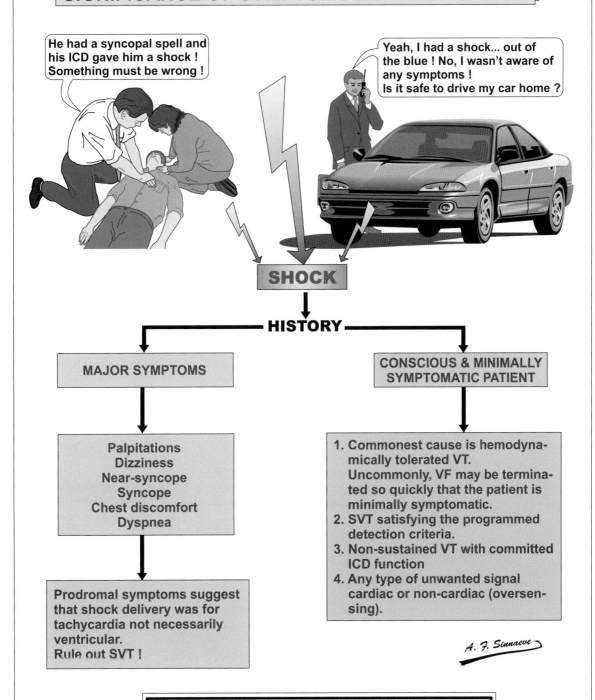

He had a syncopal spell and his ICD gave him a shock ! Something must be wrong !

Yeah, I had a shock... out of the blue ! No, I wasn't aware of any symptoms ! Is it safe to drive my car home ?

SHOCK

HISTORY

MAJOR SYMPTOMS

Palpitations
Dizziness
Near-syncope
Syncope
Chest discomfort
Dyspnea

Prodromal symptoms suggest that shock delivery was for tachycardia not necessarily ventricular.
Rule out SVT !

CONSCIOUS & MINIMALLY SYMPTOMATIC PATIENT

1. Commonest cause is hemodynamically tolerated VT. Uncommonly, VF may be terminated so quickly that the patient is minimally symptomatic.
2. SVT satisfying the programmed detection criteria.
3. Non-sustained VT with committed ICD function
4. Any type of unwanted signal cardiac or non-cardiac (oversensing).

A. F. Sinnaeve

REMEMBER

1. About 30% of shocks are inappropriate !
2. A shock does not prove the patient had VT or VF !
3. The total absence of symptoms does not rule out an appropriate shock !

Figure 10.02

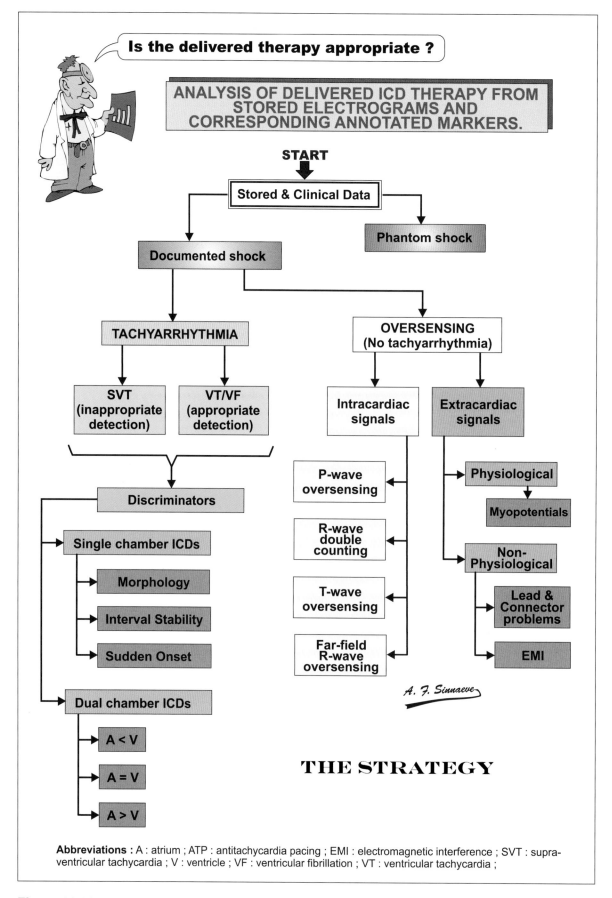

Is the delivered therapy appropriate ?

ANALYSIS OF DELIVERED ICD THERAPY FROM STORED ELECTROGRAMS AND CORRESPONDING ANNOTATED MARKERS.

START

Stored & Clinical Data

Documented shock

Phantom shock

TACHYARRHYTHMIA

OVERSENSING (No tachyarrhythmia)

SVT (inappropriate detection)

VT/VF (appropriate detection)

Intracardiac signals

Extracardiac signals

Discriminators

Single chamber ICDs

Morphology

Interval Stability

Sudden Onset

Dual chamber ICDs

A < V

A = V

A > V

P-wave oversensing

R-wave double counting

T-wave oversensing

Far-field R-wave oversensing

Physiological

Myopotentials

Non-Physiological

Lead & Connector problems

EMI

A. F. Sinnaeve

THE STRATEGY

Abbreviations : A : atrium ; ATP : antitachycardia pacing ; EMI : electromagnetic interference ; SVT : supra-ventricular tachycardia ; V : ventricle ; VF : ventricular fibrillation ; VT : ventricular tachycardia ;

Figure 10.03

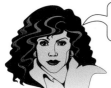

Automatic gain or automatic sensitivity adjustment ensures the ICD sensing of low amplitude and variable VEGMs during VF. This function (associated with dynamic high sensitivity) predisposes the ICD to oversensing !

OVERSENSING OF INTRACARDIAC SIGNALS

 P-wave oversensing in sinus rhythm

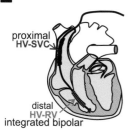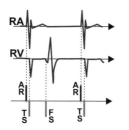

Cause :
Distal coil of an integrated bipolar lead too close to the tricuspid valve. May occur in children but is rare in adults (only if the lead is dislodged from the apex).
Inappropriate detection of VF during AF or AFL

Therapy :
* Lead revision
* Force atrial pacing (using DDDR or Dynamic Overdrive modes)

 R-wave double counting

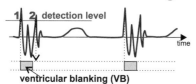

typical "railroad track" on interval plots (long-short alternation)

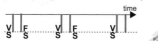

Cause :
A split or fragmented VEGM with a duration longer than the ventricular blanking (especially with use-dependency due to sodium-channel blocking drugs). Older cardiac resynchronization devices with a Y-adapter can separately sense RV and LV.

Therapy :
* Lead revision
* Increase ventricular blanking period (VB) if possible
  cave : a longer VB may impair VF/VT sensing
* Reduce the ventricular sensitivity
  cave : assure that VF/VT sensing is still adequate

 T-wave oversensing

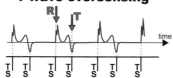

RR intervals usually alternate, but the magnitude of alternation may be small

Cause :
May be due to prolonged QT-interval, development of bundle branch block or very small R-waves (bringing about the maximum ventricular sensitivity)
T-wave oversensing may be transient (hyperglycemia, hyperkalemia) or more established.

Therapy :
* Same as for R-wave double counting
* Reprogram the "decay delay" (only SJM devices)

 Far-field R-wave oversensing

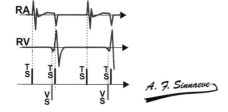

A. F. Sinnaeve

Cause :
Is the sensing of the ventricular depolarization (R wave) by the atrial channel.

May confound SVT-VT discrimination, but does not cause inappropriate detection of VT if the ventricular rate is in the sinus zone; may also cause inappropriate mode switching.

NOTE : There is also the possibility of a non-physiologic intracardiac signal due to contact of the sensing electrode with an abandoned lead fragment.

Abbreviations : AF : atrial fibrillation ; AFL : atrial flutter ; RA : right atrium ; RV : right ventricle ; SVT : supraventricular tachycardia ; VF : ventricular fibrillation ; VT : ventricular tachycardia ; VEGM = ventricular electrogram ;

Figure 10.04

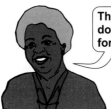

The replacement of the isoelectric baseline with high-frequency noise that does not has a constant relationship to the cardiac cycle is characteristic for oversensing of extracardial signals !

OVERSENSING OF EXTRACARDIAC SIGNALS

 External electromagnetic interference (EMI)

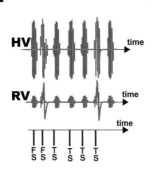

The larger the spacing between the electrodes, the larger the amplitude of the interfering signals (the high voltage EGM is widely spaced, the right ventricular EGM uses closely spaced true bipolar sensing).

Cause :
The EMI signals may be continuous or pulsating. EMI is mostly caused by medical equipment (scanners, imaging, lithotripsy, radiotherapy,...), industrial machinery (power drill, electric arc welding,...) or electronic appliances (EAS article surveillance, customs detector gates, cellular phones,...).

Therapy :
* avoid all EMI sources (keeping distance).

 Lead / Connector problems

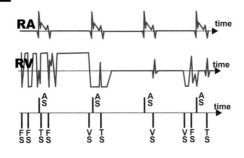

Cause :
The oversensing may be due to the header, a set-screw, an adapter or the lead itself.
The problem is mostly intermittent, only occuring during a small fraction of the cardiac cycle and usually associated with postural changes.
Often, the pacing-lead impedance is abnormal.

Therapy :
* lead revision (check set-screw and sealing plugs)

 Myopotential oversensing

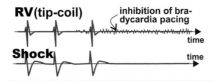

Persistent oversensing causing inhibition of pacing may give rise to inappropriate detection of VF and shock !
Clinically this may present as syncope followed by an inappropriate shock. This is an exception to the rule that syncope prior to a shock indicates an appropriate shock.

Cause :
Oversensing usually occurs after long diastolic intervals or after ventricular paced events when the amplifier sensitivity (or gain) is maximal. Diaphragmatic myopotentials are the most likely causes of inhibition. Pectoral myopotentials may be seen on a far-field EGM that includes the ICD can, but these EGMs are not used for rate-counting (one exception : VT-SVT discrimination using a morphology algorithm)

Therapy :
* reduce ventricular sensitivity (make sure that VF sensing and detection are still reliable !)

Figure 10.05

Once a tachycardia is detected by a single chamber ICD, only three detection enhancements can be used to discriminate between VT and SVT : morphology, sudden onset and interval stability.

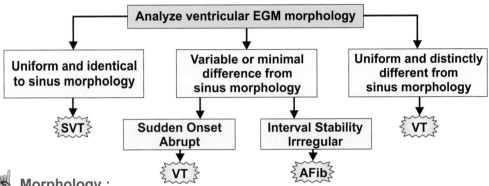

VT versus SVT
Analysis of SINGLE CHAMBER electrograms

Analyze ventricular EGM morphology

| Uniform and identical to sinus morphology | Variable or minimal difference from sinus morphology | Uniform and distinctly different from sinus morphology |

SVT

Sudden Onset Abrupt → VT

Interval Stability Irregular → AFib

VT

 Morphology :

* EGM morphology has to be analyzed from all recorded channels, ideally including a far-field dipole (i.e. RV-EGM for near field and HV-EGM for far-field). SVT cannot be discriminated from VT unambiguously using near-field EGMs in 5-10% of VTs.
* A real-time template of conducted baseline rhythm should be taken to compare morphology with that of the stored EGM (by preference in the same posture).
* Caveat ! * Rate related BBB during SVT will be classified as VT.
       * After shocks EGM morphology is distorded (lead polarization / local electroporation) and cannot be used to discriminate VT from SVT until postchock EGM distortion resolves.

 Interval Stability :

* Characteristic : * ventricular rhythm is regular during monomorphic VT
              * ventricular rhythm is irregular during atrial fibrillation.
* Exception : * RR intervals become more regular at faster ventricular rates and thus interval stability is no longer reliable at rates above ~170 bpm.
        * Conducted ventricular rhythm may regularize at slower rates due to transient organization of the atrial rhythm.
        * Amiodarone (type IC antiarrhythmic drugs) may cause monomorphic VT to become markedly irregular or polymorphic VT to slow, causing irregular intervals during true VT.

Sudden Onset :

* Characteristic : * Sinus tachycardia accelerates gradually
              * VT or paroxysmal SVT starts abruptly
* Caveat ! * If VT starts abruptly, but with an initial rate below the programmed VT detection rate, the beginning of the stored EGM does not record the onset of the arrhythmia. When the VT accelerates gradually across the programmed sinus-VT boundary, it will be classified as SVT.

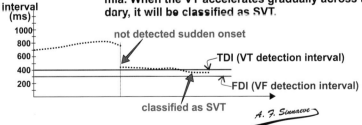

Abbreviations :
Afib = atrial fibrillation
BBB = bundle branch block
EGM = electrogram
HV = high voltage
VT = ventricular tachycardia
SVT = supraventricular tachycardia
VF = ventricular fibrillation

A. F. Sinnaeve

Figure 10.06

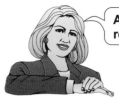

Analysis of both atrial and ventricular rates and atrio-ventricular relationships are the foundations of dual chamber rhythm analysis !

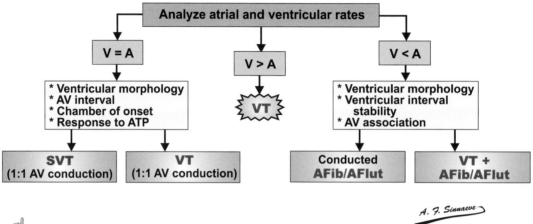

VT versus SVT
Analysis of DUAL CHAMBER electrograms

Analyze atrial and ventricular rates

V = A	V > A	V < A

V = A:
* Ventricular morphology
* AV interval
* Chamber of onset
* Response to ATP

→ **SVT** (1:1 AV conduction)
→ **VT** (1:1 AV conduction)

V > A:
→ **VT**

V < A:
* Ventricular morphology
* Ventricular interval stability
* AV association

→ **Conducted AFib/AFlut**
→ **VT + AFib/AFlut**

A. F. Sinnaeve

 Ventricular rate > atrial rate (V > A) :

* The diagnosis is always VT

 Ventricular rate = atrial rate (V = A) :

* Tachycardias with 1:1 AV relationship
    * most tachycardias with 1:1 AV relationship are SVT
    * VT with 1:1 VA conduction accounts for less than 10% of cases
    * transient AV block permits diagnosis of SVT
    * transient VA block permits diagnosis of VT
* Atrial tachycardia usually begins with a short PP interval followed by a short RR interval
* VT usually begins with a short RR interval
* Before a 1:1 AV conduction stabilizes, a few beats of AV dissociation may occur
* In sinus tachycardia, the atrial rhythm accelerates gradually with an approximately stable PR interval

 Ventricular rate < atrial rate (V < A) :

* Eliminate far-field sensing of R waves
* Most VT during paroxysmal AFib is fast enough to be classified in the VF zone
* Abnormal ventricular morphology and regular ventricular rate are most helpful for diagnosing VT during AFib
* Conducted AFlut may be diagnosed in the presence of abnormal ventricular morphology if consistent 2:1 AV association or Mobitz 1 AV block is present
* VT during AFlut is diagnosed based on abnormal ventricular morphology and AV dissociation.

Abbreviations : AFib = atrial fibrillation ; AFlut = atrial flutter ; AV = atrioventricular ; SVT = supraventricular tachycardia ; VT = ventricular tachycardia ;

Figure 10.07

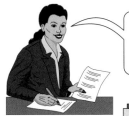

Clinical circumstances, the response to therapy and information from the patient's arrhythmia history may provide supportive data when analysis of stored EGMs is inconclusive. The patient should be asked about the occurence of shocks or syncope !

VT versus SVT
Diagnostic data ancillary to stored EGMs

 Clinical data :

* Inappropriate therapy for SVT does not occur in patients with complete heart block (AVB III)
* A history of rapidly conducted atrial fibrillation suggests inappropriate therapy for atrial fibrillation
* Multiple ineffective shocks during vigorous exercise suggests inappropriate therapy for sinus tachycardia (if the integrity of electrodes is verified)
* Shocks without antecedent symptoms do not distinguish SVT from VT

 Response to therapy

* When atrial rate exceeds ventricular rate (A > V) :
    * Termination of a tachycardia by a single trial of antitachycardia pacing (ATP) favors the diagnosis of VT
    * During AFib, retrograde concealed conduction from ventricular ATP may result in post pacing pauses and/or slowing of antegrade conduction that must be distinguished from true termination of VT
* In tachycardias with 1:1 association :
    * Transient AV block permits the diagnosis of SVT, while transient VA block permits the diagnosis of VT
    * Success of ventricular ATP is not helpful because pacing terminates > 50% of inappropriately detected 1:1 pathological SVTs
    * Atrial tachycardia is terminated by ventricular ATP only if the atrial rate accelerates during pacing
    * VT can be diagnosed if high-grade VA block occurs at the onset of ATP without acceleration of the atrial rate
    * If the atrial cycle length is unchanged by ventricular ATP, the diagnosis is SVT (since the atrial tachycardia does not depend on retrograde conduction)
    * If the atrial rate accelerates to the ventricular rate during ventricular ATP, an AAV response when the tachycardia resumes, is diagnostic for SVT
* Since the vast majority of VTs are terminated by one or two shocks, failure of multiple high-ouput shocks to terminate a regular tachycardia suggests a sinus tachycardia. The converse is not true !
* A regular tachycardia during AFib may be identified as VT, if a tachycardia with the same rate and morphology occured during sinus rhythm.

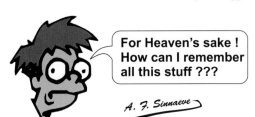

For Heaven's sake ! How can I remember all this stuff ???

A. F. Sinnaeve

Abbreviations : AFib = atrial fibrillation; ATP = anti-tachycardia pacing ; AV = atrioventricular (antegrade) ; AVB III = atrioventricular block of third degree ; EGM = electrogram ; SVT = supraventricular tachycardia ; VA = ventriculoatrial (retrograde) ; VT = ventricular tachycardia ;

Figure 10.08

FOLLOW-UP OF ICDs: part 1

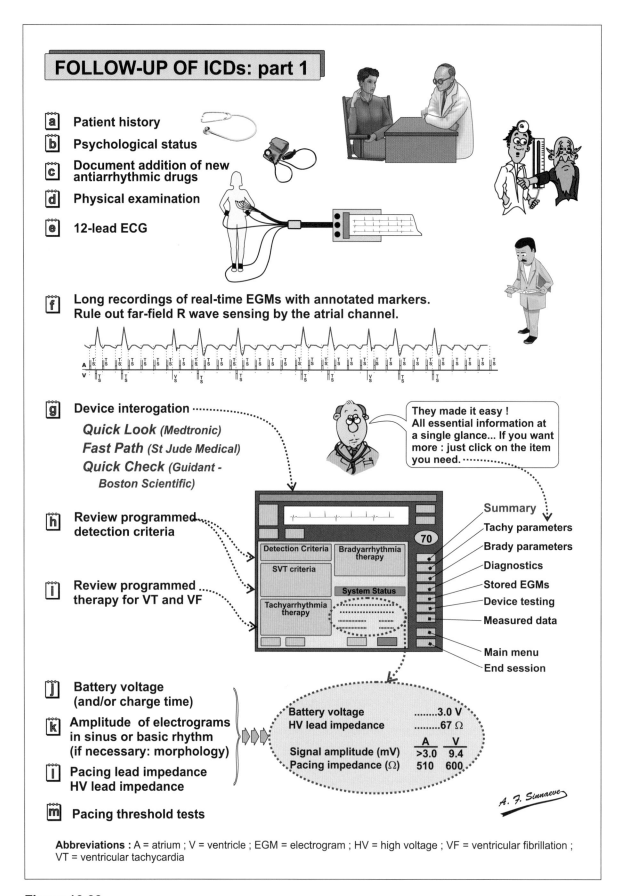

a Patient history

b Psychological status

c Document addition of new antiarrhythmic drugs

d Physical examination

e 12-lead ECG

f Long recordings of real-time EGMs with annotated markers. Rule out far-field R wave sensing by the atrial channel.

g Device interrogation ·····
  Quick Look (Medtronic)
  Fast Path (St Jude Medical)
  Quick Check (Guidant - Boston Scientific)

They made it easy !
All essential information at a single glance... If you want more : just click on the item you need. ·····

h Review programmed detection criteria

i Review programmed therapy for VT and VF

Detection Criteria
SVT criteria
Tachyarrhythmia therapy
Bradyarrhythmia therapy
System Status

70

Summary
Tachy parameters
Brady parameters
Diagnostics
Stored EGMs
Device testing
Measured data

Main menu
End session

j Battery voltage (and/or charge time)

k Amplitude of electrograms in sinus or basic rhythm (if necessary: morphology)

l Pacing lead impedance HV lead impedance

m Pacing threshold tests

		A	V
Battery voltage	........3.0 V		
HV lead impedance	.........67 Ω		
Signal amplitude (mV)		>3.0	9.4
Pacing impedance (Ω)		510	600

A. F. Sinnaeve

Abbreviations : A = atrium ; V = ventricle ; EGM = electrogram ; HV = high voltage ; VF = ventricular fibrillation ; VT = ventricular tachycardia

Figure 10.09

FOLLOW-UP OF ICDs: part 2

n Diagnostic data including episode data: time of event occurrence and delivered therapy.

o RR intervals and stored electrograms of all arrhythmias causing arrhythmia detection and possible therapy. Number and causes of aborted shocks.

p Evaluate recorded SVT episodes: increase the rate cutoff and activate discriminators.

q Diagnostic data: Number and duration of mode switching episodes (surrogate for atrial arrhythmias).

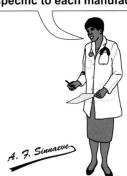

Follow-up of contemporary ICDs is not extremely complicated. The new programmers and algorithms are very helpful !
Of course, you have to know a lot of abbreviations and some jargon specific to each manufacturer.

A. F. Sinnaeve

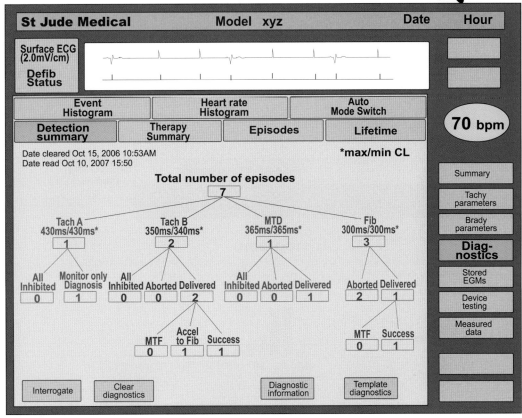

*max/min CL = maximum/minimum cycle length of the episodes
Tach A = slow ventricular tachycardia (slow VT)
Tach B = fast ventricular tachycardia (fast VT or FVT)
MTD = maximum time to diagnosis (if an arrhythmia lasts longer than the programmed MTD due to SVT discrimination, the programmable MTD therapy is delivered)
Fib = ventricular fibrillation
MTF = maximum time to fibrillation therapy (maximum time during which the device may attempt tachycardia therapies e.g. ATP)

Figure 10.10

FOLLOW-UP OF ICDs: part 3

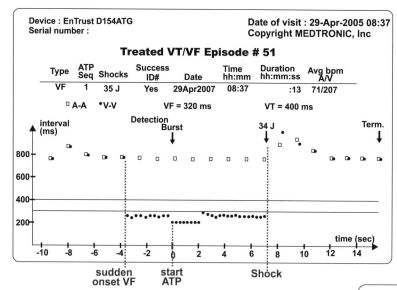

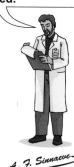

Of course, you can see every tachycardia episode in detail. You may see the effect of therapy and how the tachycardia started.

A. F. Sinnaeve

Brady status and histograms.
Reduce percentage of RV pacing if possible.

Do not forget the common pacemaker function !

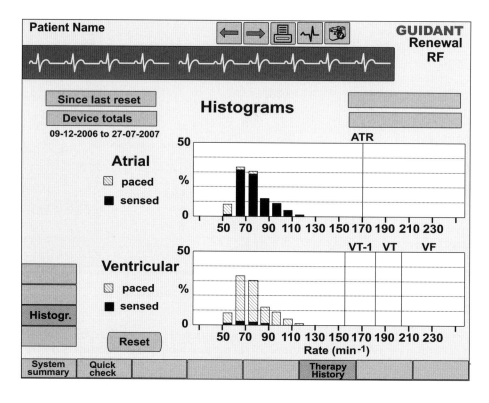

Figure 10.11

FOLLOW-UP OF ICDs: part 4

⑤ Shock impedance including value recorded with the past delivery of a shock.

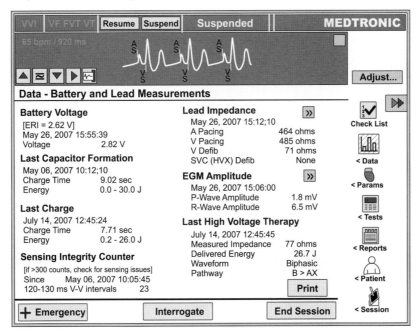

ⓣ Elective replacement indicators should be checked and documented in the chart.

ⓤ Oversensing: provocative maneuvers with simultaneous real-time EGM recordings. In suspected lead malfunction, try manipulation of ICD within the pocket to bring out false signals. Use deep respiration to bring out diaphragmatic myopotential oversensing. Diagnostic data may show recording of many nonphysiologic intervals.

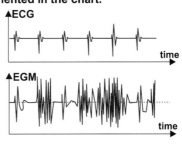

ⓥ Reprogram ICD for optimal function: detection, avoidance of sensed supraventricular tachyarrhythmias or sensing of undesired signals.

ⓦ Annual overpenetrated chest X ray to identify presence of lead disruption not identifiable by otherwise routine examination.

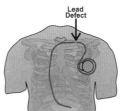

ⓧ Software updates.

ⓨ Check final settings and compare with initial parameters.

ⓩ **SPECIAL TESTING FOR CRT PATIENTS**

Assess % ventricular sensing, optimization of AV and V-V intervals, intrathoracic impedance data about status of pulmonary fluid, and exercise testing in selected patients to look for abnormalities such as atrial undersensing or threshold problem not apparent at rest.

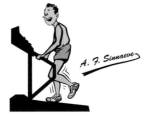

Figure 10.12

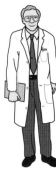

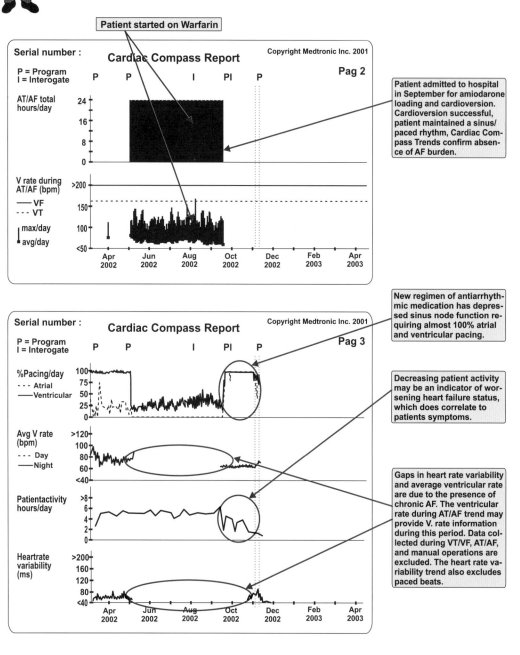

FOLLOW-UP OF ICDs: Value of diagnostics (Medtronic Cardiac Compass)

At routine follow-up in July, Cardiac Compass Trends document 100% AF burden with a controlled ventricular response. The patient returned in October for evaluation of progressive and refractory congestive heart failure. Cardiac Compass showed that the cardioversion performed in September had continued to be successful, but that he was completely paced.
Based on the symptoms and confirmation through Cardiac Compass, the device was upgraded to a biventricular ICD. In January, he returned to the clinic with markedly improved symptoms while his functional class was improved to NYHA Class II.

Figure 10.13

WIRELESS PROGRAMMING

A wireless programmer is easier to handle and less cumbersome. It gives greater speed and even added security and safety !

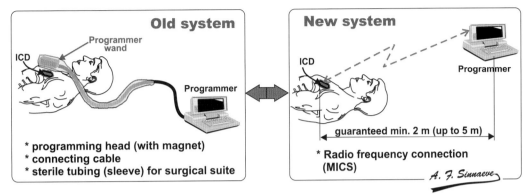

Old system

* programming head (with magnet)
* connecting cable
* sterile tubing (sleeve) for surgical suite

New system

guaranteed min. 2 m (up to 5 m)

* Radio frequency connection (MICS)

A. F. Sinnaeve

Advantages : * More convenient (less infections, no more sterile sleeves, physician can close wound while the device is being programmed at a distance)
* Faster retrieval of data
* Device optimization during follow-up (treadmill testing, etc.)

MICS (Medical Implant Communications System)

⭐ Special frequency band approved by FCC (Federal Communications Committee).

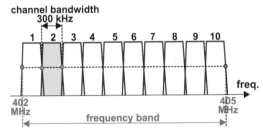

channel bandwidth 300 kHz

freq.

402 MHz · 405 MHz

frequency band

* the MICS frequency band operates from 402 MHz to 405 MHz and is conducive to transmitting radio signals in the human body
* effective isotropic radiated power max. 25 µW
* 10 channels are available with a max. bandwidth of 300 kHz
* no voice transmission is allowed
* the *Medtronic* application of MICS is called *"Conexus Wireless Telemetry"* and works with the latest devices

⭐ To extend the operating life of the battery, an ultra low-power RF transceiver is applied and a wake-up mode of operation is used.

* the transceiver inside the ICD is normally "asleep" and its current drain from the battery is extremely small (less than 1 µA)
* a handheld *activator* is used to "wake-up" the circuit and to enable the communication with the programmer

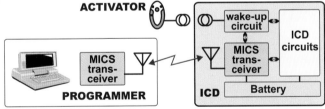

⭐ To avoid interference, the system scans all 10 channels in the MICS band prior to establishing a telemetry session. The channel with the lowest ambient signal level (i.e. the least noisy channel) or the first channel with an ambient level below a certain threshold, will be chosen for the telemetry session (LBT = Listen Before Talk).
Medtronic uses *"Smart Radio"*, a protocol that chooses the least interfered channel for its "Conexus Wireless Telemetry". This protocol allows multiple simultaneous programming sessions to be collected without interference.

NOTE :

1. An initial handshake with the programmer wand is needed to activate the telemetry.
2. The "Invisi-Link" Wireless Telemetry (St Jude Medical) also uses the 402-405 MHz frequency band.
3. Boston Scientific (Guidant) has a similar system called "ZIP wandless telemetry", working in the ISM band at 914 MHz. (ISM : industrial-Scientific-Medical).

Figure 10.14

INTERNET-BASED REMOTE MONITORING OF ICDs - 1

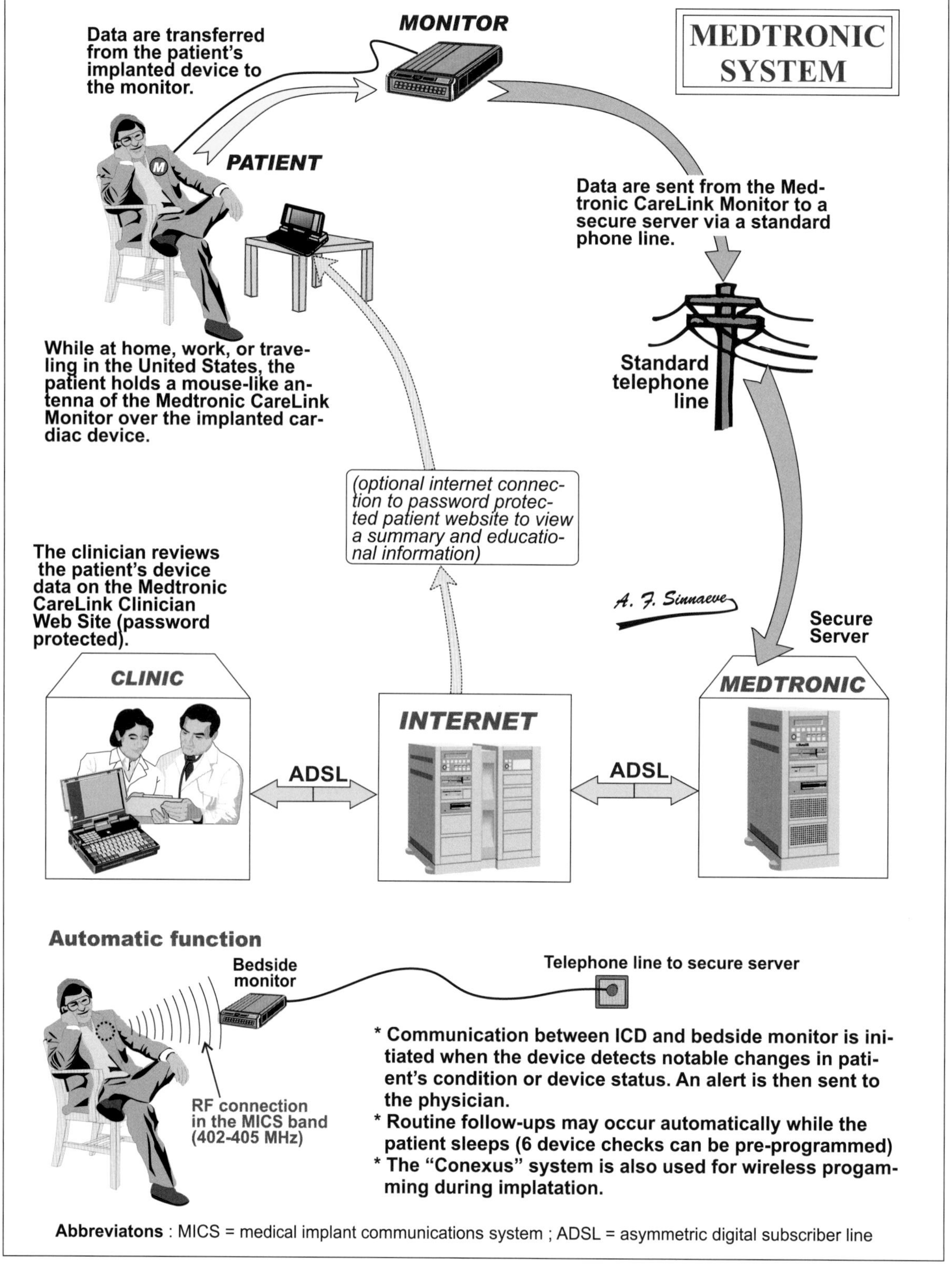

MONITOR

MEDTRONIC SYSTEM

Data are transferred from the patient's implanted device to the monitor.

PATIENT

Data are sent from the Medtronic CareLink Monitor to a secure server via a standard phone line.

While at home, work, or traveling in the United States, the patient holds a mouse-like antenna of the Medtronic CareLink Monitor over the implanted cardiac device.

Standard telephone line

(optional internet connection to password protected patient website to view a summary and educational information)

A. F. Sinnaeve

The clinician reviews the patient's device data on the Medtronic CareLink Clinician Web Site (password protected).

Secure Server

CLINIC

INTERNET

MEDTRONIC

ADSL

ADSL

Automatic function

Bedside monitor

Telephone line to secure server

* Communication between ICD and bedside monitor is initiated when the device detects notable changes in patient's condition or device status. An alert is then sent to the physician.
* Routine follow-ups may occur automatically while the patient sleeps (6 device checks can be pre-programmed)
* The "Conexus" system is also used for wireless progamming during implatation.

RF connection in the MICS band (402-405 MHz)

Abbreviatons : MICS = medical implant communications system ; ADSL = asymmetric digital subscriber line

Figure 10.15

INTERNET-BASED REMOTE MONITORING OF ICDs - 2

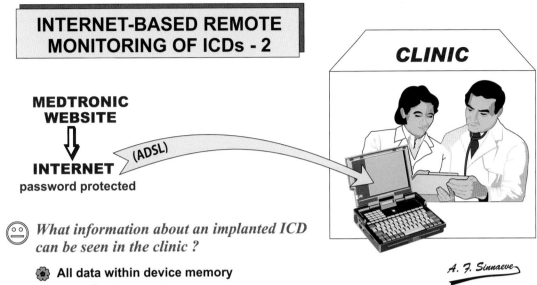

MEDTRONIC WEBSITE

⇩

INTERNET (ADSL)
password protected

CLINIC

A. F. Sinnaeve

😐 *What information about an implanted ICD can be seen in the clinic ?*

🏵 **All data within device memory**
* patient parameters
* device parameters (ICD status, lead information, ...)
* stored episodes (VF - FVT - VT - SVT - NST - mode switch - % pacing - ...)

🏵 **All diagnostics**
* stored intracardiac electrograms
* 10 seconds real-time electrogram of presenting rhythm

☹ *What cannot be done by the remote monitoring ?*

🏵 Direct communication with and interrogation of the ICD is impossible.

🏵 Transtelephonic reprogramming of the device is not a present reality.

😊 *What are the advantages ?*

🏵 Remote follow-up is easy to use and convenient for the patient as it may reduce the frequency of clinic visits.

🏵 The remote follow-up provides the clinician with the same information that is available at an office visit used to assess the appropriateness of device therapies and operation.

🏵 Internet-based follow-up may serve as a triage tool to determine which patients need further medical attention.

🏵 The tremendous wealth of physiological data collected by implanted devices may also be important in the discovery of undocumented and asymptomatic arrhythmias, new disease processes, and the management of chronic diseases including drug initiation and titration.

🏵 Remote follow-up offers an alternative for the overcrowded and overwhelmed clinics.

Figure 10.16

INTERNET-BASED REMOTE MONITORING OF ICDs - 3

BIOTRONIK HOME MONITORING SYSTEM

The criteria for data transmission are entirely programmable by the clinician, allowing for customized reports based on each patients needs.

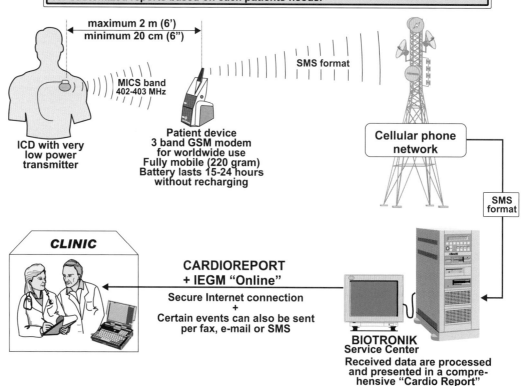

maximum 2 m (6')
minimum 20 cm (6")

SMS format

MICS band
402-403 MHz

ICD with very low power transmitter

Patient device
3 band GSM modem
for worldwide use
Fully mobile (220 gram)
Battery lasts 15-24 hours
without recharging

Cellular phone network

SMS format

CLINIC

CARDIOREPORT + IEGM "Online"

Secure Internet connection
+
Certain events can also be sent
per fax, e-mail or SMS

BIOTRONIK
Service Center
Received data are processed
and presented in a comprehensive "Cardio Report"

The use of daily "Home Monitoring" communication may shorten the device battery life for max. 2 months (conservative estimate assuming daily transmission through "Cardio Messenger", occasional event reports and 12 IEGMs per year)

Trend Reports
* Time controlled transmission (any time between 0:00 and 23:50) (recommended between 0:00 and 4:00 while the patient is asleep)
* Monitoring interval : 1 day
* Data are presented in graphs and tables. When viewing reports on the internet, Cardio Reports can be individually configured for each patient

Event Reports
* Event controlled messages are sent upon termination of detection
* Event triggered messages are also sent when a measurement range is exceeded

Home Monitoring Scope of Functions
* Monitoring system integrity
  - Battery status, battery voltage
  - Detection and therapy activation
* Monitoring lead integrity
  - Atrial and ventricular pacing impedances
  - Shock impedance
* Bradycardia & tachycardia rhythm and therapy monitoring
  - Sensing/pacing counters
  - Detected episodes
  - SVT frequency
  - Delivered therapies
  - Success of ATPs & shocks

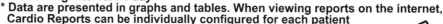

impedance

fracture ?

days

A. F. Sinnaeve

Abbreviations : ATP = antitachycardia pacing; GSM = global system for mobile communications; IEGM = internal electrogram; MICS = medical implant communications system; SMS = short message service; SVT = supraventricular tachycardia

Figure 10.17

MANAGEMENT OF ICD PATIENTS UNDERGOING ELECTROSURGERY

Preoperative

* Ask the surgeon to consider alternative tools which do not generate EMI (knife and ligatures, ultrasonic or laser scalpel)
* Check device
    (programming, telemetry, thresholds, battery status, etc.)

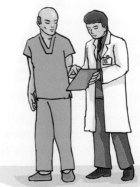

In the operating room

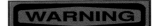

* *Disable* ICD tachyarrhythmia therapies
    (e.g. by using a magnet)
* Deactivate rate-responsive function
* If the patient is pacemaker-dependent :
    > Decrease the maximum sensitivity
    > Program the noise reversion mode to asynchronous (DOO, VOO)
        (with Guidant devices the asynchronous mode requires conti-
        nuous application of the programmer wand during surgery)
    > Preapply external transthoracic pacing system
    > Have available equipment for temporary transvenous pacing
* Monitor peripheral pulse, oximeter, or intra-arterial blood pressure
    (ECG is probably obscured by cautery artifact)
* Position the ground plate to keep the active-to-dispersive current
    pathways as far as possible and perpendicular from the pulse
    generator to electrode pathway)
* Use bipolar cautery whenever possible
* Limit cutting current to short bursts interrupted by pauses of at
    least 10 seconds
* Use the lowest effective cutting or coagulation power output
* Do not use cautery near device

WARNING

DOCUMENTATION
All progamming chan-
ges (device activated or
deactivated) must be
immediately documen-
ted in the chart. This is
a major problem in cli-
nical practice as it is
often not done leading
to important errors
in management !!!

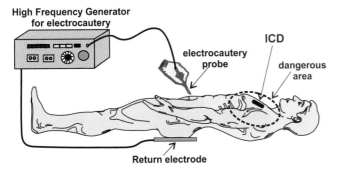

High Frequency Generator
for electrocautery

ICD

electrocautery
probe

dangerous
area

Return electrode

POSSIBLE COMPLICATIONS DUE TO ELECTROCAUTERY

* Oversensing of EMI
    - inappropriate shocks
    - multiple shocks
* Inhibition of pacing
* Disabling of detection
* Power-on reset and errone-
    ous end-of-life indication
* Induction of VF (rare)
* High chronic pacing thres-
    hold (rare)
* Major component failure

Postoperative

* *Reactivate* tachyarrhythmia therapy as soon as possible
* Check device (programming, telemetry, thresholds, battery status, etc.)
* Replace generator if circuit damage is documented
* Replace lead(s) if pacing threshold(s) is too high

Figure 10.18

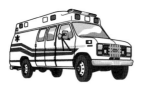

MANAGEMENT OF ICD PATIENTS IN THE EMERGENCY ROOM

A single shock without associated major symptoms does not constitute an emergency and patients are generally advised not to go to the ER (emergency room). The device should be interrogated in 24 - 48 hrs.

The management of the shocked ICD patient who comes to the ER does not lend itself easily to an algorithmic approach. Criteria for admission/discharge and immediate/elective device interrogation are not standardized. Assessment in the ER should focus primarily on identifying patients who are at risk for acute cardiac decompensation.

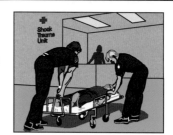

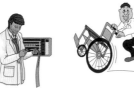 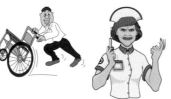

Patients who can be discharged

Many patients present to the ER looking and feeling well after sustaining a single shock. If this is the first shock or the pattern of shocks is unchanged and the physical examination, monitored rhythm, ECG, chest X-ray and potassium level are all normal or unchanged, it is reasonable to send the patient home. The ICD does not necessarily need interrogation in the ER, as long as the arrangements are made for follow-up in the ICD clinic in the next day or two.

NEED TO KNOW

Remember that some patients experience "phantom shocks", which usually occur at night and are sensations that represent anxiety rather than actual ICD discharges.

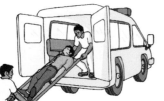

Patients who require admission

More than 3 shocks in a day represents an electrophysiologic emergency !

All patients who have had *multiple ICD shocks* require admission. In the hospital, cardiac status can be reassessed, and their ICD and medical therapy adjusted accordingly.
Patients with a frank syncopal spell, or a near syncopal event, even after a single shock, generally require admission. They may have been shocked multiple times without realizing it, a pattern suggesting a new cardiac event or ICD malfunction.

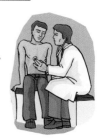

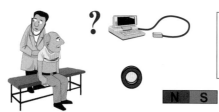

? N S

Inappropriate shocks for SVT can be treated by suspending tachycardia detection with a magnet placed over the generator until the device is interrogated an reprogrammed.

A. F. Sinnaeve

ABBREVIATIONS : ECG = electrocardiogram; SVT = supraventricular tachycardia

Figure 10.19

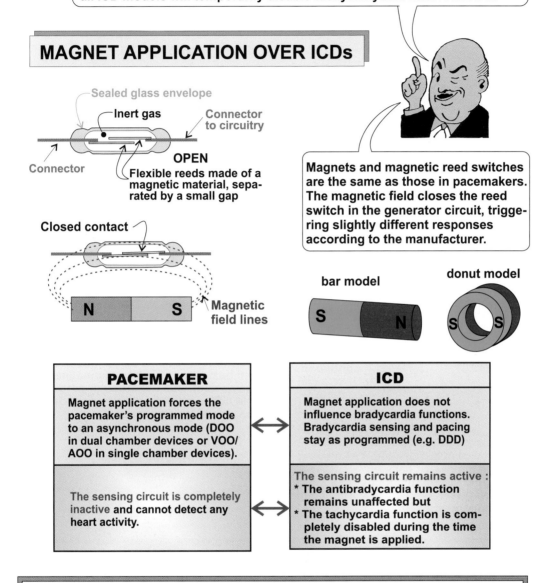

MAGNET APPLICATION OVER ICDs

When the specific programmer is not available, a magnet placed on top of all ICD models will temporarily disable tachyarrhytmia intervention !!!

Sealed glass envelope

Inert gas

Connector to circuitry

Connector

OPEN

Flexible reeds made of a magnetic material, separated by a small gap

Magnets and magnetic reed switches are the same as those in pacemakers. The magnetic field closes the reed switch in the generator circuit, triggering slightly different responses according to the manufacturer.

Closed contact

N   S

Magnetic field lines

bar model

S   N

donut model

S   S

PACEMAKER	ICD
Magnet application forces the pacemaker's programmed mode to an asynchronous mode (DOO in dual chamber devices or VOO/ AOO in single chamber devices).	Magnet application does not influence bradycardia functions. Bradycardia sensing and pacing stay as programmed (e.g. DDD)
The sensing circuit is completely **inactive** and cannot detect any heart activity.	The sensing circuit remains active : * The antibradycardia function remains unaffected but * The tachycardia function is completely disabled during the time the magnet is applied.

The magnet response is useful in emergencies when shocks must be aborted. In the case of multiple shocks (in situations suggesting inappropriate therapy) the magnet can be applied by medical personnel provided the patient is being monitored to determine the underlying rhythm.
The magnet can also be applied in the operating room where electrocautery is used during surgery. This may be preferable to deactivation of the device during surgery in case an arrhythmia has to be treated.
As a rule, the magnet should not be given to the patient unless it is to be used only in the presence of medical personnel.

Figure 10.20

216

DEACTIVATING A GUIDANT ICD USING A MAGNET

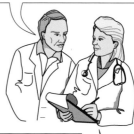

What do you mean by listening to the ICD ? Are you really going to talk to the device ?

Place donut magnet over device

Do you hear tones ?

yes / no → Check magnet position. If still no tones : a Guidant programmer is required or the device may not be manufactured by Guidant

Are tones continuous ?

no → R-wave synchronous tones (discontinuous sounds !)

yes

Not exactly ! I'm just applying a donut magnet and I'm listening to the tones. The device reveals its status !

Hold magnet over device for at least 30 seconds

Is tone continuous (like a dial tone)?

no → Therapy will be temporarily inhibited if the magnet is taped in place (R-wave synchronous tones, i.e. discontinuous sounds, will be heard as long as the magnet is over the device). Due to particular programming, it is not possible to permanently deactivate the device using a magnet.

yes

The device is deactivated. The magnet may be removed from the device. To turn the device back on :
* Reapply the magnet longer than 30 seconds.
* Listen for tones to change from continuous to R-wave synchronous (discontinuous sounds).

A. F. Sinnaeve

* Magnet application does not affect bradycardia pacing !!!
* 'Enable Magnet Use' is the master switch. When programmed 'OFF', the magnet has no effect. A programmer is needed to turn the 'Tachy Mode' ON/OFF. 'Enable Magnet Use' to OFF may be useful for patients exposed to strong magnetic fields.
* If 'Enable Magnet Use' is programmed 'ON', and 'Change Tachy Mode with Magnet' is 'OFF', a magnet will inhibit any tachy therapy as long as the magnet is applied and the device will beep synchronously with the heart rate. Normal operation will resume 2 seconds after removal of the magnet. This is useful during surgical interventions,as it allows to fix a magnet over the device to inhibit tachy therapy during cauterization, but in case an arrhythmia occurs, by simply removing the magnet the device will return to active status.
* If both 'Enable Magnet Use' and 'Change Tachy Mode with Magnet' are programmed 'ON', a magnet will inhibit Tachy Therapy, but if applied > 30 seconds, the Tachy Mode will be switched 'OFF'.
* 'Patient Triggered Monitor' : when programmed 'ON', the application of a magnet will trigger storage of EGM and intervals, time stamps and A & V rates while other magnet operations (beeping and tachy therapy inhibition) are deactivated.
* NEW : Recent and future ICD models will continue to have the 'Enable Magnet Use' as a programmable feature, however, 'Change Tachy Mode with Magnet' will no longer be available.

Figure 10.21

* Causes of delivered or aborted shocks due to oversensing
    - part 1 : intracardiac signals
    - part 2 : extracardiac signals

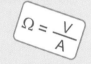

* Testing for lead problems

* Pacing impedance vs shocking impedance

* Management of patients with multiple ICD shocks

* ICDs and electromagnetic interference (EMI): essential elements

* Electromagnetic spectrum and sources of EMI

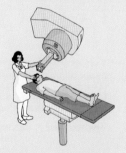

* Potential sources of EMI: an overview

* EMI situations in the hospital

* EMI situations in a industrial environment

* Interference by 60 (50) Hz leakage current

Shock

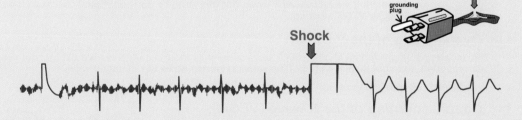

Figure 11.00

CAUSES OF DELIVERED OR ABORTED SHOCKS DUE TO OVERSENSING : part 1 INTRACARDIAC SIGNALS

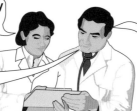

Does the clinical history help in the diagnosis of oversensing ?

Not much except in the diagnosis of over-sensing some causes of EMI.

Remember that oversensing of the VEGM by T wave sensing or double counting of the QRS can be identified by characteristic alteration of intervals and EGM morphology (e.g. TQ vs. QT intervals) separated by a clear isoelectric line.

1. PHYSIOLOGIC

(a) *Oversensing of the spontaneous T wave.*

Automatic gain or autoadjusting sensitivity ensures ICD sensing of low-amplitude and variable VGEMs during VF. This function (associated with dynamic high sensitivity) predisposes the ICD to uninten-ded sensing of the T wave. For this reason a small R wave (VGEM) more commonly causes T wave sensing than a larger one. T wave oversensing is more common in integrated ICD leads.

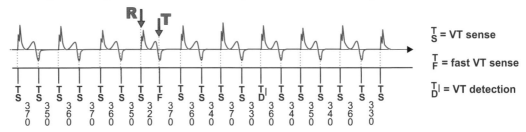

T_S = VT sense

T_F = fast VT sense

T_D^I = VT detection

T wave oversensing may be related to a small or large VEGM, and may be transient (hyperglycemia, hyperkalemia) or more established. Predisposing factors include : low-amplitude R wave, prolonged QT interval and occasionally the development of bundle branch block. All in the setting of sinus tachycardia allow "double counting" of ventricular events to a critical ventricular rate detected by the ICD with the risk of delivering an inappropriate shock.

Treatment :
a. Decrease the sensitivity of the ventricular channel and then document (with VF induction) appropriate VT/VF sensing at the lower sensitivity setting.
b. Occasionally the sensing lead needs to be repositioned or replaced to achieve larger amplitude R waves which in turn may prevent T wave oversensing.
c. Some ICDs allow programming of a longer ventricular sensing blanking period to contain the oversensed T wave, but this must be done cautiously because it may impair VT/VF sensing.

(b) *Oversensing of the P wave.*

This is rare; an inappropriate shock from P wave sensing is theoretically possible but has not yet been reported. Rule out displacement of the sensing lead towards the tricuspid valve.

Treatment : Repostion the lead

(c) *Double counting of the R wave (VEGM).*

A split or fragmented VEGM may be counted twice if its duration is longer than the ventricular blanking period after sensing.

Treatment : as for T wave oversensing

    N.B. Older cardiac resynchronization devices with a Y-adapter can separately sense the RV and the LV electrograms.

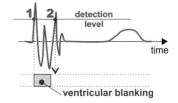

2. NONPHYSIOLOGIC

Contact of sensing lead with abandoned lead fragment.

Treatment : removal of inactive lead

ABBREVIATIONS : EMI = electromagnetic interference; VEGM = ventricular electrogram; VF = ventricular fibrillation; VT = ventricular tachycardia

Figure 11.01

CAUSES OF DELIVERED OR ABORTED SHOCKS DUE TO OVERSENSING : part 2 EXTRACARDIAC SIGNALS

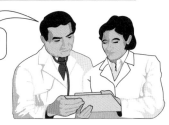

Look, not all signals causing oversensing are generated by the heart !!!

1. PHYSIOLOGIC SIGNALS (MYOPOTENTIALS)

a Lead insulation failure with sensing of myopotentials (usually pectoral)

insulation — contact with muscle

b Diaphragmatic myopotentials.

The ICD interprets interference either as unsustained or sustained VT. The interference typically generates low amplitude high frequency signals on the EGM sensing lead.

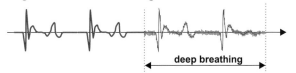

deep breathing

Diagnosis : Reproduce diaphragmatic myopotentials with deep breathing, Valsalva maneuver, cough, etc.

Treatment : Decrease sensitivity and retest the ICD for capability to sense VF ; reposition lead or use a true bipolar lead to replace an integrated one.

Take a deep breath and cough and try to laugh !

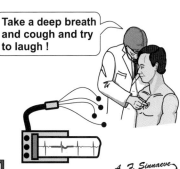

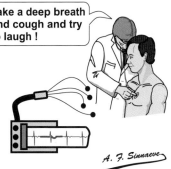

A. F. Sinnaeve

2. NONPHYSIOLOGIC SIGNALS FROM ICD SYSTEM

a Lead fracture.

Diagnosis :

A high pacing impedance indicates complete or partial electrical interuption of the sensing lead. X-ray is often unhelpful in diagnosis !

moving the left arm (spurious signals resulting from conductor fracture of RV sensing lead)

b Lead insulation defect :

Lead may show a pacing impedance below 200 Ω. X ray is often unhelpful in diagnosis.

Beware : * Pacing impedance may not be altered
* Impedance is an insensitive measure of insulation problem
* Pacing capture may be maintained !

c Loose set-screw or adapter

d "Chatter" in an active fixation lead

3. ELECTROMAGNETIC INTERFERENCE

Electrocautery, lithotripsy, MRI, poorly shielded equipment, etc.
Diagnosis :

Noise effects both atrial and ventricular channels and the ICD may interpret the disturbance as a double tachycardia (atrial and ventricular).

REMEMBER !!!

1. The "make and break" signals of a defective lead or a connection problem are often intermittent. Such signals are often oversensed by the ICD as R-R intervals close to the sensed ventricular blanking period (120-140 ms). Such short intervals do not occur with VF/VT. Some ICDs record the number of these suspicious short R-R intervals providing data helpful in the diagnosis of an occult lead problem but double counting of the QRS complex (VPCs) will also increment the short R-R counter

If you see many NSVT episodes, suspect a lead problem creating false signals !!!

2. Perform physical maneuvers. The evaluation of lead or connector related oversensing should include changes in body position, pocket manipulation, isometric exercise, various motions of the ipsilateral arm while telemetering the VEGM so as to bring out the abnormalities.

ABBREVIATIONS : *VEGM = ventricular electrogram; VF = ventricular fibrillation; VT = ventricular tachycardia; NSVT = non-sustained ventricular tachycardia; MRI = magnetic resonance imaging;*

Figure 11.02

ICD TROUBLESHOOTING : TESTING FOR LEAD PROBLEMS

1 Study the *near-field* and *far-field* (shocking) *electrograms* carefully.

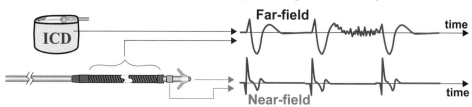

Comparing near-field and far-field EGMs can help determine which conductor is affected. Noise only on the far-field EGM suggests that the defect involves the shocking lead and not the sensing lead.

Look for abnormalities with changes in body position, deep respiration, coughing, movement of the ipsilateral arm, pocket manipulation and Valsalva maneuver. Differentiate myopotentials from false signals but the two may coexist.
A slight decrease in sensitivity (0.3 to 0.45 mV) may eliminate myopotentials but is unlikely to eliminate false signals.
Note that an insulation defect may set the stage for oversensing pectoral myopotentials.

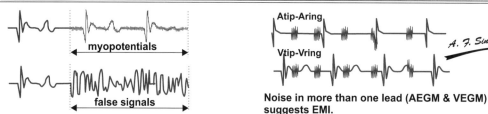

Noise in more than one lead (AEGM & VEGM) suggests EMI.

2 Verify the *pacing impedance* and the *high-voltage* (shocking pathway) *impedance*.

The *HV shocking impedance* measures between 20 and 100 ohms. This shocking impedance is always recorded when a shock is delivered. A high value indicates a fracture, a low value an insulation defect. In the past this was determined by deliberate delivery of a small shock. In contemporary devices, it is a painless measurement with a small test pulse. In some ICDs, these painless pulses are delivered periodically to construct a trend plot.

The *pacing impedance* is related to lead design. Values lower than 200 ohms indicate an insulation defect, while values higher than 2000 ohms indicate a fracture, a loose set screw or a defective adapter (*Note that high impedance leads do not cause pacing impedances above 2000 ohms*).
A change in impedance larger than 30% in a mature lead suggests malfunction. The trend of lead impedance can be useful in the diagnosis of fracture.
Occasionally a lead problem is associated with a normal impedance.

3 *Remember*

* Numerous aborted shocks due to oversensing suggest a lead problem.
* Multiple shocks without prior symptoms may also be caused by lead problems.
* Ineffectual shocks for VT/VF may occur if the problem involves the shocking electrode.
* Audible "Patient Alert" system may be activated by a lead problem.

ABBREVIATIONS : AEGM = atrial electrogram; EMI = electromagnetic interference; VEGM = ventricular electrogram; VF = ventricular fibrillation; VT = ventricular tachycardia; HV = high voltage

Figure 11.03

PACING IMPEDANCE vs SHOCKING IMPEDANCE

A LOW VOLTAGE IMPEDANCE

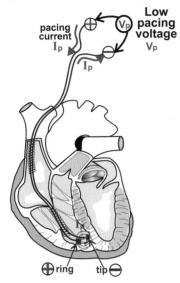

pacing current I_p

Low pacing voltage V_p

⊕ ring   tip ⊖

PACING IMPEDANCE : (lead + tissue)
$R_p = \dfrac{\text{Pacing voltage } V_p}{\text{Pacing current } I_p}$

INSULATION DEFECT < 250 Ω	NORMAL PACING IMPEDANCE ca. 500 Ω	LEAD FRACTURE > 2000 Ω

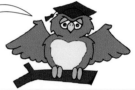

JUST REMEMBER OHM's LAW !!!

All impedances are measured according Ohm's law. However different voltages are used between the different electrodes !

$$\text{Impedance (ohm)} = \frac{\text{Voltage (volt)}}{\text{Current (ampere)}}$$

$$R\ (\Omega) = \frac{U\ (V)}{I\ (A)}$$

A. F. Sinnaeve

B HIGH VOLTAGE IMPEDANCE

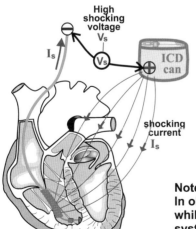

High shocking voltage V_s

I_s

ICD can

shocking current I_s

SHOCKING IMPEDANCE (lead + tissue)
$R_s = \dfrac{\text{Shocking voltage } V_s}{\text{Shocking current } I_s}$

INSULATION DEFECT < 20 Ω	NORMAL PACING IMPEDANCE 20 - 100 Ω	LEAD FRACTURE > 100 Ω

Note :
In older systems, the shocking impedance was measured while delivering a real shock to the heart. In contemporary systems a painless reduced voltage (V_s) is used (altough higher than the pacing voltage).

Figure 11.04

MANAGEMENT OF PATIENTS WITH MULTIPLE ICD SHOCKS

Multiple shocks (3 or more dischar-ges in 24 hrs) cause significant psy-chological stress to the patient and consequently they constitute a me-dical emergency ! What are the cau-ses for multiple shocks and what can be done to keep them under control ?

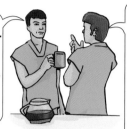

The causes of multiple ICD shocks are numerous. Accurate differential diagno-sis is needed for correct management ! Since analysis of retrieved data and sto-red EGMs facilitates elucidation of com-plex arrhythmic events, the device has to be interrogated as soon as possible. Initial evaluation of patients experien-cing multiple shocks, should be perfor-med in a setting with 12 lead ECG moni-toring where advanced cardiac resusci-tation is immediately available !

APPROPRIATE MULTIPLE SHOCKS

Frequently recurring VT or VF (electrical storm ; incessant VT)
Acute treatment : * Intravenous antiarrhythmic or beta blockade therapy
           * Consider temporary device deactivation
Definitive management : * Optimization of oral antiarrhythmic drugs
           * Antitachycardia pacing
           * VT ablation

Failure to terminate VT or VF reliably
Causes : * Programming of inappropriate low shock output
       * Antiarrhythmic drug effect
       * Shocking lead dislodgment or failure
       * Ipsilateral pneumothorax
Acute treatment : * External cardioversion/defibrillation
           * Avoid class I antiarrhythmic drugs
Defintive management : * Device reprogramming
           * Optimization of oral antiarrhythmic drugs
           * Surgical revision

ECG

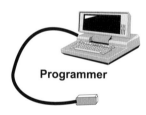

INAPPROPRIATE (SPURIOUS) SHOCKS

"Committed shocks" for nonsustained ventricular arrhythmias
Acute treatment : * Intravenous antiarrhythmic drugs
           * Consider temporary device deactivation
Definitive management : * Device reprogramming
           * Optimization of oral antiarrhythmic drugs

AA drugs

Supraventricular tachyarrhythmias
Acute treatment : * Temporary device deactivation
           * AV nodal blocking drugs
           * Pharmacologic or electrical cardioversion
Definitive management : * Device reprogramming
             * Optimization of oral antiarrhythmic drugs
             * Catheter ablation of arrhythmic substrate
             * Catheter ablation of AV junction

Programmer

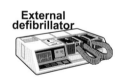

Oversensing during baseline rhythm
Causes : * Oversensing of intracardiac signals (T wave sensing)
       * Oversensing of diaphragmatic myopotentials
       * Sensing lead failure
       * External electromagnetic interference (EMI)
Acute treatment : * Temporary device deactivation
Definitive management : * Device reprogramming
           * Surgical revision
           * Avoidance and elimination of the EMI source(s)

External defibrillator

A. F. Sinnaeve

WARNING !

NOTE : Shocks result in substantial battery consumption ! ICDs designed to last years, can become nearly depleted within days by incessant discharges !

Multiple shocks may cause damage to the heart tissue !!!

Figure 11.05

ICDs and ELECTROMAGNETIC INTERFERENCE (EMI)

EMI is a complicated matter with 3 essential elements :
- ☆ a CULPRIT or electromagnetic source emitting some electro-magnetic energy
- ☆ a VICTIM (here an implanted ICD) that cannot function properly due to the reception of some unwanted EM energy
- ☆ a COUPLING PATH between them that allows the source to interfere with the receptor

Most EMI situations in daily life are benign for ICDs

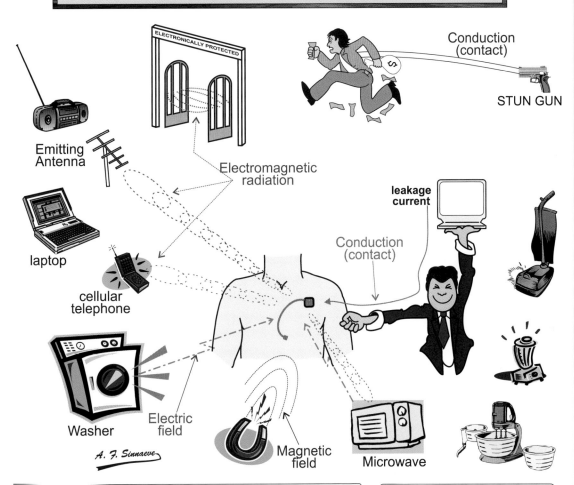

Conduction (contact) — STUN GUN

Emitting Antenna

Electromagnetic radiation

leakage current

Conduction (contact)

laptop

cellular telephone

Washer

Electric field

Magnetic field

Microwave

A. F. Sinnaeve

Several coupling methods are possible :
- * Pure electromagnetic radiation (e.g. from HF electronic equipment)
- * Conduction (e.g. touching leaking appliances - 60 or 50 Hz)
- * By magnetic fields (e.g. close to strong magnets or devices using strong alternating currents)
- * By electric fields (e.g. in the vicinity of alternating high voltages)

EMI depends upon :
- * Intensity of the field (power of the EMI source).
- * Wavelength (spectrum) of EMI
- * Distance to the EMI source
- * Type and programming of the ICD (parameter settings)
- * Type and position of the leads

Abbreviations : HF = high frequency ; LF = low frequency.

Figure 11.06

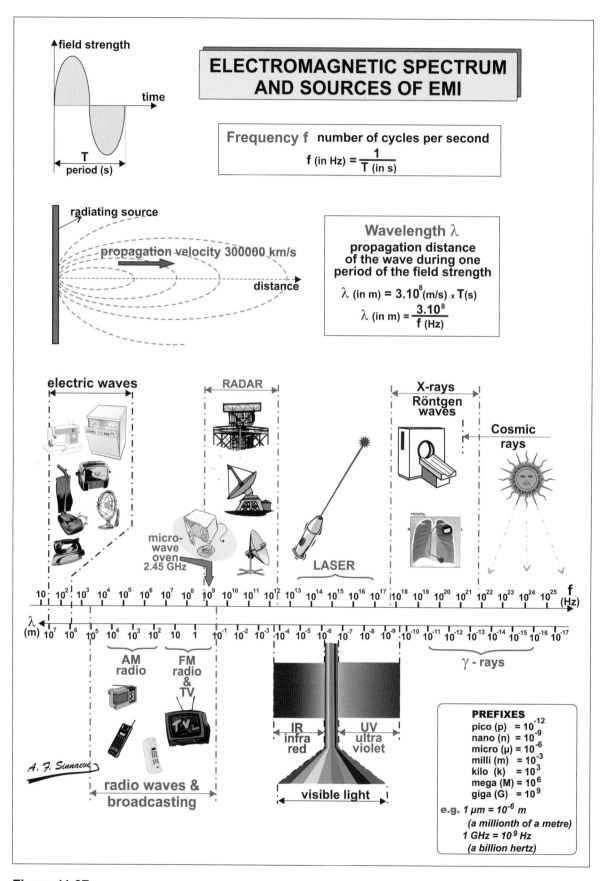

field strength

time

T
period (s)

ELECTROMAGNETIC SPECTRUM AND SOURCES OF EMI

Frequency f number of cycles per second

$$f \text{ (in Hz)} = \frac{1}{T \text{ (in s)}}$$

radiating source

propagation velocity 300000 km/s

distance

Wavelength λ
propagation distance of the wave during one period of the field strength

$$\lambda \text{ (in m)} = 3.10^8 \text{(m/s)} \times T \text{(s)}$$

$$\lambda \text{ (in m)} = \frac{3.10^8}{f \text{ (Hz)}}$$

electric waves

RADAR

X-rays
Röntgen waves

Cosmic rays

micro-wave oven 2.45 GHz

LASER

FRONTAL

γ - rays

f
10 10^2 10^3 10^4 10^5 10^6 10^7 10^8 10^9 10^{10} 10^{11} 10^{12} 10^{13} 10^{14} 10^{15} 10^{16} 10^{17} 10^{18} 10^{19} 10^{20} 10^{21} 10^{22} 10^{23} 10^{24} 10^{25} (Hz)

λ
(m) 10^7 10^6 10^5 10^4 10^3 10^2 10 1 10^{-1} 10^{-2} 10^{-3} 10^{-4} 10^{-5} 10^{-6} 10^{-7} 10^{-8} 10^{-9} 10^{-10} 10^{-11} 10^{-12} 10^{-13} 10^{-14} 10^{-15} 10^{-16} 10^{-17}

AM radio

FM radio & TV

IR infra red

UV ultra violet

A. F. Sinnaeve

radio waves & broadcasting

visible light

PREFIXES
pico (p) $= 10^{-12}$
nano (n) $= 10^{-9}$
micro (μ) $= 10^{-6}$
milli (m) $= 10^{-3}$
kilo (k) $= 10^3$
mega (M) $= 10^6$
giga (G) $= 10^9$

e.g. 1 μm = 10^{-6} m
(a millionth of a metre)
1 GHz = 10^9 Hz
(a billion hertz)

Figure 11.07

ELECTROMAGNETIC INTERFERENCE : OVERVIEW

Electromagnetic interference (or EMI) occurs when electrical signals of noncardiac or nonphysiological origin affect or disturb the proper function of implanted electronic devices (e.g. ICDs).

For clinical purposes, it is useful to recognize the different sources of EMI :

Radiated EMI can be :

* **intended** (as for communication purposes, e.g. cellular phones)
* **unintended** (e.g. motor operation in electric razor)

Conducted EMI galvanic currents introduced in the body :

* **therapeutically** (e.g. transcutaneous electrical nerve stimulation (TENS))
* by **accidental physical contact** with improperly grounded electrical equipment (mostly at power frequencies 50 Hz (Europe) or 60 Hz (USA))

POTENTIAL SOURCES OF EMI

ELECTROMAGNETIC FIELDS

Daily life :
* Cellular telephones
* Electronic article surveillance (EAS) devices
* Airport security devices
* Metal detectors (handheld and walkthrough)
* Radiofrequency (RF) remote controls (e.g. toys)
* Houshold appliances (mixers, razors, induction ovens,...)
* Improperly grounded appliances and tools in close contact to the body
* Slot machines
* Large stereo speakers

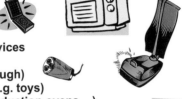
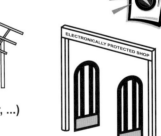

Work and industrial environment :
* High voltage power lines
* Industrial transformers and motors
* Electric melting furnaces (induction)
* Electric welding equipment (arc)
* Large RF transmitters (broadcasting, radar, ...)
* Degaussing coils

Medical environment :
* Magnetic resonance image scanners
* Electrosurgical equipment
* Therapeutic diathermy
* Pacemaker programmers
* External defibrillators
* Neurostimulators and TENS
* Radiofrequency (RF) catheter ablation

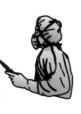
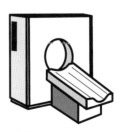

IONIZING RADIATION
Medical environment : radiotherapy (e.g. used in oncology)

ACOUSTIC RADIATION
Medical environment : lithotripsy
(shock waves to disintegrate kidney and gallbladder stones)

A. F. Sinnaeve

Figure 11.08

ICDs AND EMI IN HOSPITALS

A lot of EMI situations in the hospital are dangerous for ICDs

Pay attention! Some medical procedures are to be avoided for ICD patients, for some others we have to act very carefully!

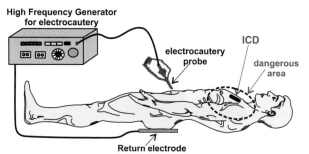

High Frequency Generator for electrocautery

electrocautery probe — ICD — dangerous area

Return electrode

Electrosurgery & electrocautery :
* Avoid it if possible and keep a distance of a few inches from ICD and leads
* Disable tachyarrhythmia detection/therapy
* Deactivate rate response features
* Close monitoring of ECG is necessary
* An external defibrillator should be at hand
* After the procedure, all function have to be restored and the ICD should be interrogated and checked thoroughly!

Cardioversion or defibrillation :
* Internal cardioversion via the implanted ICD is preferable
* If external defibrillation is to be used, a programmer and an external pacemaker should be available
* External cardioversion has to be done with a biphasic wave form and the lowest effective energy
* A posterior-anterior position of the paddles should be employed
* After external cardioversion a complete analysis of the ICD and all its functions is imperative

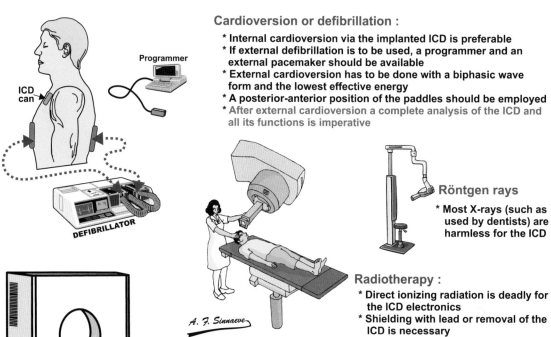

ICD can — Programmer — DEFIBRILLATOR

A. F. Sinnaeve

Röntgen rays
* Most X-rays (such as used by dentists) are harmless for the ICD

Radiotherapy :
* Direct ionizing radiation is deadly for the ICD electronics
* Shielding with lead or removal of the ICD is necessary

Magnetic resonance imaging (MRI) :
is absolutely contraindicated for patients with an ICD !

Lithotripsy :
is possible if the shock wave does not comes in the vicinity of the ICD

Endoscopy with wireless video-capsule :
The Pill-Cam© emits signals at 434.09 MHz. Most ICDs are not disturbed, but some over-sensing and inappropriate therapy have been noted.

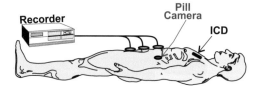

Recorder — Pill Camera — ICD

Figure 11.09

ICDs and EMI in an INDUSTRIAL ENVIRONMENT

Not all industrial situations or workplaces are dangerous! We have to be careful if strong radiation, high voltage or strong electrical current are involved. In general :
* field strength decreases rapidly when distance increases : so *keep your distance* from suspected sources.
* ICD patients working in an industrial environment should be equipped with *true (dedicated) bipolar sensing* to minimize EMI pick-up.

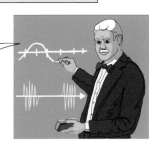

Industrial EMI situations ask for on-site evaluation.
The device manufacturer should be contacted !

RADAR & BROADCASTING TRANSMITTORS

HIGH VOLTAGE POWER LINES

ELECTRIC WELDING (ARC)

HEAVY MACHINERY

ELECTRIC MOTORS

ELECTRIC MELTING FURNACES (INDUCTION)

These modulated waves are activating my ICD !

Modulated high frequency (HF) waves are more dangerous than continuous waves with a constant amplitude. The low frequency modulation (i.e. large variations of the amplitude) might be detected by the electronics and might trigger the ICD functions.

Pulse modulation

time

Amplitude modulation

time

A. F. Sinnaeve

Figure 11.10

INTERFERENCE BY 60 (50) Hz LEAKAGE CURRENT

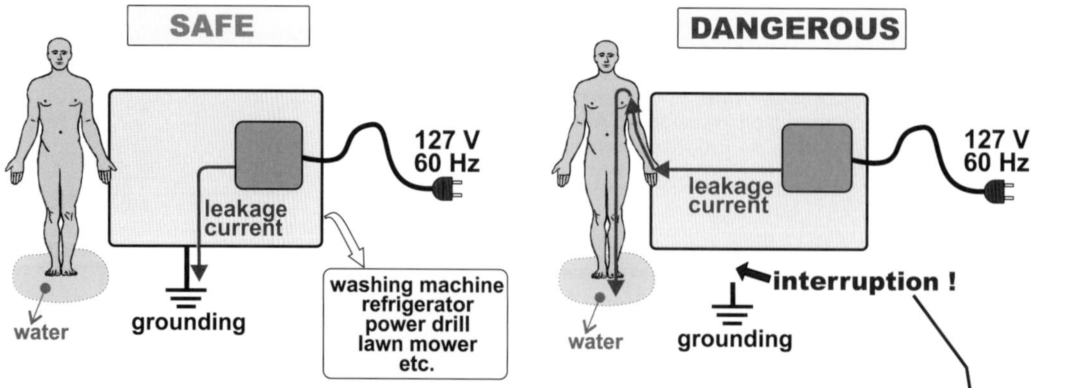

SAFE

DANGEROUS

127 V
60 Hz

leakage
current

grounding

washing machine
refrigerator
power drill
lawn mower
etc.

water

127 V
60 Hz

leakage
current

water

grounding

interruption !

grounding
plug

frayed
power cord

A leakage current through the patient due to an interrupted grounding is mostly caused by a frayed power cord, a broken plug, a loose screw, ...
The leakage current may provoke inappropriate shocks from the ICD but is also a hazard for the patient (possible electrocution). Since water is a good conductor, the danger is greater when the patient is connected to the ground via water (under a shower, feet in a swimming pool, etc.)

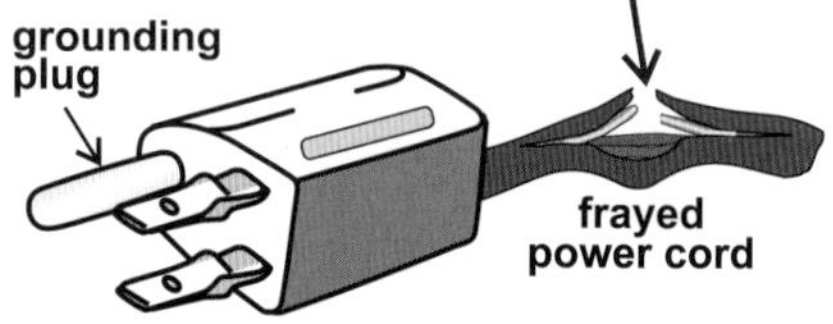

Inappropriate VF detection and cessation after shock

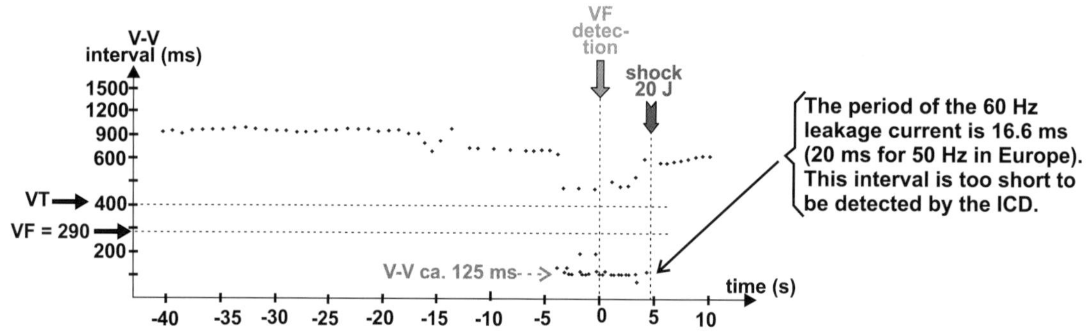

V-V
interval (ms)

VF
detec-
tion

shock
20 J

1500
1200
900
600

VT → 400
VF = 290 →

200

V-V ca. 125 ms- - >

time (s)

-40 -35 -30 -25 -20 -15 -10 -5   0   5   10

The period of the 60 Hz leakage current is 16.6 ms (20 ms for 50 Hz in Europe). This interval is too short to be detected by the ICD.

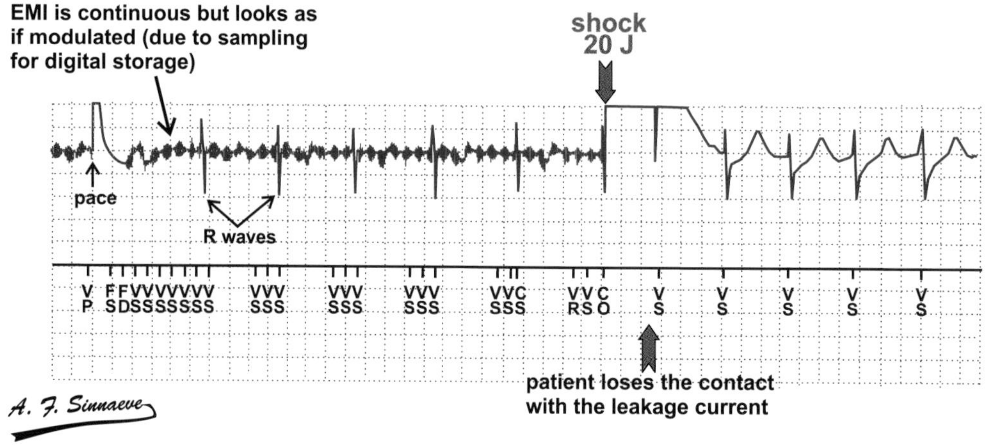

EMI is continuous but looks as if modulated (due to sampling for digital storage)

shock
20 J

pace

R waves

V FFVVVVVVVV   VVV   VVV   VVV   VVC   VVC   V   V   V   V   V
P SDSSSSSSSS   SSS   SSS   SSS   SSS   RSO   S   S   S   S   S

patient loses the contact
with the leakage current

A. F. Sinnaeve

Figure 11.11

12 SPECIAL ICD FUNCTIONS AND RESYNCHRONIZATION THERAPY

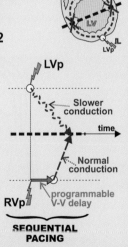

* ICDs for atrial and ventricular therapy and biventricular ICDs
* Left ventricular dyssynchrony and response to CRT
* Biventricular pacing systems and ventricular lead polarity
* Diaphragmatic stimulation
* Causes of poor clinical response to CRT
* Frontal plane axis during single chamber ventricular pacing and biventricular pacing
* Monochamber LV pacing in a patient with a biventricular pacemaker
* ECG from a patient with a biventricular pacemaker with the RV lead in the apex
* ECG from a patient with a biventricular pacemaker with the RV lead in the RVOT
* Lack of a dominant R wave in lead V1 during BiV pacing
* BiV pacing and ventricular fusion with the spontaneous QRS
* BiV pacing systems : effect of RV anodal stimulation
* RV anodal capture with monochamber LV pacing : parts 1 & 2
* Electrical desynchronization in biventricular pacemakers
* P wave tracking and ventricular desynchronization
* Atrial tracking recovery : a Medtronic algorithm
* Upper rate limitation in CRT : parts 1 & 2
* Optimal programming of biventricular pacemakers
* Optimization of AV and VV intervals : parts 1 - 4
* Device monitoring of lung fluid

Figure 12.00

SPECIAL ICD FUNCTIONS

Some ICDs provide both ventricular and atrial defibrillation using the standard leads for ventricular defibrillation. However, detection and therapy of atrial fibrillation are independent of the ventricular detection and defibrillation system.
Other ICDs also provide ventricular resynchronization by pacing in the left as well as in the right ventricle in patients with left ventricular dyssynchrony.

ATRIAL & VENTRICULAR ICD PROVIDING ATP AND DEFIBRILLATION TO BOTH ATRIUM AND VENTRICLE

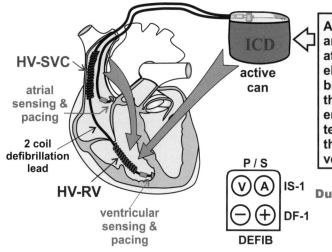

HV-SVC
atrial sensing & pacing
2 coil defibrillation lead
HV-RV
ventricular sensing & pacing

ICD
active can

Additional capability for atrial ATP and defibrillation. The shock for atrial defibrillation uses the same electrodes as for ventricular defibrillation. Atrial sensing and atrial therapy sequence (ATP and shock energy) are programmable separately from ventricular detection and therapy (ATP, shock energy) for ventricular tachyarrhythmias.

P / S
(V) (A) IS-1
(−) (+) DF-1
DEFIB

Dual chamber ICD Active can

BIVENTRICULAR ICD

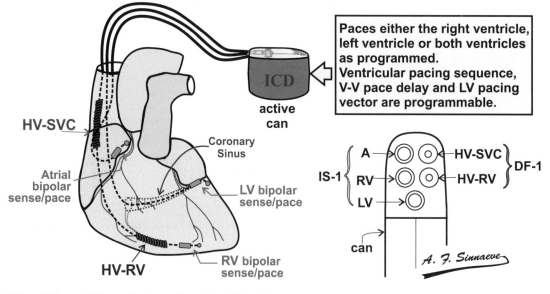

HV-SVC
Atrial bipolar sense/pace
Coronary Sinus
LV bipolar sense/pace
HV-RV
RV bipolar sense/pace

ICD
active can

Paces either the right ventricle, left ventricle or both ventricles as programmed.
Ventricular pacing sequence, V-V pace delay and LV pacing vector are programmable.

A → ⊙ ← HV-SVC
IS-1 { RV → ⊙ ← HV-RV } DF-1
LV → ⊙
can

A. F. Sinnaeve

Abbreviations : ATP = antitachycardia pacing ; HV = high voltage ; LV = left ventricle ; RV = right ventricle ; SVC = superior vena cava ; V-V delay = time interval between the pacing pulse in the RV and the one in the LV ;

Figure 12.01

LEFT VENTRICULAR DYSSYNCHRONY AND RESPONSE TO CRT

CRT has become increasingly accepted as a treatment modality for patients with heart failure (HF), low ejection fraction (EF) and LV wall contraction dyssynchrony. However, it has become clear that up to 30% of patients do not respond to CRT. Hence, identification of potential responders to CRT before implantation of an ICD is extremely important !

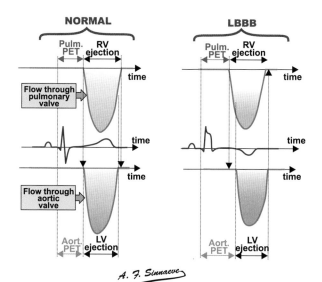

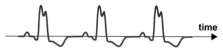

Interventricular dyssynchrony due to left bundle branch block (LBBB). The LV is delayed with respect to the RV.

Normally, the pre-ejection time (PET) of the pulmonary artery and the aortic artery are almost equal. With complete LBBB, there a distinct prolonging of the aortic pre-ejection time is noted.

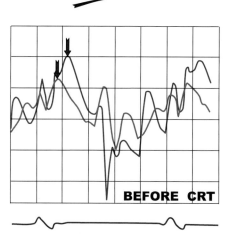

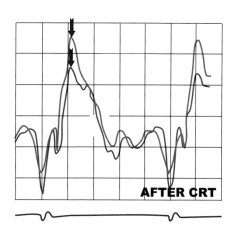

Intraventricular or LV mechanical dyssynchrony : in the example Tissue Doppler Imaging (TDI) shows a patient with the basal posterior wall delayed with respect to the basal anteroseptal wall of 90 ms; the delay was totally abolished after CRT. The peak systolic velocity during ejection phase in each view is shown by arrows.

Studies showed that patients with extensive LV dyssynchrony respond well to CRT.

Figure 12.02

BIVENTRICULAR PACING SYSTEMS
VENTRICULAR LEAD POLARITY

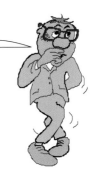

Both RV and LV leads may be unipolar as well as bipolar in BiV pacing systems ! Moreover, unipolar systems may use the can or a shared common ring ! It is confusing !?
And when is RV anodal stimulation possible in a BiV system ?

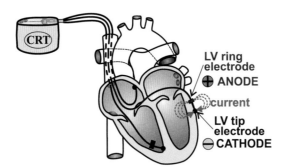

Device can
⊕ ANODE

CRT

current

LV tip electrode
⊖ CATHODE

Dual Ventricular Unipolar

* both leads are unipolar
* during LV pacing there is an electric current between LV tip electrode and the ICD can
* NO RV ANODAL capture possible

CRT

LV ring electrode
⊕ ANODE

current

LV tip electrode
⊖ CATHODE

Dual Ventricular Bipolar

* both leads are bipolar
* during LV pacing there is an electric current between LV tip electrode and the LV ring electrode
* NO RV ANODAL capture possible

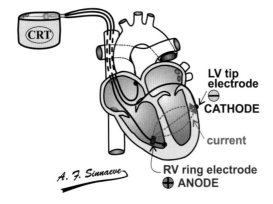

CRT

LV tip electrode
⊖ CATHODE

current

A. F. Sinnaeve

RV ring electrode
⊕ ANODE

Shared Common Ring Bipolar

* LV lead is unipolar ; RV lead is bipolar and the RV ring is shared
* during LV pacing there is an electric current between LV tip electrode and the shared RV ring electrode
* RV ANODAL CAPTURE POSSIBLE if the LV pulse amplitude is large enough

Note :
1. the normal RV threshold is lower than the LV threshold (due to better contact)
2. anodal capture is caused by the high current density generated at the RV anode by the high LV output. The threshold for RV anodal stimulation is variable and it may be higher or lower than the LV pacing threshold.

Abbreviations : CRT = cardiac resynchronization therapy ; BiV = biventricular ; LV = left ventricle ; RV = right ventricle .

Figure 12.03

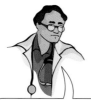

PHRENIC NERVE STIMULATION

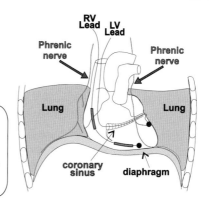

Phrenic nerve stimulation is not uncommon (5-10% of patients) in LV pacing due to :
* close vicinity of the epicardial coronary venous lead to the left phrenic nerve when the LV lead is implanted in a posterior or posterolateral coronary vein. It may also be caused by lead dislodgment
* constraints of coronary venous anatomy

HOW TO AVOID DIAPHRAGMATIC STIMULATION

1 Another site should be sought to avoid phrenic stimulation (but the LV pacing threshold may be higher !)

2 Reduce the LV output if both ventricular outputs are separately programmable

3 Change to "Electronic Repositioning" (Guidant - Boston Scientific) i.e. from extended bipolar (unipolar) to dedicated bipolar LV lead :

LV Tip to RV Coil	LV Ring to RV Coil	LV Tip to LV Ring	LV Ring to LV Tip
Extended Bipolar Pacing Vector	Extended Bipolar Pacing Vector	Dedicated Bipolar Pacing Vector	Dedicated Bipolar Pacing Vector

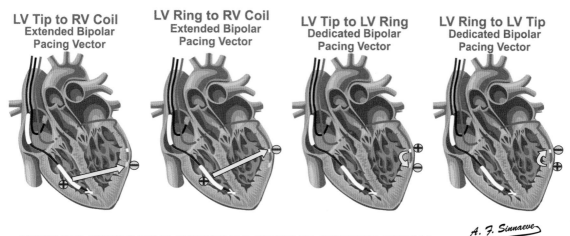

A. F. Sinnaeve

HOW TO TEST FOR PHRENIC NERVE STIMULATION

1 *AT IMPLANTATION :*
Phrenic nerve stimulation at implantation is assessed with a high voltage output at 10 volts and deep breathing maneuvers.

2 *AFTER IMPLANTATION :*
The occurence of phrenic nerve stimulation early after LV lead implantation may be due to LV lead displacement even if inapparent on the chest X-ray.
If the LV capture threshold is far below that of the phrenic nerve stimulation threshold, a reduction of LV pacing amplitude (volts) below the phrenic nerve stimulation threshold may simply solve the problem. This approach runs the risk of loss of LV capture so that lead repositioning is often necessary. Increasing the pulse duration to maintain LV capture with a low voltage output rarely works.
Recently, some bipolar pacing LV leads and devices (Guidant - Boston Scientific) allow reprogramming of the LV lead pacing configuration that may decrease phrenic nerve stimulation without the need of an invasive procedure for correction.

Abbreviations : LV = left ventricle ; RV = right ventricle

Figure 12.04

CAUSES OF POOR CLINICAL RESPONSE TO CRT

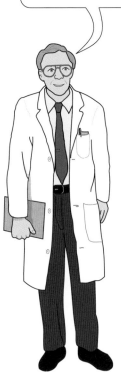

Some of my patients are nonresponders to CRT !
A lot of causes are possible and therefore a careful
examination of patient and system is necessary !

➤ LV lead dislodgment or high threshold

➤ LV lead in the anterior or middle cardiac vein

➤ LV lead on nonviable myocardium

➤ No LV dyssynchrony despite wide QRS

➤ Irreversible mitral regurgitation

➤ Long AV delay

➤ Suboptimal AV delay and/or VV delay

➤ Atrial tachyarrhythmias with fast ventricular rate

➤ Frequent VPCs

➤ ??? Severely impaired myocardial function

➤ Comorbidities

➤ Delayed LV activation : Increased LV latency or severe local intramyocardial conduction delay or both

➤ Too strict definition of positive response

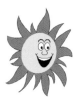

Contrast-enhanced MRI has promising potential for identifying scar and potentially viable tissue !

Abbreviatons : AV = atrioventricular ; CRT = cardiac resynchronisation therapy ; LV = left ventricle ; MRI = magnetic resonance imaging ; VPC = ventricular premature complex ; VV delay = interventricular delay ;

Figure 12.05

FRONTAL PLANE AXIS DURING SINGLE CHAMBER VENTRICULAR AND BIVENTRICULAR PACING

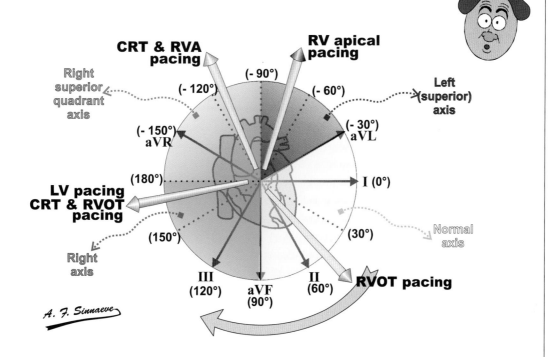

① **Monochamber RV pacing**
During RV outflow tract/septal pacing, the axis may be in the "normal" site in the left inferior quadrant and it moves to the right inferior quadrant (right axis deviation) as the site of stimulation moves superiorly towards the pulmonary valve.

② **Monochamber LV pacing from target site in the coronary venous system**
The axis points to the right inferior quadrant (right axis deviation) and less commonly to the right superior quadrant. In an occasional patient the axis may point to the left inferior or left superior quadrant. The reasons for these unusual axis locations are unclear.

③ **Biventricular pacing (coronary venous system) with RV apical stimulation**
The axis usually moves superiorly from the left (monochamber RV apical pacing) to the right superior quadrant (biventricular pacing) in an anticlockwise fashion. The axis may occasionally reside in the left superior rather than the right superior quadrant during uncomplicated biventricular pacing.

④ **Biventricular pacing (coronary venous system) with RV outflow tract/septal stimulation**
The axis is often directed to the right inferior quadrant (right axis deviation).

Figure 12.06

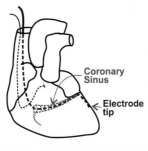

Coronary Sinus

Electrode tip

MONOCHAMBER LV PACING IN A PATIENT WITH A BiV PACEMAKER

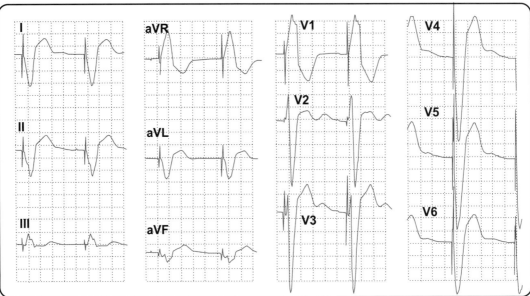

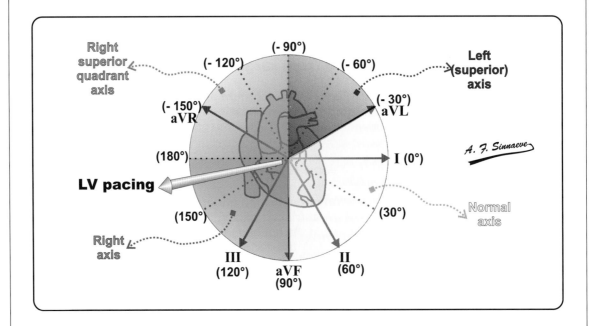

Abbreviations : BiV = biventricular ; LV = left ventricle ; RVOT = right ventricular outflow tract ;

Figure 12.07

ECG FROM A PATIENT WITH A BIVENTRICULAR PACEMAKER WITH RV LEAD IN THE APEX

Monochamber RV apical pacing

QRS
duration = 243 ms

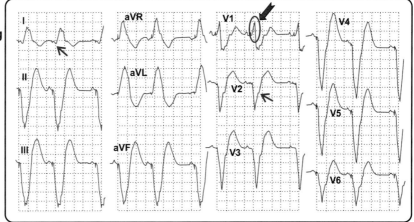

Monochamber LV pacing

QRS
duration = 240 ms

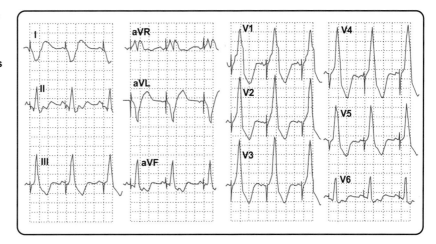

BiV pacing LV & RV apex

QRS
duration = 170 ms

Dominant R in lead V1 is common if RV pacing at apex.

Right superior axis is typical; occasionally left superior axis is possible.

A. F. Sinnaeve

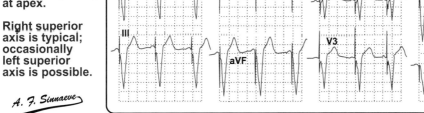

Abbreviations : BiV = biventricular ; LV = left ventricle ; RV = right ventricle ;

Figure 12.08

ECG FROM A PATIENT WITH A BIVENTRICULAR PACEMAKER WITH RV LEAD IN THE RVOT

Monochamber RVOT Pacing

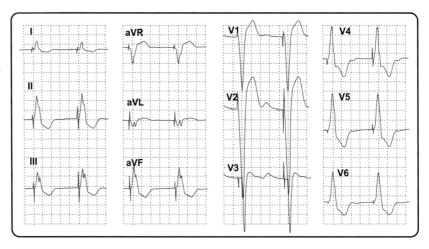

Monochamber LV Pacing
(RVOT Off)

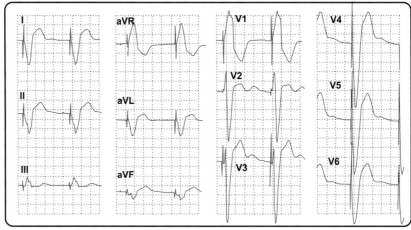

Biventricular Pacing LV & RVOT

Note right axis in frontal plane and LBBB in lead V1

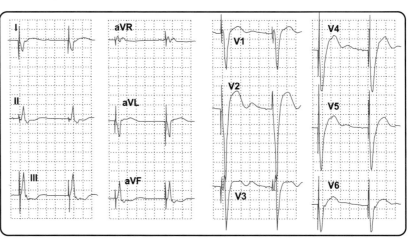

Abbreviations : BiV = biventricular ; LBBB = left bundle branch block ; LV = left ventricle ; RV = right ventricle ; RVOT = right ventricular outflow tract ;

Figure 12.09

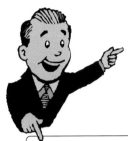

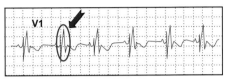

LACK OF A DOMINANT R WAVE IN LEAD V1 DURING BiV PACING

A dominant R wave in lead V1 is common during BiV pacing if RV pacing is at the apex. However, a lack of a dominant R wave in lead V1 may be normal during uncomplicated BiV pacing with RV apical stimulation !

This may be due to different activation of an heterogeneous biventricular substrate (ischemia, scar, His-Purkinje participation in view of the varying patterns of LV activation in spontaneous LBBB, etc.)

But the following situations must be ruled out :

1. RVOT & LV pacing

2. Incorrect placement of lead V1 (too high on the chest)

3. Lack of LV capture

4. LV lead displacement

5. Marked LV latency (exit block or delay from the LV stimulation site)

6. Ventricular fusion with conducted QRS complex

7. Pacing via the middle cardiac vein or anterior interventricular vein

8. Unintended placement of 2 leads in the RV

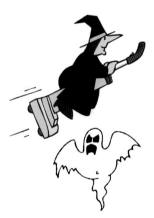

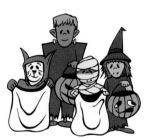

A. F. Sinnaeve

Abbreviations : BiV = biventricular ; LBBB = left bundle branch block ; LV = left ventricle ; RV = right ventricle ; RVOT = right ventricular outflow tract ;

Figure 12.10

BiV pacing with Fusion
Initial ECG ; As-Vp = 100ms
QRS narrowing too good
to be true

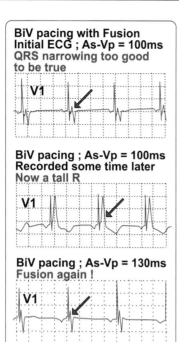

BiV pacing ; As-Vp = 100ms
Recorded some time later
Now a tall R

BiV pacing ; As-Vp = 130ms
Fusion again !

BiV Pacing and Ventricular Fusion with the Spontaneous QRS

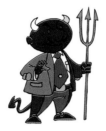

* In patients with sinus rhythm and a relatively short PR interval, a ventricular fusion phenomenon may lead to misinterpretation of the ECG. This is a frequent pitfall with BiV pacing in the presence of a relatively short PR interval and a more narrow paced QRS complex

* Ventricular fusion may be intermittent and present only in situations associated with enhanced AV conduction (increased catecholamines) !

A. F. Sinnaeve

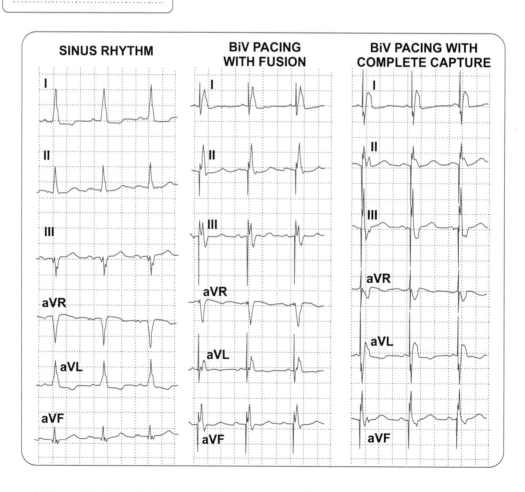

| SINUS RHYTHM | BiV PACING WITH FUSION | BiV PACING WITH COMPLETE CAPTURE |

Abbreviations : BiV = biventricular ; As = atrial sense ; Vp = ventricular pace ;

Figure 12.11

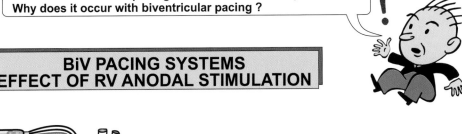

We never saw anodal pacing with conventional RV pacemakers. Why does it occur with biventricular pacing ?

BiV PACING SYSTEMS
EFFECT OF RV ANODAL STIMULATION

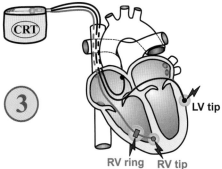

Triple site ventricular pacing

* Simultaneous ventricular capture from both LV and RV tip plus RV ring *(RV anodal capture at the ring)*.
* Triple pacing produces a 12-lead ECG configuration somewhat different from the pure 2 site pacing without anodal capture.

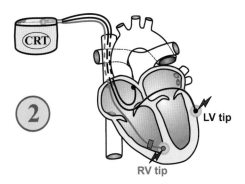

Two site ventricular pacing

* As the LV output is decreased, RV anodal capture often disappears.
* In 2 site pacing, the 12-lead ECG configuration will be identical to the ECG during pure unipolar RV and unipolar LV with the anode on the pacemaker can where RV anodal capture is impossible.

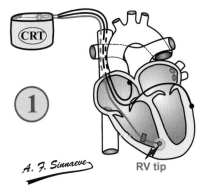

Single site ventricular pacing

* Decreasing the ventricular output will almost always cause loss of LV pacing with preservation of RV capture because LV pacing threshold is often higher than that of the RV.

Abbreviations : Ap = atrial pacing ; LV = left ventricle ; RV = right ventricle ; Vp = ventricular pacing ;

Figure 12.12

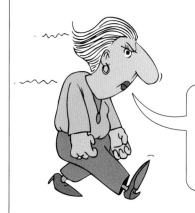

RV ANODAL CAPTURE WITH MONOCHAMBER LV PACING - 1

It's a mad world !
Monochamber LV pacing (i.e. from LV tip to RV ring) mimics the standard BiV pacing !
The pattern of LV depolarization cannot be ascertained if the LV threshold is high because RV anodal stimulation (via the RV ring electrode) prevents pure LV activation.

BiV pacing

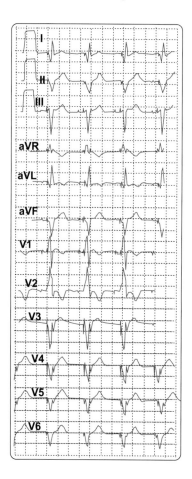

High output monochamber LV pacing (RV output off) RV anodal capture. AV = 90 ms

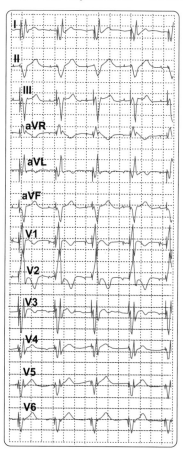

A. J. Sinnaeve

Abbreviations : AV = atrioventricular ; BiV = biventricular ; LV = left ventricle ; RV = right ventricle ;

Figure 12.13

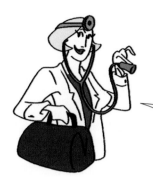

RV ANODAL CAPTURE WITH MONOCHAMBER LV PACING - 2

* The RV anodal threshold can be determined by lowering the LV output.
* Pacing from LV to can to show pure LV activation is not available in BiV ICDs.

High output monochamber LV pacing (RV output off) RV anodal capture. AV = 90 ms

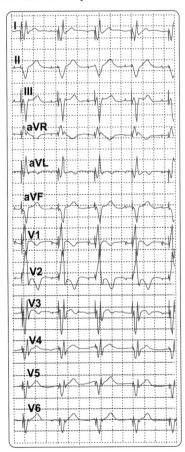

LV output at 3.5 V (RV output off) 2:1 anodal RV stimulation intermittent RV capture

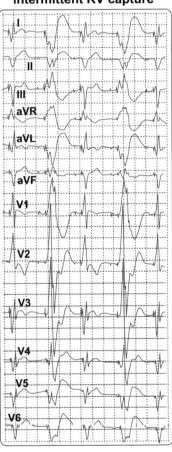

LV output at 2.8 V (RV output off) Pure LV pacing LV stimulation only

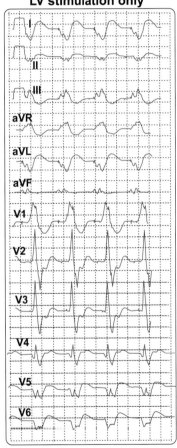

A. F. Sinnaeve

Abbreviations : AV = atrioventricular ; BiV = biventricular ; LV = left ventricle ; RV = right ventricle ;

Figure 12.14

ELECTRICAL DESYNCHRONIZATION IN BIVENTRICULAR PACEMAKERS

> CRT is another example where one must know the timing cycles of the device to understand its function

1 Loss of resynchronization below the programmed upper rate and locking of P waves inside the PVARP due to a long P-R interval

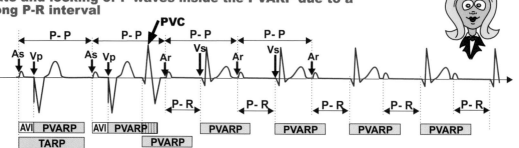

NOTE :
The same locking of P waves inside the PVARP can be caused by T wave oversensing

2 No locking of P waves inside the PVARP if the P-R interval is shorter

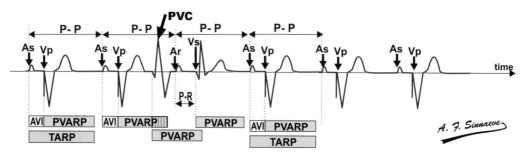

A. F. Sinnaeve

3 Sinus tachycardia can produce desynchronization even when the P-R interval is relatively short

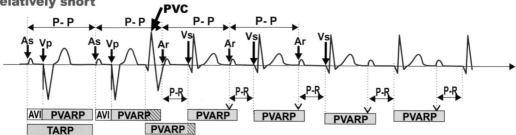

Development of electrical desynchronization may be favored by :

- ⚙ Relatively fast sinus rhythms
- ⚙ First-degree AV block (long P- R interval)
- ⚙ Relatively long programmed PVARP

"Locking" of the P waves can often be prevented by :

- ⚙ Elimination of the initiating mechanism (e.g. reduce ventricular sensitivity to avoid T wave sensing)
- ⚙ Programming a shorter PVARP
- ⚙ Slowing the sinus rate with drugs
- ⚙ Refractory cases (marked 1st degree AV block) can be treated by AV junctional ablation

---

Abbreviations : AVI = programmed AV interval ; As = sensed atrial event ; Ar = sensed atrial event during refractory period ; P-P = period between two consecutive P waves ; P-R = period between a P wave and its following R wave ; PVARP = post-ventricular atrial refractory period ; PVC = premature ventricular complex ; TARP = total atrial refractory period ; Vp = paced ventricular event ; Vs sensed ventricular event .

Figure 12.15

P WAVE TRACKING AND VENTRICULAR DESYNCHRONIZATION

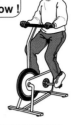

If I'm exercising too hard, my CRT-ICD device cannot follow !

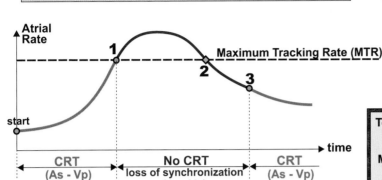

Total atrial refractory period :

$$TARP = AVI + PVARP$$

Maximum tracking rate :

$$MTR = \frac{60,000}{TARP}$$

✿ From start to point 1 : As - Vp sequence

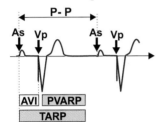

P-P > TARP ⟶ atrial rate < MTR

The spontaneous atrial rate is lower than the maximum tracking rate. Since both ventricles are paced, adequate CRT is delivered.

✿ From point 1 to point 2 : Ar - Vs sequence

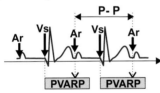

P-P < TARP ⟶ atrial rate > MTR

As soon as the atrial rate exceeds the MTR, the P wave falls within the PVARP and ventricular resynchronization is lost.

Note : (Ar - Vs) > AVI (= As - Vp)

✿ From point 2 to point 3 : Ar - Vs sequence

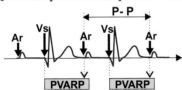

P-P > TARP ⟶ atrial rate < MTR

The timing cycles of the device force the continuation of the Ar - Vs sequences as long as P-P < [(Ar - Vs) + PVARP]

At point 3 the atrial rate is decreased far enough as to make P-P = [(Ar - Vs) + PVARP]

✿ From point 3 to the end : As - Vp sequence

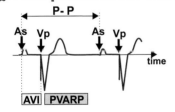

P-P > [(Ar - Vs) + PVARP] and ventricular synchronized pacing restarts

P-P > TARP ⟶ atrial rate < MTR
Same ECG as between points 1 and 2

A. F. Sinnaeve

> **Note : The actual "Total atrial refractory period" generated by Ar-Vs sequences is longer than the programmed TARP because Ar-Vs > programmed As-Vp (=AVI) !**

Abbreviations : As = atrial sensed event ; Ar = atrial event sensed in the atrial refractory period where tracking cannot occur ; AVI = programmed AV interval ; CRT = cardiac resynchronization therapy ; MTR = maximum tracking rate ; P-P = interval between to consecutive P waves ; PVARP = postventricular atrial refractory period ; TARP = total atrial refractory period ; Vp = biventricular paced event ; Vs = ventricular sensed event.

Figure 12.16

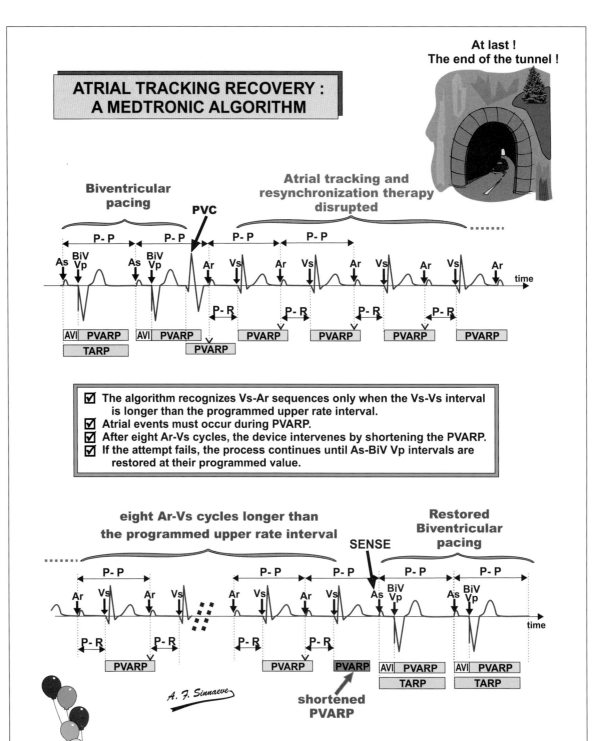

At last !
The end of the tunnel !

ATRIAL TRACKING RECOVERY : A MEDTRONIC ALGORITHM

☑ The algorithm recognizes Vs-Ar sequences only when the Vs-Vs interval is longer than the programmed upper rate interval.
☑ Atrial events must occur during PVARP.
☑ After eight Ar-Vs cycles, the device intervenes by shortening the PVARP.
☑ If the attempt fails, the process continues until As-BiV Vp intervals are restored at their programmed value.

Note : GUIDANT has a similar algorithm for restoring AV synchrony.

Abbreviations : AVI = programmed AV interval ; As = sensed atrial event ; Ar = sensed atrial event during refractory period ; P-P = period between two consecutive P waves ; P-R = period between a P wave and its following R wave ; PVARP = post-ventricular atrial refractory period ; PVC = premature ventricular complex ; TARP = total atrial refractory period ; BiV Vp = biventricular paced event ; Vs sensed ventricular event .

Figure 12.17

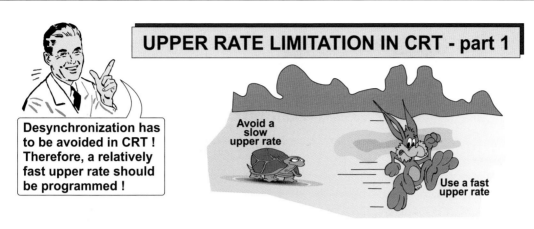

UPPER RATE LIMITATION IN CRT - part 1

Desynchronization has to be avoided in CRT ! Therefore, a relatively fast upper rate should be programmed !

Avoid a slow upper rate

Use a fast upper rate

Normal upper rate response of the Wenckebach type

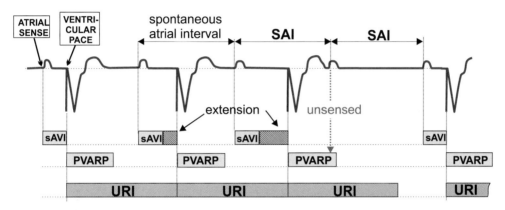

The pre-empted Wenckebach behavior with short sAVI

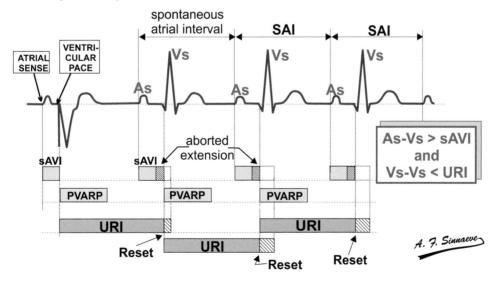

As-Vs > sAVI and Vs-Vs < URI

A. F. Sinnaeve

Abbreviations : As = atrial sense, Vs = ventricular sense, CRT = cardiac resynchronization therapy ; sAVI = AV delay after sensing, PVARP = postventricular atrial refractory period, URI = upper rate interval ; SAI = spontaneous atrial interval

Figure 12.18

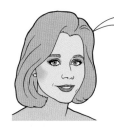

CRT devices that memorize episodes of ventricular sensing together with preceding events have facilitated the diagnosis of pacemaker upper rate behavior. The long-term stored data in CRT devices are diagnostically far superior than conventional 24 hr Holter recordings !

UPPER RATE LIMITATION IN CRT - part 2

Normal BiV pacing : AS - BV

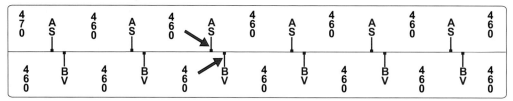

Pre-empted Wenckebach upper rate response : AS - VS
Programmed upper rate = 130 ppm :
VS - VS < upper rate interval 460 ms

AS is beyond PVARP

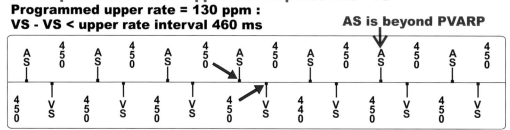

Cardiac Resynchronization Therapy : Wenckebach upper rate response

A standard Wenckebach upper rate response terminates with uiniform AR-VS sequences with every P in the PVARP. Note that the sequence with AR-VS combinations occurs when the spontaneous AR-AR or VS-VS intervals are shorter than the TARP (see a similar response in the bottom recording). In this situation there are no blocked or unsensed P waves in a 2:1 fashion as in traditional fixed-ratio upper rate response because of normal AV conduction. All P waves are in the PVARP and they all conduct to the ventricle (VS)

AS - VP lengthens
P in PVARP

P in PVARP

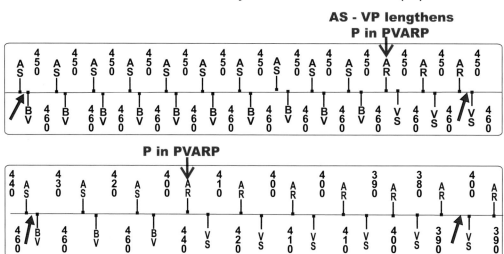

Abbreviations : AS = atrial sense ; AR = atrial sense during refractory period ; BV = biventricular pace ; PVARP = postventricular atrial refractory period ; VP = ventricular pace ; VS = ventricular sense ; TARP = total atrial refractory period.

A. F. Sinnaeve

Figure 12.19

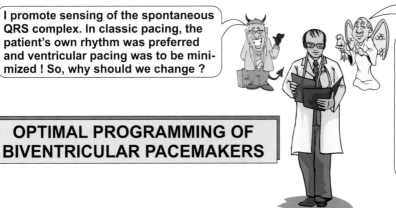

I promote sensing of the spontaneous QRS complex. In classic pacing, the patient's own rhythm was preferred and ventricular pacing was to be minimized ! So, why should we change ?

On the contrary ! CRT must show virtually 100% pacing ! So, for biventricular devices ventricular pacing has to be maximized to maintain cardiac resynchronization !

OPTIMAL PROGRAMMING OF BIVENTRICULAR PACEMAKERS

PARA-METERS	MANAGEMENT
AV & VV delay	1. A long AV delay should not be used. 2. Optimize the As - Vp delay and generally try to avoid ventricular fusion with the spontaneous conducted QRS complex. 3. Program rate-adaptive (dynamic) AV delay "OFF" during temporary testing (with VDD mode slower than sinus rate to sense atrial activity). 4. Programming rate-adaptive AV delay for long-term pacing is controversial. 5. Program VV delay at the optimal As - LVp delay
Atrial Sensing & PVARP	1. Program a short PVARP (aim for 250 ms). (may have to use algorithms for the automatic termination of endless loop tachycardia). 2. Program "OFF" the post-PVC PVARP extension and the pacemaker-mediated tachycardia termination algorithm based on one cycle of PVARP extension. 3. Program "OFF" automatic mode switching in devices using a relatively long PVARP mandated by the mode switching algorithm.
Upper rate	Program a relatively fast upper rate so patients do not have "break-through" ventricular sensing within their exercise zone. Initial upper rate of 140 bpm is often appropriate in the absence of myocardial ischemia during pacing at this rate.
AV conduction	1. Use drugs that impair AV conduction to avoid ventricular fusion or double counting in devices with a common sensing channel. 2. Consider ablation of the AV junction in patients with a long PR interval or intra- or interatrial conduction delay difficult to manage. 3. AV junctional ablation in patients with permanent atrial fibrillation.

A. F. Sinnaeve

Abbreviations : As = atrial sensed event ; AV = atrioventricular ; bpm = beats per minute ; CRT = cardiac resynchronization therapy ; LVp = left ventricular pacing ; PVARP = postventricular atrial refractory period ; PVC = premature ventricular complex ; Vp = ventricular pacing ; VV = interval between left and right ventricular pacing ;

Figure 12.20

OPTIMIZATION OF AV AND VV INTERVALS - 1

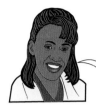

The influence of the AV delay appears to be less important than the proper choice of LV pacing site. Nevertheless, programming of the left-sided AV delay is important in CRT patients. Appropriate AV interval timing can maximize the benefit of CRT, and if programmed poorly, it has the potential to curtail the beneficial effects.

AVD OPTIMAL

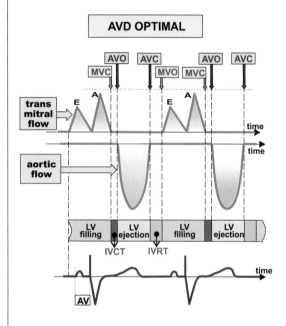

The optimal AV delay in CRT patients exhibits great variability from patient to patient. An empirically programmed AV delay interval is sub-optimal in many patients. Optimized AV synchrony is achieved by the AV delay setting that provides the best left atrial contribution to LV filling, the maximum stroke volume, shortening of the isovolumic contraction time, and the longest diastolic filling time in the absence of diastolic mitral regurgitation (in patients with a long PR interval).

The optimal AV delay is often performed by determining the aortic velocity time integral (VTI) i.e. the surface area under the aortic flow curve.

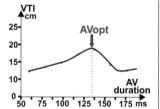

AVO = aortic valve opening ; AVC = aortic valve closure
MVO = mitral valve opening ; MVC = mitral valve closure
IVCT = isovolumic contraction time
IVRT = isovolumic relaxation time
E : early diastolic maximum velocity of mitral inflow
A : atrial systolic maximum velocity of mitral inflow

AVD SHORT

AVD LONG

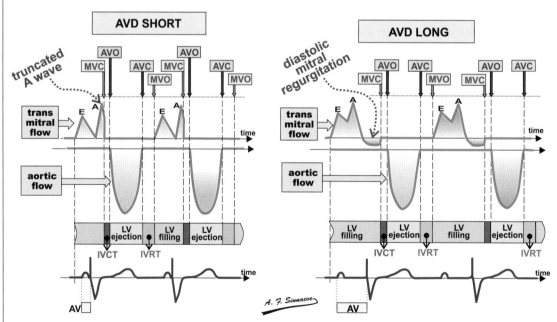

A. F. Sinnaeve

Abbreviations : AVD = AV delay ; AVopt = optimal AV delay ; CRT = cardiac resynchronization therapy ; LV = left ventricle ;

Figure 12.21

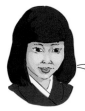

OPTIMIZATION OF AV AND VV INTERVALS - 2

AV optimization in DDD(R) pacemakers has traditionally been achieved using noninvasive Doppler echocardiography which still remains widely used in CRT patients for acute and long-term hemodynamic assessment.
The same technique is used for the VV optimization.

Schematic representation of resynchronization via tissue Doppler

Doppler probe

heart

A. F. Sinnaeve

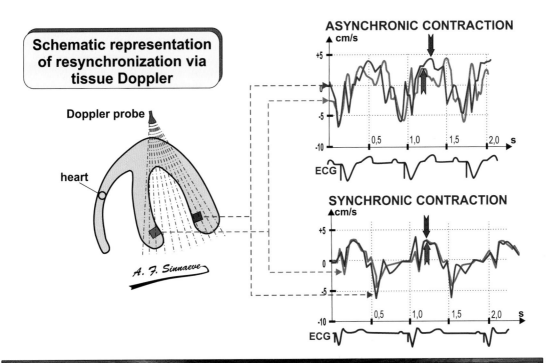

ASYNCHRONIC CONTRACTION

SYNCHRONIC CONTRACTION

BIVENTRICULAR PACING aims at synchronous activation of the LV from both RV and LV pacing sites. The two wave fronts should meet around the middle of the LV; if the conduction from one ventricle (e.g. LV) is delayed, than the other one (e.g. RV) should be stimulated after a VV delay.

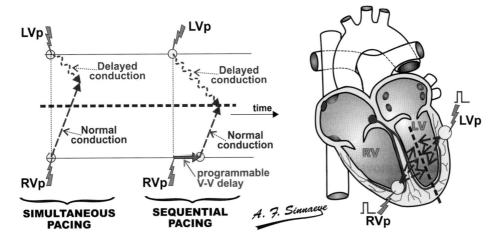

Abbreviations : AV = atrioventricular ; CRT = cardiac resynchronization therapy ; LVp = left ventricular pace ; RVp = right ventricular pace ; VV = time interval between LVp and RVp ;

Figure 12.22

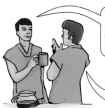

Tissue Doppler echocardiography is very efficient for AV and VV optimization but it is time consuming !

OPTIMIZATION OF AV AND VV INTERVALS - 3

Yes, it is! But there is an alternative. SJM recently introduced QuickOpt, a new algorithm that can do the job in a couple of minutes without the need for expensive equipment !

1 QUICK-OPT - part 1 : optimization of the PV and AV intervals

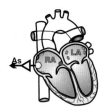

Measurement of the duration of the sensed P wave (PWD) in the RA is the cornerstone of the AV optimization.
The RA-EGM is sampled and the PWD is the average of 8 measurements within 15 seconds. Each measurement starts at the first sample which is larger than 0.2 mV and stops at the end of the third sample smaller than 0.2 mV

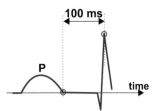

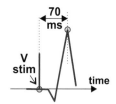

It has been shown that the peak of the QRS complex always follows 100 ms after the end of a spontaneous P wave and 70 ms after ventricular stimulation.

In CRT, the ventricles are always paced and the atrioventricular delay should be optimal

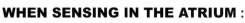

WHEN SENSING IN THE ATRIUM :

If PWD > 100ms :

PVopt = PWD + 100 ms - 70 ms

PVopt = PWD + 30 ms

If PWD < 100 ms :

PVopt = PWD + 60 ms

(For PWD < 100 ms, there is under-estimation of the P wave - the first part may be missed).

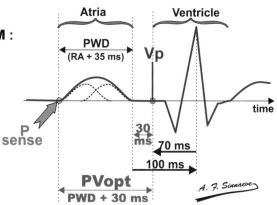

WHEN PACING IN THE ATRIUM :

AVopt = PVopt + (AVD - PVD)

AVopt = PVopt + 50 ms

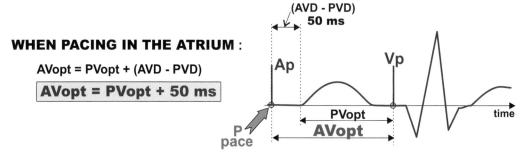

Abbreviations : AV = atrioventricular ; CHF = congestive heart faillure ; LA = left atrium ; RA =right atrium ; PVopt = optimal delay between a sensed atrial event and the succeeding ventricular stimulus ; AVopt = optimal delay between atrial and ventricular stimuli ; PWD = P wave duration

Figure 12.23

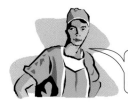

OPTIMIZATION OF AV AND VV INTERVALS - 4

The QuickOpt algorithm provides a reliable and simple method for VV optimization and correlates extremely well with the standard aortic velocity time integral (VTI) method

2 QUICK-OPT - part 2 : optimization of VV interval

Measurement of intrinsic interventricular depolarization delay Δ

Δ = time difference between the LV and the RV sensing after a paced or sensed atrial event

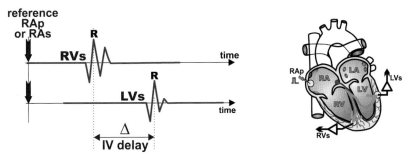

Measurement of interventricular conduction delays (IVCD)

ε = difference between the conduction times from right to left (RL) and from left to right (LR)

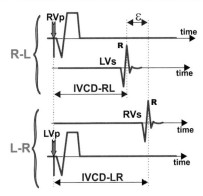

$$\varepsilon = (IVCD\text{-}LR) - (IVCD\text{-}RL)$$

ε is a correction term depending upon the wavefront velocity in both LV and RV

BIVENTRICULAR PACING aims at synchronously activating the LV from the RV and LV pacing sites. Therefore the two wave fronts should meet in the middle of the LV. It follows that :

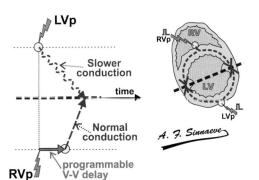

A. F. Sinnaeve

$$\boxed{VV_{opt} = 0.5 \times (\Delta + \varepsilon)}$$

The LV is activated first if VV > 0 if VV < 0 the RV isstimulated first.

SEQUENTIAL PACING

Abbreviations : LVs = left ventricular sense ; RVs = right ventricular sense ; LVp = left ventricular pace ; RVp = right ventricular pace ;

Figure 12.24

DEVICE MONITORING OF LUNG FLUID

Volume overload is a major complication in patients with moderate-to-severe heart failure and is a frequent cause of hospitalizations

The *OptiVol Fluid Status Monitoring (Medtronic)* **works by measuring intrathoracic impedance many times a day. A small subthreshold electrical impulse travels between the RV coil and the can of the ICD and the impedance is calculated according Ohm's law. Since body fluids are good conductors, the impedance decreases when fluid accumulates in the lungs.**

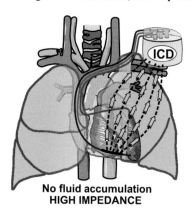

**No fluid accumulation
HIGH IMPEDANCE**

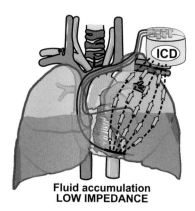

**Fluid accumulation
LOW IMPEDANCE**

The *"Thoracic Impedance Trend"* **is a plot of daily average impedance values. The data are stored on a 14-month basis and can be viewed in the reports.**

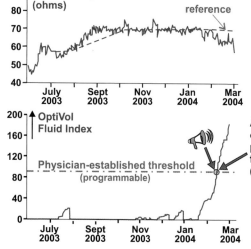

An *"OptiVol Fluid Index"* **is calculated based on the intrathoracic impedance. As the fluid accumulates in the lungs the impedance decreases below the reference and fluid index increases. If the condition is not resolved and the fluid index crosses a threshold, an observation will be triggered. When the fluid buildup has been resolved and the daily impedance value is trending at or above the reference impedance, the fluid index will return to zero.**

An *audible warning* **will sound from the implanted device once per day for 30 seconds at a time specified by the physician. The alert will continue to sound daily until the fluid index drops below the threshold.
(the audible tone may be turned off)**

A → fluid buildup ; impedance decreases below reference ; fluid index increases
B → fluid index reaches threshold ; patient alarm starts
C → therapy is started
D → problem is solved

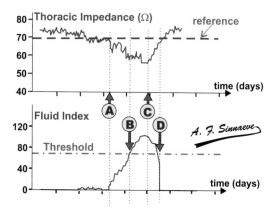

Abbreviations : CHF = congestive heart failure ;
RV = right ventricle

Figure 12.25

ICD FUNCTION with emphasis on STORED ELECTROGRAMS

 Medtronic Markers for ICDs

Guidant Marker Channel for ICDs

St Jude Medical Event Markers for ICDs

Representative examples of ICD function from 1 to 65

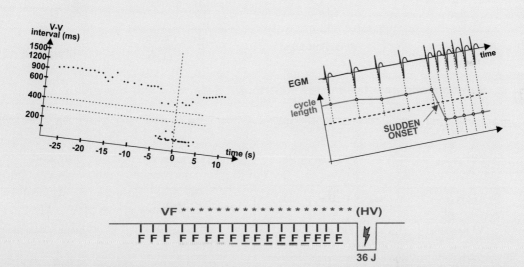

Figure 13.00

Difficult to memorize, you know !!!

MEDTRONIC MARKERS for ICDs

Symbols and annotations for bradyarrhythmia

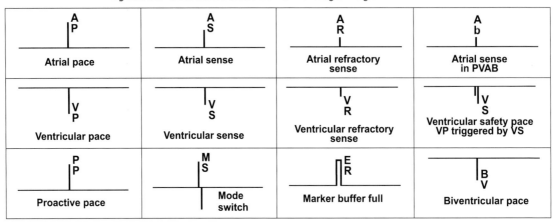

A P — Atrial pace	A S — Atrial sense	A R — Atrial refractory sense	A b — Atrial sense in PVAB
V P — Ventricular pace	V S — Ventricular sense	V R — Ventricular refractory sense	V S — Ventricular safety pace VP triggered by VS
P P — Proactive pace	M S — Mode switch	E R — Marker buffer full	B V — Biventricular pace

Symbols and annotations for atrial detection and therapies

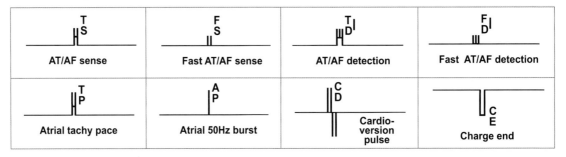

T S — AT/AF sense	F S — Fast AT/AF sense	T D — AT/AF detection	F D — Fast AT/AF detection
T P — Atrial tachy pace	A P — Atrial 50Hz burst	C D — Cardioversion pulse	C E — Charge end

Symbols and annotations for ventricular detection and therapies

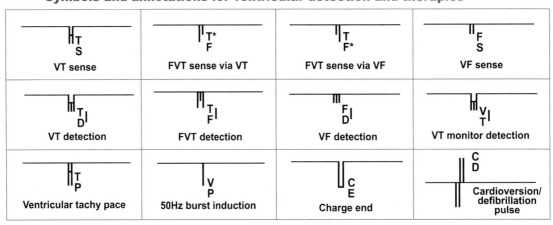

T S — VT sense	T* F — FVT sense via VT	T F* — FVT sense via VF	F S — VF sense
T D — VT detection	T F — FVT detection	F D — VF detection	V T — VT monitor detection
T P — Ventricular tachy pace	V P — 50Hz burst induction	C E — Charge end	C D — Cardioversion/ defibrillation pulse

Abbreviations : AF = atrial fibrillation; AT = atrial tachycardia; FVT= fast ventricular tachycardia; PVAB = postventricular atrial blanking; VF = ventricular fibrillation; VT = ventricular tachycardia;

Figure 13.01

GUIDANT MARKER CHANNEL for CRT-Devices (CRT-D)

ANNOTATIONS FOR THE ATRIAL CHANNEL

AS	A. Sense after refractory and AFR window
AS-Hy	A. Sense in hysteresis offset
AS-Fl	A. Sense in AFR window
(AS)	A. Sense during TARP
[AS]	A. Sense during blanking
AP	A. Pace - lower rate
AP↓	A. Pace - rate smoothing down
AP↑	A. Pace - rate smoothing up
AP-FB	A. Pace - fallback (in ATR)
AP-Hy	A. Pace at hysteresis rate
AP-Sr	A. Pace at sensor rate
AP→	A. Pace inserted after AFR
AP-Ns	A. Pace - noise (asynchronous pacing)
AP-Tr	A. Pace - trigger mode
AF	AF zone Sense
AN	Atrial rate noise
ATR↓	Atrial tachy sense - count down
ATR↑	Atrial tachy sense - count up
ATR-Dur	ATR Duration started
ATR-FB	ATR Fallback started
ATR-End	ATR Fallback ended
AFib	A Fib criteria met

ANNOTATIONS FOR THE VENTRICULAR CHANNEL

All the following annotations are preceded by an "R" for RIGHT or a "L" for LEFT.

VS	V. Sense after refractory
[VS]	V. Sense during blanking
VP	V. Pace at lower rate or atrial tracked
VP↓	V. Pace - rate smoothing down
VP↑	V. Pace - rate smoothing up
VP-FB	V. Pace - fallback (in ATR)
VP-Sr	V. Pace - sensor rate
VP-Hy	V. Pace at hysteresis rate
VP-MT	V. Pace - atrial tracked at MTR
VP-Ns	V. Pace - noise (asynchronous pacing)
VP-Tr	V. Pace - trigger mode
VP-VRR	V. Pace - ventricular rate regulation
VN	Ventricular rate noise

Inh-LVP	Left ventr. pace inhibited due to LVPP

PVC	PVC after refractory	Epsd	Start/End episode
VT-1	VT-1 Zone Sense	Dur	Duration met
VT	VT Zone Sense	Detct	Detection met
VF	VF Zone Sense	Chrg	Start/End charge
TN	Telemetry noise	Dvrt	Therapy diverted
VN	Ventricular rate noise	Shock	Shock delivered
PVP→	PVARP after PVC	SRD	Sustained rate duration expired
PMT-B	PMT termination	--	Unclassified event
V>A	Ventr. rate faster than atrial rate	#.#V	Amplitude threshold test
Stb	Stable	#.##ms	Pulse width threshold test
Unstb	Unstable	####	Interval (A-A or V-V or RV-LV)
Suddn	Sudden onset	>2s	Interval greater than 2 seconds
Gradl	Gradual onset	>10s	Interval greater than 10 seconds

Abbreviations :
AFR = atrial flutter response ; ATR = atrial tachy response ; MTR = maximum tracking rate ; PMT = pacemaker mediated tachycardia ; PVARP = postventricular atrial refractory period ; PVC = premature ventricular complex ; TARP = total atrial refractory period (AVI + PVARP) ; LVPP = left ventricular protection period

Figure 13.02

258

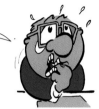

All manufacturers say their system is very logical and self-explanatory. But they are all different and I cannot afford any mistakes when I am using different systems. So I have to study them very carefully !

St JUDE MEDICAL MARKERS for ICDs

Symbols and annotations for bradyarrhythmia

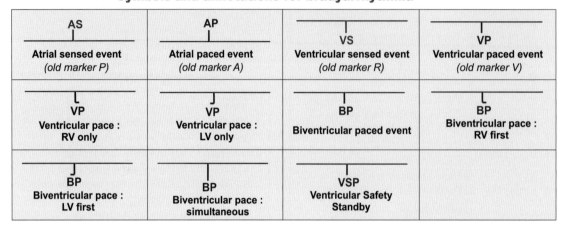

AS — Atrial sensed event *(old marker P)*	AP — Atrial paced event *(old marker A)*	VS — Ventricular sensed event *(old marker R)*	VP — Ventricular paced event *(old marker V)*
VP — Ventricular pace : RV only	VP — Ventricular pace : LV only	BP — Biventricular paced event	BP — Biventricular pace : RV first
BP — Biventricular pace : LV first	BP — Biventricular pace : simultaneous	VSP — Ventricular Safety Standby	

Bradyarrhythmia : special events markers

AMS .... Automatic mode switching
AFx .... AF suppression algorithm operation
SIR .... Activity sensor-indicated rate
HYS .... Rate hysteresis started by search timer or sensed event
Neg-HYS..... Negative AV-hysteresis search started
VIP.............. VIP search started

(VIP = Ventricular Intrinsic Preference : an algorithm which allows the ICD to search for intrinsic conduction.)

Episode trigger event markers

If an event triggers EGM storage, a vertical bar with a 'Trigger' flag appears at the trigger point

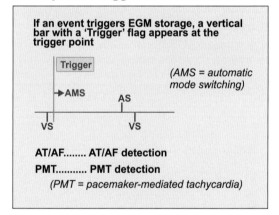

(AMS = automatic mode switching)

AT/AF........ AT/AF detection
PMT.......... PMT detection
(PMT = pacemaker-mediated tachycardia)

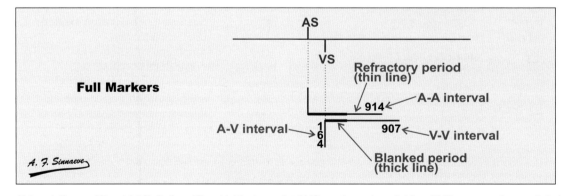

Full Markers — AS, VS, Refractory period (thin line), A-A interval, 914, A-V interval → 164, 907, V-V interval, Blanked period (thick line)

A. F. Sinnaeve

Abbreviations : AF = atrial fibrillation; AT = atrial tachycardia; AMS = auto mode switching; PMT = pacemaker mediated tachycardia; VF = ventricular fibrillation; VT = ventricular tachycardia;

Figure 13.03

Lucky me ! The marker legend is available in the technical manual or by a special command in the programmer.

St JUDE MEDICAL MARKERS for ICDs - con'd

Symbols and annotations for tachyarrhythmia

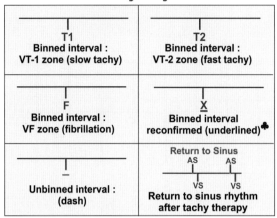

T1 Binned interval : VT-1 zone (slow tachy)	**T2** Binned interval : VT-2 zone (fast tachy)
F Binned interval : VF zone (fibrillation)	**X̲** Binned interval reconfirmed (underlined)♣
— Unbinned interval : (dash)	**Return to Sinus** AS AS VS VS **Return to sinus rhythm after tachy therapy**

♣ *Binned interval reconfirmed : "during charging"*

Morphology markers

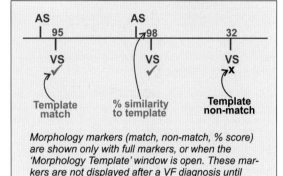

Template match — % similarity to template — Template non-match

Morphology markers (match, non-match, % score) are shown only with full markers, or when the 'Morphology Template' window is open. These markers are not displayed after a VF diagnosis until return to sinus is confirmed.

Tachy charge delivery markers

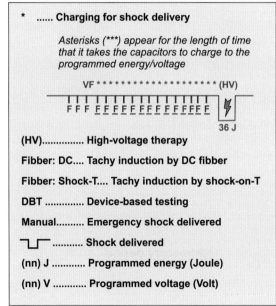

***** ...... Charging for shock delivery

Asterisks (***) appear for the length of time that it takes the capacitors to charge to the programmed energy/voltage

VF ******************** (HV)
F F F F̲ F̲ F̲ F̲ F̲ F̲ F̲ F̲ F̲ F̲ F̲ F̲ F̲ F̲ ⚡ 36 J

(HV).............. High-voltage therapy
Fibber: DC.... Tachy induction by DC fibber
Fibber: Shock-T.... Tachy induction by shock-on-T
DBT .... Device-based testing
Manual.......... Emergency shock delivered
⊓̅ .... Shock delivered
(nn) J .... Programmed energy (Joule)
(nn) V .... Programmed voltage (Volt)

A. F. Sinnaeve

Tachy detection, diagnosis, therapy

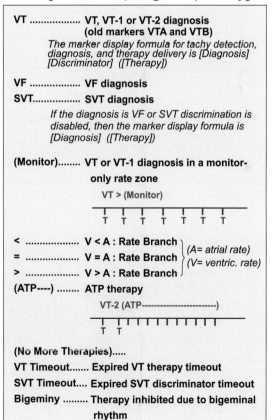

VT .... VT, VT-1 or VT-2 diagnosis (old markers VTA and VTB)
The marker display formula for tachy detection, diagnosis, and therapy delivery is [Diagnosis] [Discriminator] ([Therapy])

VF .... VF diagnosis
SVT................. SVT diagnosis
If the diagnosis is VF or SVT discrimination is disabled, then the marker display formula is [Diagnosis] ([Therapy])

(Monitor)........ VT or VT-1 diagnosis in a monitor-only rate zone
VT > (Monitor)
T T T   T   T   T   T

< .... V < A : Rate Branch
= .... V = A : Rate Branch   (A= atrial rate)
> .... V > A : Rate Branch   (V= ventric. rate)
(ATP----) .... ATP therapy
VT-2 (ATP--------------------------)
T T

(No More Therapies).....
VT Timeout....... Expired VT therapy timeout
SVT Timeout.... Expired SVT discriminator timeout
Bigeminy .... Therapy inhibited due to bigeminal rhythm

Figure 13.04

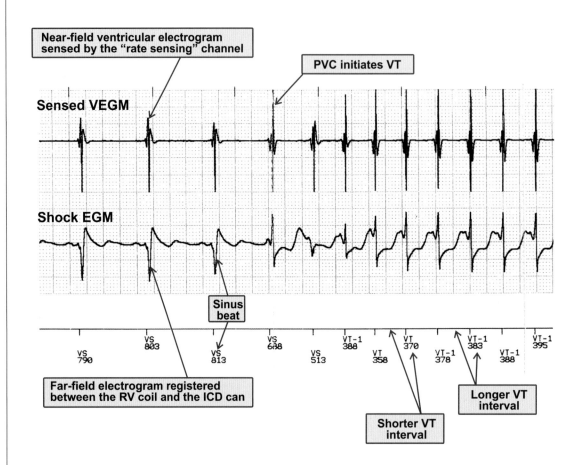

PVC STARTS VT IN A SINGLE CHAMBER ICD - CASE 1

Near-field ventricular electrogram sensed by the "rate sensing" channel

PVC initiates VT

Sensed VEGM

Shock EGM

Sinus beat

VS 790
VS 803
VS 813
VS 688
VS 513
VT-1 388
VT 358
VT 370
VT-1 378
VT-1 383
VT-1 388
VT-1 395

Far-field electrogram registered between the RV coil and the ICD can

Shorter VT interval

Longer VT interval

COMMENT :

The first three R waves are sensed sinus conducted beats (marked VS). A P wave precedes the R wave as seen on the shock EGM. A late PVC with a different morphology occurs 688 ms after the third R wave and starts a VT. The fourth R wave may be a fusion beat. The VT with a rate of approximately 150 bpm shows slight cycle length variation. A short cycle falls within the VT zone (labeled VT) and the longer cycles fall in the VT-1 zone.

Figure 13.05

T WAVE SENSING DURING EXERCISE - CASE 2

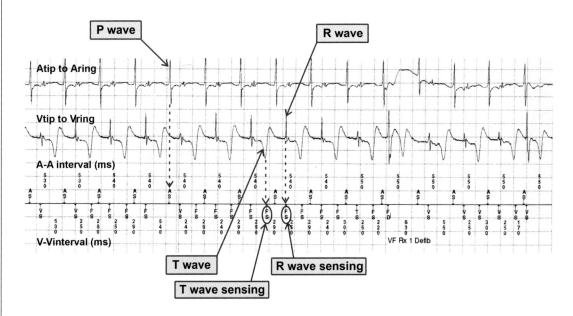

The top tracing, recorded from the atrial channel, shows a regular sinus rhythm. The middle tracing is recorded between the tip and the ring of the pacing/sensing lead. As the T wave is sensed, there is double counting (R waves and T waves) resulting in short V-V intervals interpreted by the device as ventricular fibrillation (labeled FS).

VT/VF Episode #8 Report

ID#	Date/Time	Type	V. Cycle	Last Rx	Success	Duration
8	Jun 19 14:11:56	VF	250 ms	VF Rx 5	Yes	6.1 min

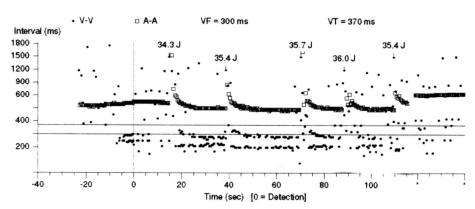

As the T waves were counted just as R waves, the resulting short intervals were interpreted as ventricular fibrillation and treated by multiple shocks.

Figure 13.06

DUAL TACHYCARDIA   AF & VF   -   CASE 3

The top tracing is the atrial EGM and shows atrial fibrillation (AF). A premature ventricular contraction (PVC) started a ventricular tachycardia (VT) that deteriorated into ventricular fibrillation (VF).

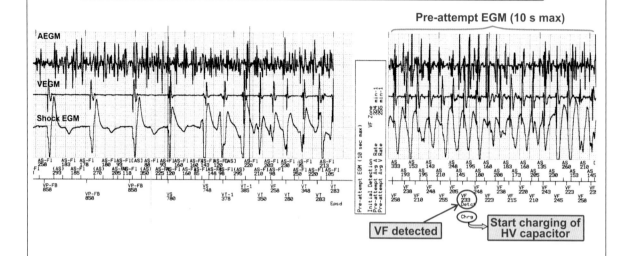

Pre-attempt EGM (10 s max)

VF detected

Start charging of HV capacitor

Two tachycardias were present : atrial fibrillation (AF) and ventricular fibrillation (VF). After detection of VF the ICD delivered a shock restoring sinus rhythm.

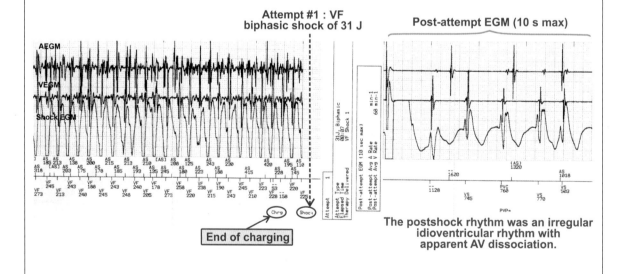

Attempt #1 : VF biphasic shock of 31 J

Post-attempt EGM (10 s max)

End of charging

The postshock rhythm was an irregular idioventricular rhythm with apparent AV dissociation.

Figure 13.07

ANTITACHYCARDIA PACING (ATP) - CASE 4

(Medtronic - GEM 7227)

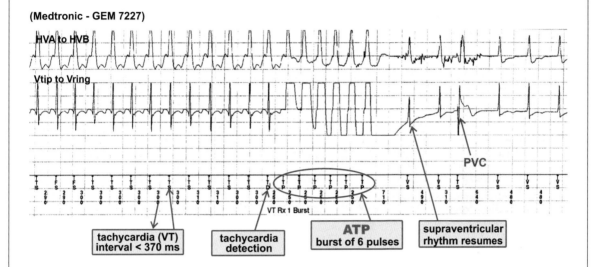

tachycardia (VT) interval < 370 ms

tachycardia detection

ATP burst of 6 pulses

supraventricular rhythm resumes

PVC

VT Rx 1 Burst

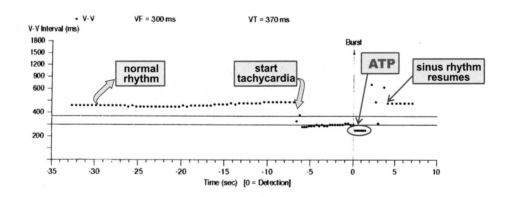

ICD Model: Gem 7227

VT/VF Episode #5 Report

ID#	Date/Time	Type	V. Cycle	Last Rx	Success	Duration
5	May 03 14:30:04	VT	300 ms	VT Rx 1	Yes	9 sec

normal rhythm

start tachycardia

ATP

sinus rhythm resumes

COMMENT :

The top tracing (HVA to HVB) was recorded between the can and the distal coil (shock EGM)
The lower tracing was recorded between the tip and the ring of the sensing lead (VEGM).
The VT zone was programmed with a cutoff rate of 162 bpm (370 ms) and a VF cutoff rate of
200 bpm (300 ms). The number of intervals to detect (NID) was 16.
The tiered therapy for tachycardias detected in the VT zone was 3 sequences of burst pacing
(ATP) followed by 5 shocks of 35 J with a configuration AX > B, i.e. from CAN (anode) to RV
(cathode).
In this case a VT with a cycle length of 300 ms was detected and successful treated with the
first burst consisting of 6 pacing pulses. The first paced beat of the burst started with a R-S1
interval of 84% of the preceding interval (300 ms x 0.84 = 252 ms round off to 250 ms).
The first burst stopped the tachycardia and restored sinus rhythm.

Figure 13.08

NOISE DETECTED AS VF - CASE 5

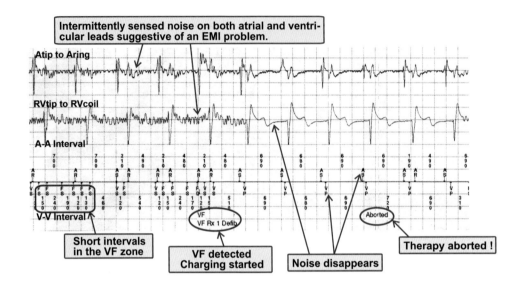

Intermittently sensed noise on both atrial and ventricular leads suggestive of an EMI problem.

Atip to Aring

RVtip to RVcoil

A-A Interval

V-V Interval

Short intervals in the VF zone

VF detected
Charging started

Noise disappears

Therapy aborted !

ICD Model: InSync Marquis 7277
Serial Number:

VT/VF Episode #3 Report

ID#	Date/Time	Type	V. Cycle	Last Rx	Success	Duration
3	Nov 24 11:45:12	VF	170 ms	(No Rx Delivered)		7 sec

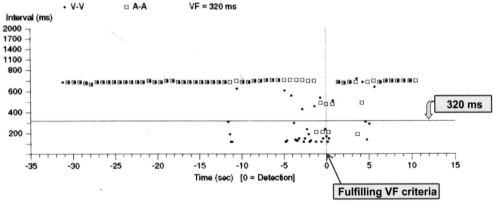

• V-V   □ A-A   VF = 320 ms

Interval (ms)

Time (sec) [0 = Detection]

320 ms

Fulfilling VF criteria

Figure 13.09

ATRIAL FIBRILLATION - CASE 6

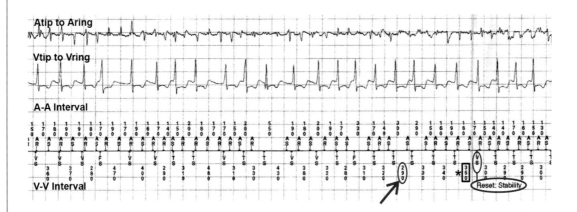

COMMENT :

The atrial channel shows atrial fibrillation with short A-A intervals. There is a varying degree of conduction to the ventricles. Since the ventricular rhythm is irregular, no therapy is delivered. In the Medtronic algorithm an interval is declared unstable if the difference between it and any of the 3 previous intervals is greater than the programmed stability interval. The ICD does not apply the stability option until the VT count reaches at least 3. When the ICD classifies an interval as unstable, it is indicated with a VS marker closing the cycle. The VS marker resets the VT count to zero.

The TS-VS cycle on the right (*) was declared an unstable cycle by the device. Note that its cycle length is 350 ms which is shorter than the tachycardia detection interval of 360 ms. Yet, the ICD did not declare the 350 ms cycle as a tachycardia sense cycle. Rather, the stability algorithm labeled the 350 ms cycle as unstable thereby terminating it with a VS marker and resetting the VT counter to zero.

ICD Model: Maximo DR 7278
Serial Number.

SVT/NST Episode #69 Report

ID#	Date/Time	A. Cycle	V. Cycle	Duration	Reason
69	Aug 18 17:59:36	160 ms	290 ms	15 sec	Stability

• V-V   ▫ A-A   VF = 290 ms   VT = 360 ms

Interval (ms)

labeled as VF

labeled as VT

360 ms

290 ms

Time (sec) [0 = Collection Start]

Figure 13.10

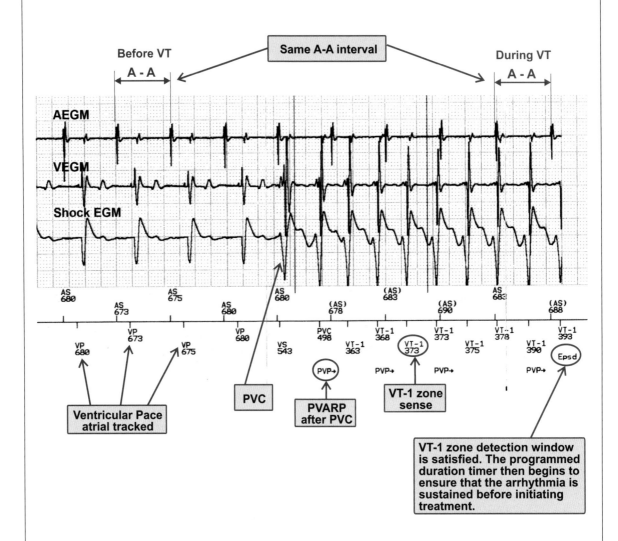

VENTRICULAR TACHYCARDIA (VT)
AV DISSOCIATION - CASE 7

Same A-A interval

Before VT — A - A

During VT — A - A

AEGM

VEGM

Shock EGM

AS 680 | AS 673 | AS 675 | AS 680 | AS 680 | (AS) 678 | (AS) 683 | (AS) 690 | AS 683 | (AS) 688

VP 680 | VP 673 | VP 675 | VP 680 | VS 543 | PVC 498 | VT-1 363 | VT-1 368 | VT-1 373 | VT-1 373 | VT-1 375 | VT-1 378 | VT-1 390 | VT-1 393 | Epsd

PVP→ | PVP→ | PVP→ | PVP→

Ventricular Pace atrial tracked

PVC

PVARP after PVC

VT-1 zone sense

VT-1 zone detection window is satisfied. The programmed duration timer then begins to ensure that the arrhythmia is sustained before initiating treatment.

COMMENT :

The atrial electrogram (AEGM) shows a regular sinus rhythm at a rate of 87 bpm.
A premature ventricular complex (PVC; different morphology) initiates a ventricular tachycardia (VT) at a rate of 152 bpm. The atrial electrogram remains unchanged during the VT and AV dissociation is observed. This proves the ventricular origin of the tachycardia.
Note that the duration timer is a feature of Boston Scientific (Guidant) devices.

Figure 13.11

1 : 1 TACHYCARDIA -   CASE 8

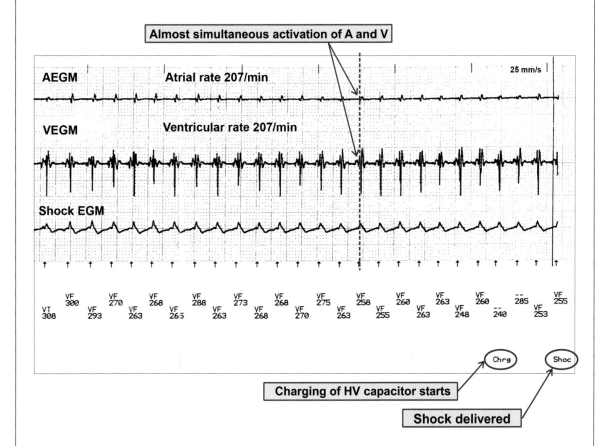

Almost simultaneous activation of A and V

AEGM   Atrial rate 207/min   25 mm/s

VEGM   Ventricular rate 207/min

Shock EGM

Charging of HV capacitor starts

Shock delivered

COMMENT :

A tachycardia at a rate of 207 bpm is detected in the VF zone triggering a shock. As the atrial rate is identical to the ventricular rate, the differential diagnosis has to be made between a VT with 1:1 retrograde VA conduction and a slow-fast AV nodal reentrant tachycardia (AVNRT) and an atrial tachycardia (AT) with first degree AV block .

The almost simultaneous activation of atria and ventricles favors the diagnosis of AVNRT.

Figure 13.12

VENTRICULAR TACHYCARDIA & ATP - CASE 9

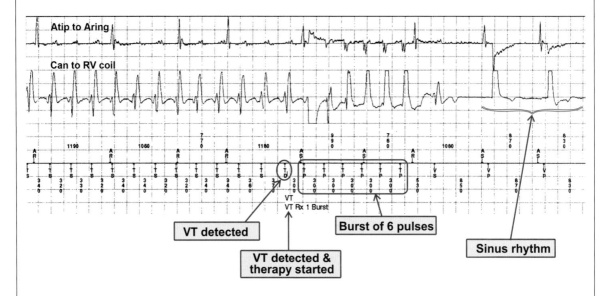

ICD Model: InSync Marquis 7277
Serial Number:

VT/VF Episode #5 Report

ID#	Date/Time	Type	V. Cycle	Last Rx	Success	Duration
5	Jul 28 20:36:04	VT	350 ms	VT Rx 1	Yes	7 sec

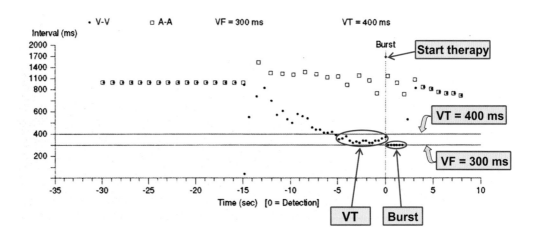

COMMENT :
Episode of ventricular tachycardia (VT) successfully treated with antitachypacing (ATP)

Figure 13.13

SINUS TACHYCARDIA (ST) - CASE 10

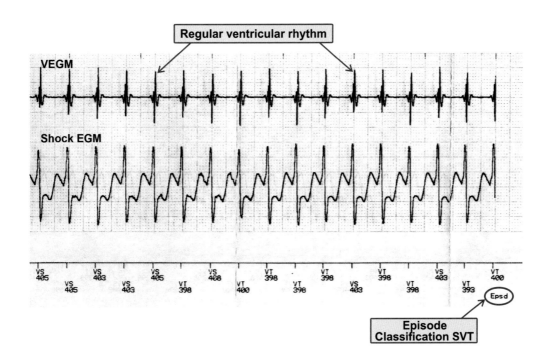

Regular ventricular rhythm

VEGM

Shock EGM

Episode
Classification SVT

COMMENT :

During exercise the rhythm accelerated to 151 bpm and was detected in the VT zone.
The episode was logged as SVT by the ICD as there was a gradual acceleration of
the rhythm.

Figure 13.14

VENTRICULAR TACHYCARDIA ACCELERATION - CASE 11

A VT was detected and a shock was delivered. The tachycardia accelerated post-shock and stopped spontaneously.

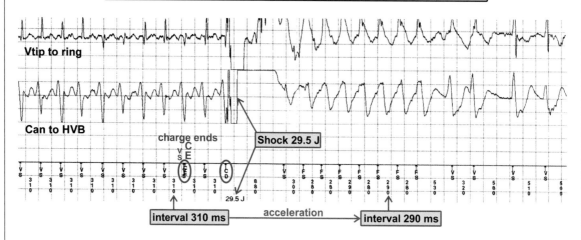

Vtip to ring

Can to HVB

charge ends
CE
V
S

Shock 29.5 J

interval 310 ms   acceleration   interval 290 ms

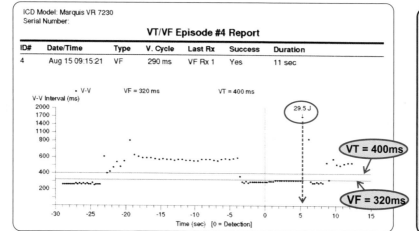

ICD Model: Marquis VR 7230
Serial Number:

VT/VF Episode #4 Report

ID#	Date/Time	Type	V. Cycle	Last Rx	Success	Duration
4	Aug 15 09:15:21	VF	290 ms	VF Rx 1	Yes	11 sec

V-V
VF = 320 ms   VT = 400 ms

V-V Interval (ms)

29.5 J

VT = 400ms

VF = 320ms

Time (sec) [0 = Detection]

Thirty minutes prior to the shock there was another episode of VT that terminated spontaneously. The last episode of VT was treated by a shock because it lasted longer. After the shock the VT accelerated and then terminated spontaneously. This VT would be best treated with ATP rather than a shock. In the setting of unsustained VT the number of intervals for detection can be increased to promote spontaneous VT termination. This approach may prevent unnecessary shocks.

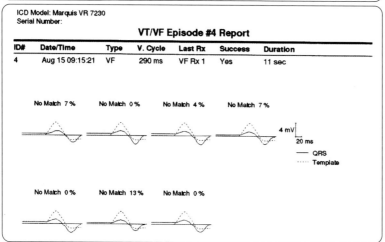

ICD Model: Marquis VR 7230
Serial Number:

VT/VF Episode #4 Report

ID#	Date/Time	Type	V. Cycle	Last Rx	Success	Duration
4	Aug 15 09:15:21	VF	290 ms	VF Rx 1	Yes	11 sec

No Match 7 %   No Match 0 %   No Match 4 %   No Match 7 %

4 mV
20 ms

— QRS
···· Template

No Match 0 %   No Match 13 %   No Match 0 %

During tachycardia the QRS complex is different from the template and the match is very low

Figure 13.15

FAR-FIELD OVERSENSING of the P WAVE - CASE 12

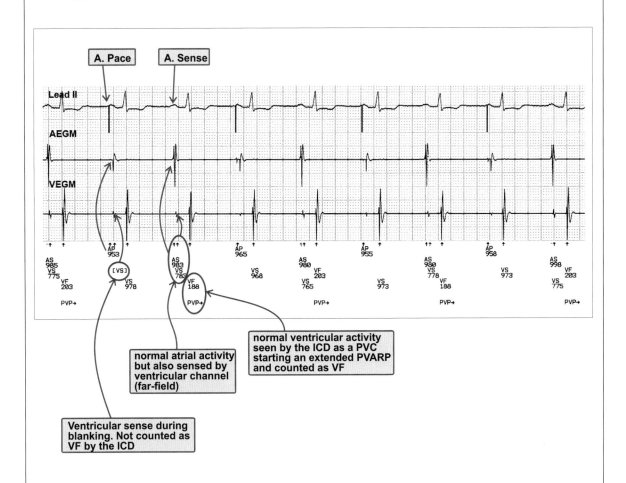

COMMENT :

Sinus (AS, VS) and atrial pacing (AP) followed by conducted QRS (VS).
There is far-field sensing of the spontaneous P wave by the ventricular channel
suggesting the distal coil of the shocking lead to be located too close to the tricuspid valve in the setting of normal atrial pacing and sensing which rules out
atrial lead displacement. This tracing shows how the high ventricular sensitivity of ICDs predisposes to ventricular sensing of small far-field atrial signals.
This form of oversensing can be catastrophic in patients with complete AV
block because of ventricular inhibition. This problem would not cause inappropriate shocks in devices using counting of consecutive short intervals or a
percentage of short intervals (x out of y).

Figure 13.16

VF INDUCTION by AC CURRENT - CASE 13

During implantation ventricular fibrillation (VF) is induced by applying alternating current (AC)

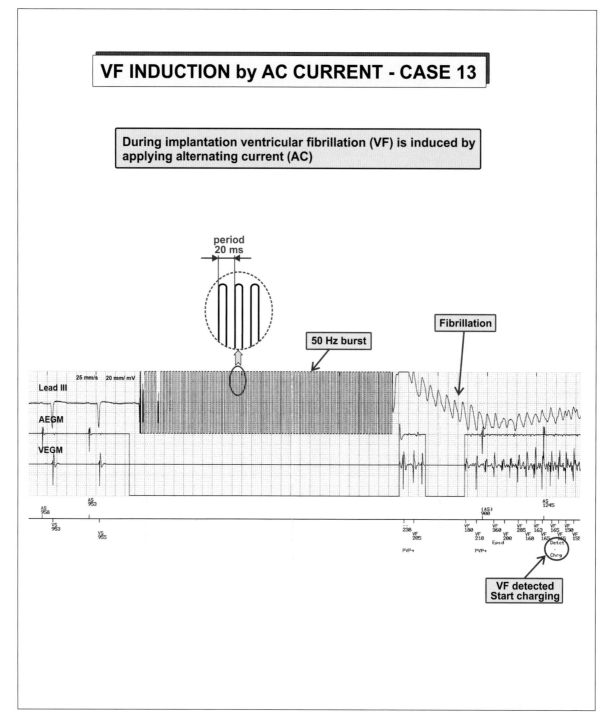

Figure 13.17

VF INDUCTION by SHOCK & ICD TESTING - CASE 14

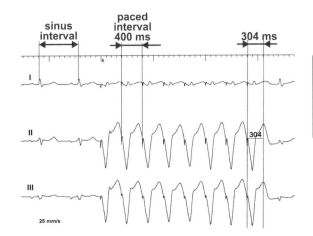

To determine the vulnerable period it is important to determine exactly the peak of the T wave.
Here, the ventricle is paced at a rate of 150 bpm. The peak of the T wave is located at 304 ms after the stimulus.

After a ventricular pacing train at 150 bpm, a shock of 1 J is delivered on the peak of the T wave inducing a tachycardia (seen as VF by the device)

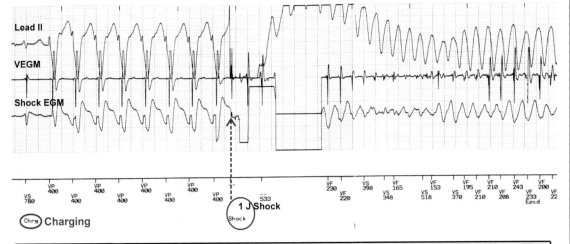

With the least value of sensitivity programmed, the VF is sensed accurately and a 20 J shock terminates the tachycardia.

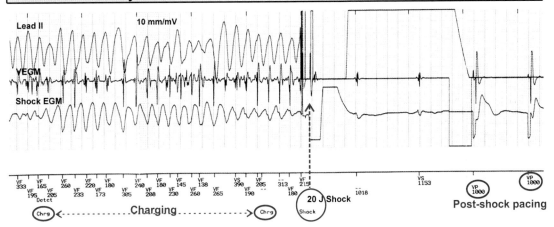

Figure 13.18

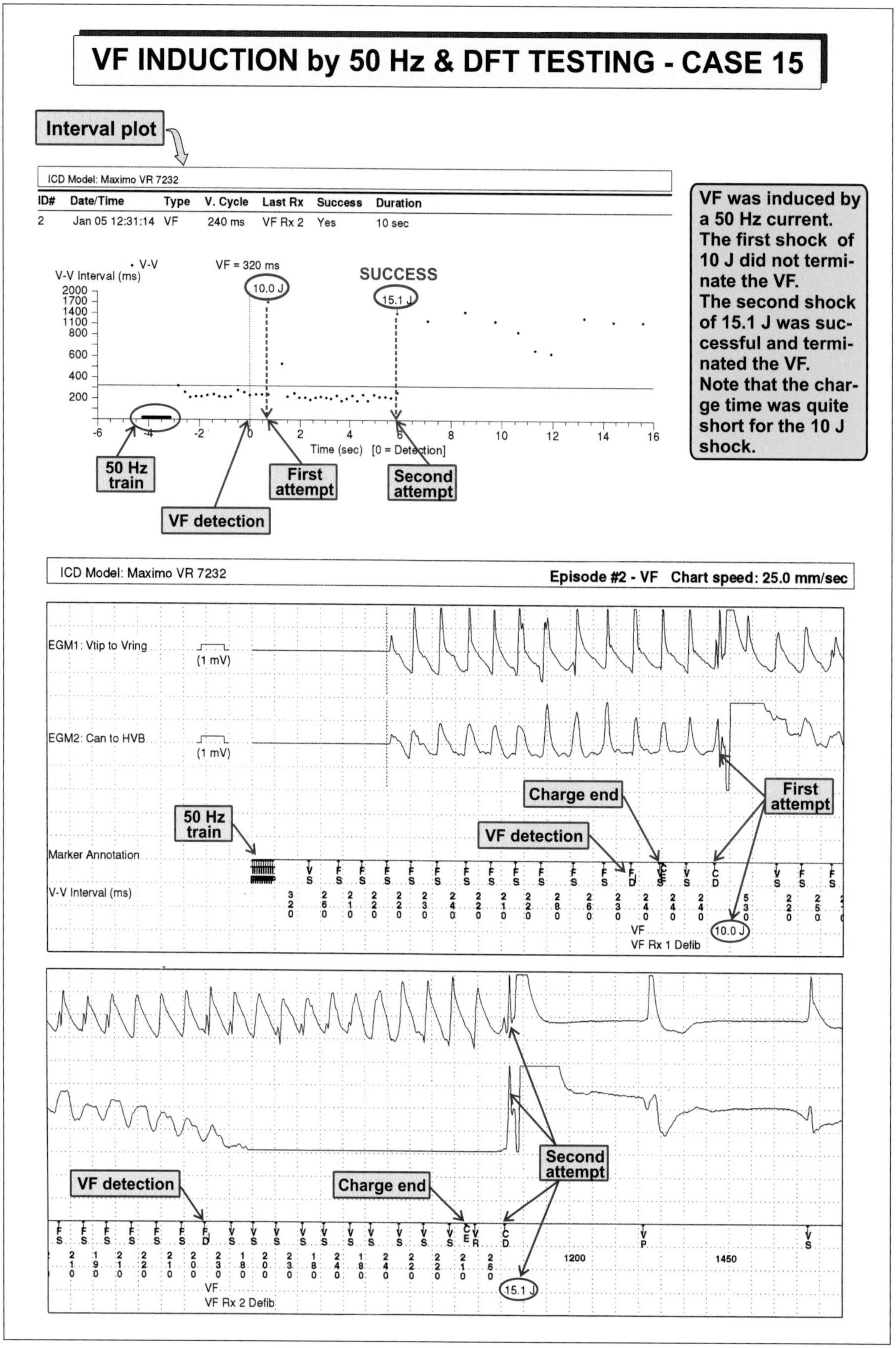

VF INDUCTION by 50 Hz & DFT TESTING - CASE 15

Interval plot

ICD Model: Maximo VR 7232

ID#	Date/Time	Type	V. Cycle	Last Rx	Success	Duration
2	Jan 05 12:31:14	VF	240 ms	VF Rx 2	Yes	10 sec

VF was induced by a 50 Hz current. The first shock of 10 J did not terminate the VF. The second shock of 15.1 J was successful and terminated the VF. Note that the charge time was quite short for the 10 J shock.

V-V Interval (ms)
• V-V
VF = 320 ms
10.0 J
SUCCESS
15.1 J

2000
1700
1400
1100
800
600
400
200

-6 -4 -2 0 2 4 6 8 10 12 14 16
Time (sec) [0 = Detection]

50 Hz train

First attempt

Second attempt

VF detection

ICD Model: Maximo VR 7232   Episode #2 - VF   Chart speed: 25.0 mm/sec

EGM1: Vtip to Vring
(1 mV)

EGM2: Can to HVB
(1 mV)

Charge end

First attempt

VF detection

50 Hz train

Marker Annotation

V-V Interval (ms)

| V S | F S | F S | F S | F S | F S | F S | F S | F S | F S | F D | C E | V S | V S | C D | V S | F S | F S |
| 320 | 260 | 220 | 220 | 220 | 230 | 240 | 220 | 210 | 280 | 260 | 230 | 240 | 240 | 530 | 200 | 220 | 250 |

VF
VF Rx 1 Defib
10.0 J

VF detection

Charge end

Second attempt

| F S | F S | F S | F S | F S | F D | V S | V S | V S | V S | V S | V S | V S | V S | C E R | V S | C D | V P | V S |
| 200 | 190 | 220 | 210 | 200 | 230 | 180 | 230 | 180 | 240 | 180 | 240 | 210 | 260 | | | | | |

VF
VF Rx 2 Defib
15.1 J
1200   1450

Figure 13.19

ELECTRICAL STORM & UNSUCCESSFUL ATP
CASE 16 - part 1

Recurrent VT during an electrical storm. After five sequences of burst pacing, the tachycardia was still not terminated. Three episodes of ramp pacing were also unsuccessful. The third sequence of ramp pacing temporarily terminated the tachycardia that restarted after a few beats.
Finally a shock of 35 joule terminated the tachycardia.

ICD Model: Maximo VR 7232
Serial Number:

VT/VF Episode #14 Report

ID#	Date/Time	Type	V. Cycle	Last Rx	Success	Duration
14	Dec 29 06:37:39	VT	350 ms	VT Rx 3	Yes	1.4 min

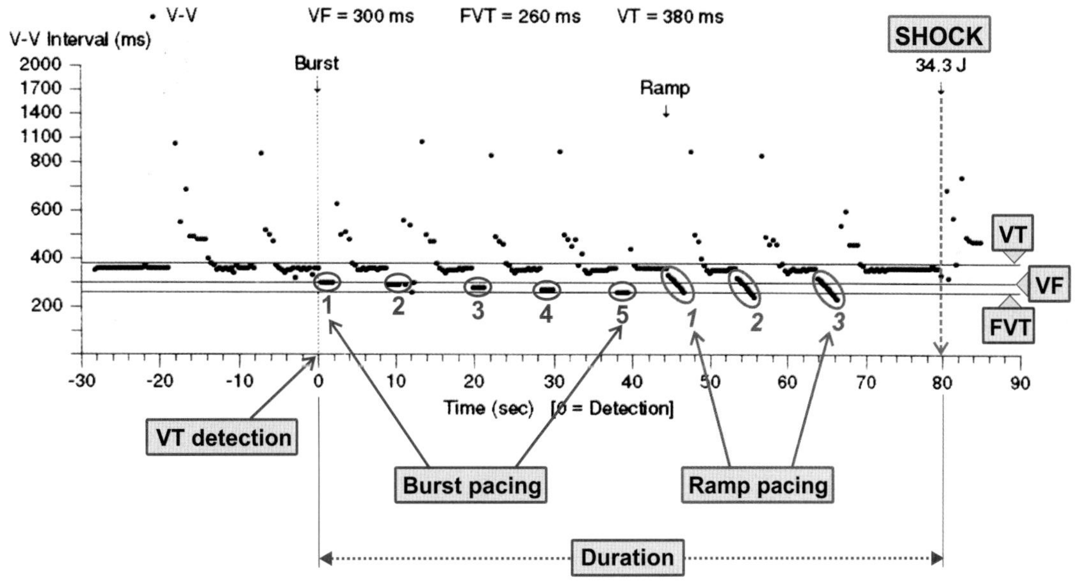

Figure 13.20

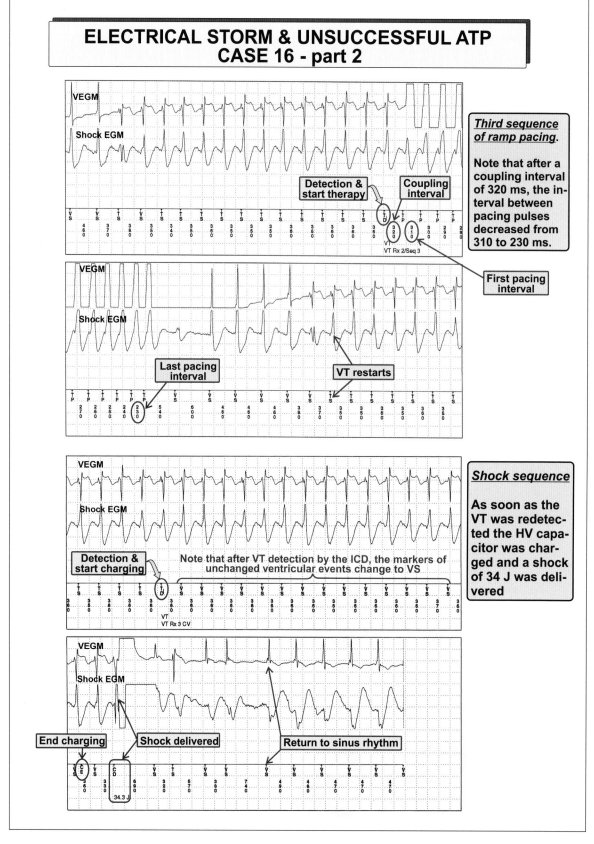

ELECTRICAL STORM & UNSUCCESSFUL ATP
CASE 16 - part 2

Figure 13.21

SINUS TACHYCARDIA
THERAPY WITHHELD BY PR LOGIC - CASE 17

A tachycardia was sensed in the VT zone but was labeled sinus tachycardia (ST) by the PR Logic (Medtronic).

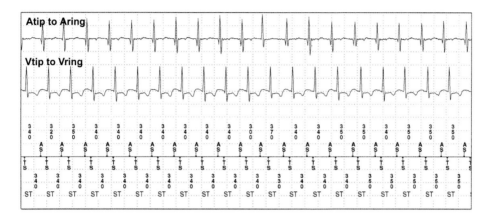

SVT/NST Episode #32 Report

ICD Model: Intrinsic 7288   Serial Number:

ID#	Date/Time	A. Cycle	V. Cycle	Duration	Reason
32	Apr 15 10:23:34	350 ms	340 ms	2.3 min	Sinus Tach

Interval plot

Therapy was withheld by the PR logic although the tachycardia was detected in the VT zone.

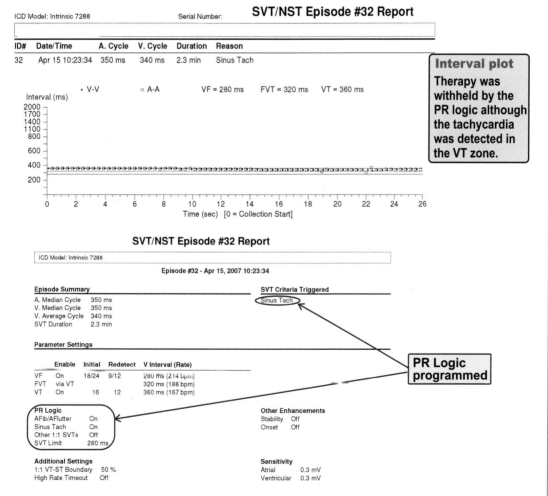

• V-V   □ A-A   VF = 280 ms   FVT = 320 ms   VT = 360 ms

Interval (ms)

Time (sec) [0 = Collection Start]

SVT/NST Episode #32 Report

ICD Model: Intrinsic 7288

Episode #32 - Apr 15, 2007 10:23:34

Episode Summary

A. Median Cycle	350 ms
V. Median Cycle	350 ms
V. Average Cycle	340 ms
SVT Duration	2.3 min

SVT Criteria Triggered

Sinus Tach

Parameter Settings

	Enable	Initial	Redetect	V Interval (Rate)
VF	On	18/24	9/12	280 ms (214 bpm)
FVT	via VT			320 ms (188 bpm)
VT	On	16	12	360 ms (167 bpm)

PR Logic

AFib/AFlutter	On
Sinus Tach	On
Other 1:1 SVTs	Off
SVT Limit	280 ms

PR Logic programmed

Other Enhancements

Stability	Off
Onset	Off

Additional Settings

1:1 VT-ST Boundary	50 %
High Rate Timeout	Off

Sensitivity

Atrial	0.3 mV
Ventricular	0.3 mV

Figure 13.22

SINUS TACHYCARDIA WITH LONG PR MISINTERPRETED AS VT - CASE 18

The PR-Logic algorithm (Medtronic) separates the 1:1 VT-ST boundary into anterograde and retrograde zones. Its nominal value is set at 50%. The tachycardia was misinterpreted as VT and therapy was delivered. Increasing the setting to 66% no longer resulted in inappropriate therapy.

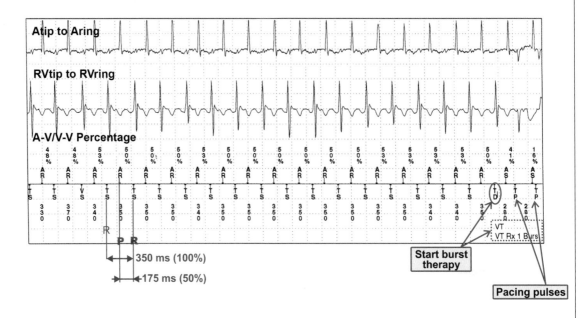

Sinus tachycardia with a relatively long PR interval (175 ms) for this fast rate and circomstances was misclassified as VT by the PR-Logic. Inappropriate therapy was delivered consisting of ATP and shocks until exhaustion of therapy. Increasing the setting to 66% no longer resulted in inappropriate therapy.

ICD Model: InSync Sentry 7298
Serial Number:

VT/VF Episode #4 Report

ID#	Date/Time	Type	V. Cycle	Last Rx	Success	Duration
4	Jan 23 12:52:07	VT	340 ms	VF Rx 1	No	4.7 min

Figure 13.23

ATRIAL FLUTTER TREATED AS VT - CASE 19

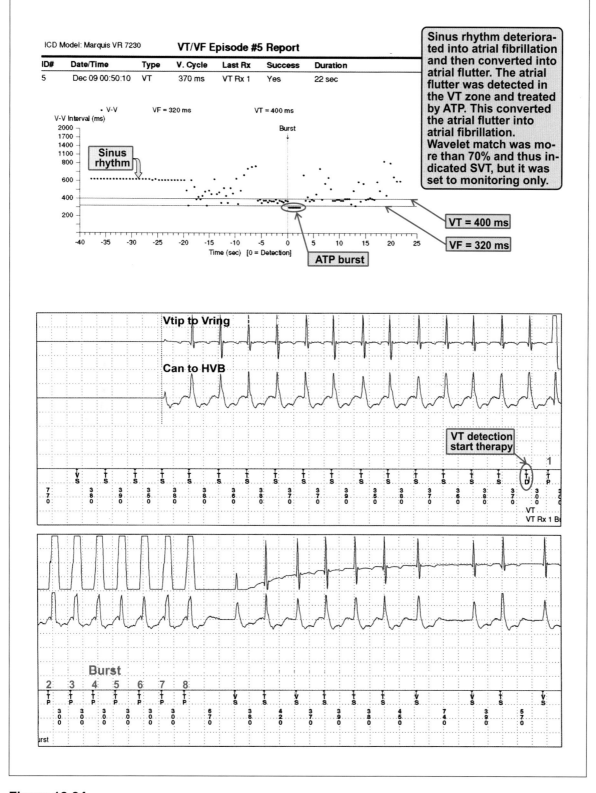

Figure 13.24

VT with RETROGRADE CONDUCTION - CASE 20

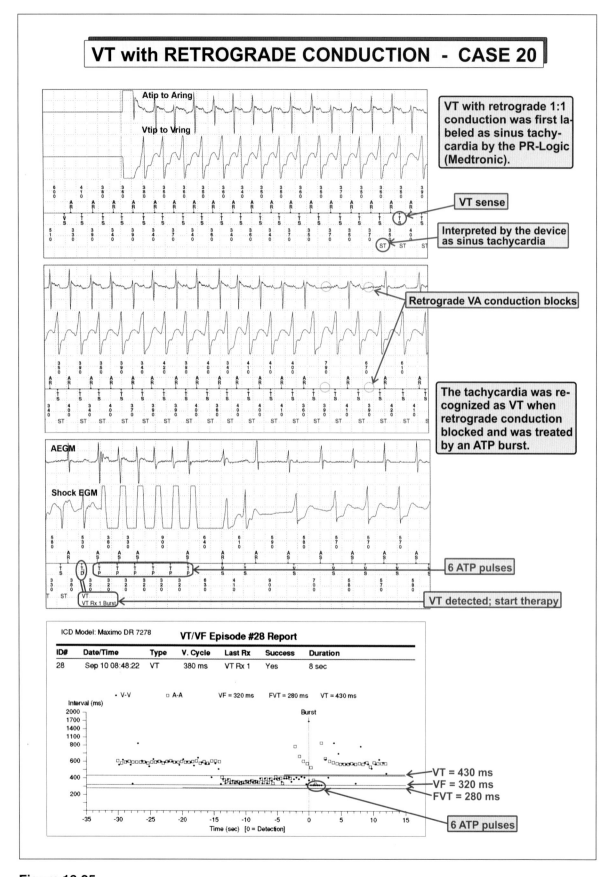

Figure 13.25

VT ACCELERATED BY ATP - CASE 21

A ventricular tachycardia (VT) was treated by ATP that accelerated the VT

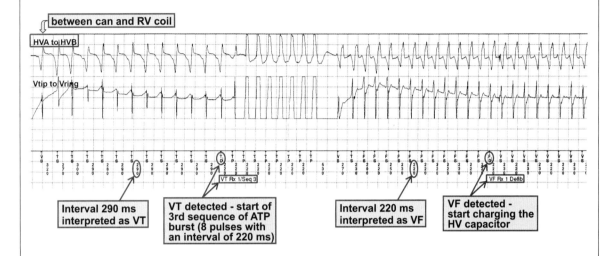

between can and RV coil

HVA to HVB

Vtip to Vring

VT Rx 1/Seq 3

VF Rx 1 Defib

Interval 290 ms interpreted as VT

VT detected - start of 3rd sequence of ATP burst (8 pulses with an interval of 220 ms)

Interval 220 ms interpreted as VF

VF detected - start charging the HV capacitor

A VT was treated by 3 bursts of ATP with each fixed burst showing a progressively shorter coupling interval/pacing interval compared to the previous burst. The last sequence of ATP (i.e. the fastest burst) accelerated the VT into the VF zone and finally it was successfully treated by a 35 J shock.

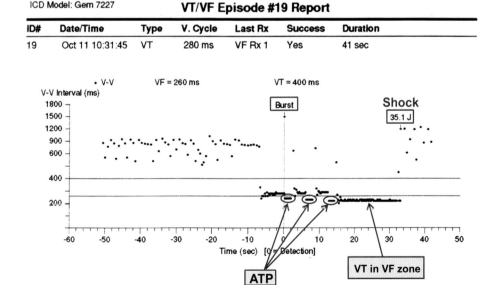

ICD Model: Gem 7227

VT/VF Episode #19 Report

ID#	Date/Time	Type	V. Cycle	Last Rx	Success	Duration
19	Oct 11 10:31:45	VT	280 ms	VF Rx 1	Yes	41 sec

• V-V   VF = 260 ms   VT = 400 ms

V-V Interval (ms)

Burst

Shock

35.1 J

Time (sec) [0 = Detection]

ATP

VT in VF zone

Figure 13.26

ICD RESPONSE TO EMI - CASE 22 - part 1

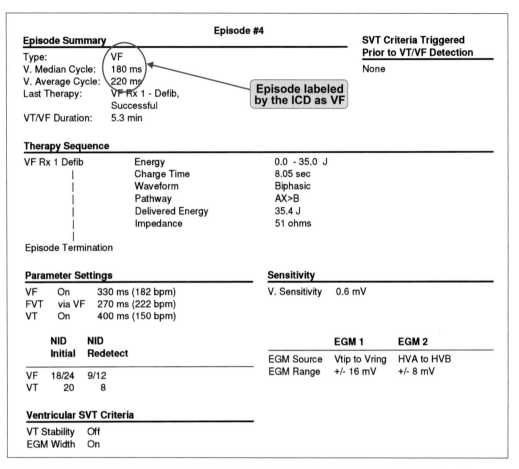

Episode #4

Episode Summary

Type: VF
V. Median Cycle: 180 ms
V. Average Cycle: 220 ms
Last Therapy: VF Rx 1 - Defib,
                    Successful
VT/VF Duration: 5.3 min

Episode labeled by the ICD as VF

SVT Criteria Triggered Prior to VT/VF Detection

None

Therapy Sequence

VF Rx 1 Defib   Energy   0.0 - 35.0 J
                     Charge Time   8.05 sec
                     Waveform   Biphasic
                     Pathway   AX>B
                     Delivered Energy 35.4 J
                     Impedance   51 ohms

Episode Termination

Parameter Settings

VF   On   330 ms (182 bpm)
FVT   via VF 270 ms (222 bpm)
VT   On   400 ms (150 bpm)

	NID Initial	NID Redetect
VF	18/24	9/12
VT	20	8

Ventricular SVT Criteria

VT Stability   Off
EGM Width   On

Sensitivity

V. Sensitivity   0.6 mV

	EGM 1	EGM 2
EGM Source	Vtip to Vring	HVA to HVB
EGM Range	+/- 16 mV	+/- 8 mV

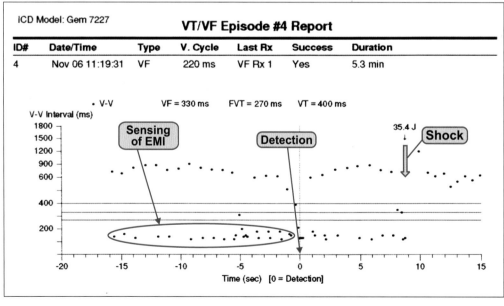

ICD Model: Gem 7227

VT/VF Episode #4 Report

ID#	Date/Time	Type	V. Cycle	Last Rx	Success	Duration
4	Nov 06 11:19:31	VF	220 ms	VF Rx 1	Yes	5.3 min

• V-V   VF = 330 ms   FVT = 270 ms   VT = 400 ms

Sensing of EMI   Detection   35.4 J   Shock

Figure 13.27

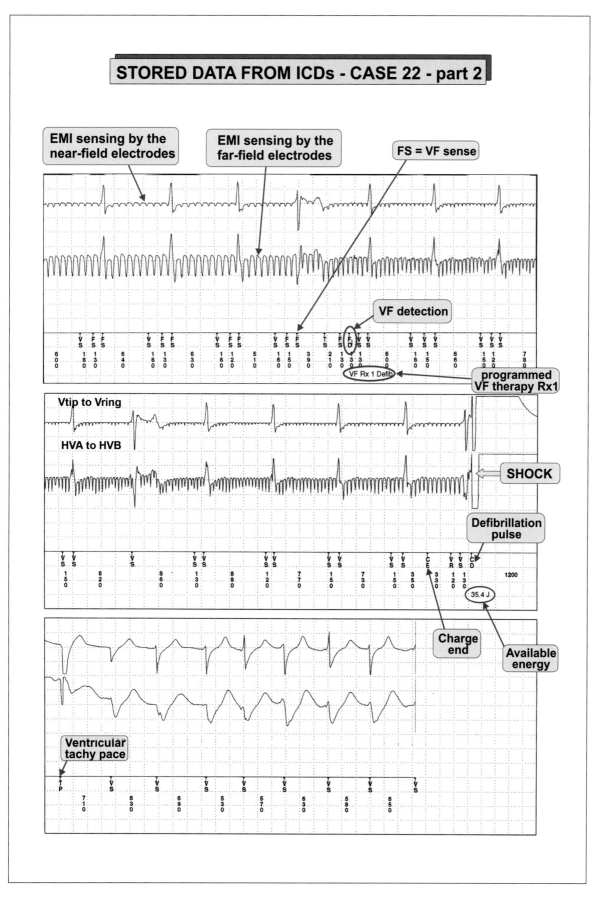

STORED DATA FROM ICDs - CASE 22 - part 2

EMI sensing by the near-field electrodes

EMI sensing by the far-field electrodes

FS = VF sense

VF detection

programmed VF therapy Rx1

Vtip to Vring

HVA to HVB

SHOCK

Defibrillation pulse

Charge end

Available energy

Ventricular tachy pace

Figure 13.28

ICD RESPONSE TO EMI - CASE 22 - part 3

Comment :

The EMI was due to contact with a vacuum cleaner with a defective grounding causing an excessive leakage current. After delivery of the shock the patient loosed contact with the defective device and the EMI stoped.

After VF detection (FD marker) the ICD started a reconfirmation process based upon a calculated interval i.e. : the programmed VT interval + 60 ms or the VF interval + 60 ms if no VT zone was programmed. Since a VT zone (400 ms) was programmed, detection during reconfirmation was based on a detection interval of 400 + 60 ms. Detected intervals longer than 460 ms are labeled "normal", shorter intervals are labeled "arrhythmic". After each new ventricular event, the ICD looks to the last 5 intervals. To abort the shock, 4 out of the last 5 intervals must be labeled "normal", i.e. longer than 460 ms. In the reconfirmation episode there were never more than 3 intervals out of 5 that are longer than 460 ms. Therefore, after charging the HV capacitor (CE marker) the shock was delivered (CD marker).

Figure 13.29

ICD TESTING AT IMPLANTATION - CASE 23

VF was induced by a pacing train of 8 ventricular stimuli at a rate of 150 bpm. The eighth stimulus coincided with a PVC. A shock of 311V on the T wave of the PVC (280 ms after the R wave) induced VF. VF was appropriately sensed at the least programmable sensitivity (12 cycles in VF zone, marked F) .

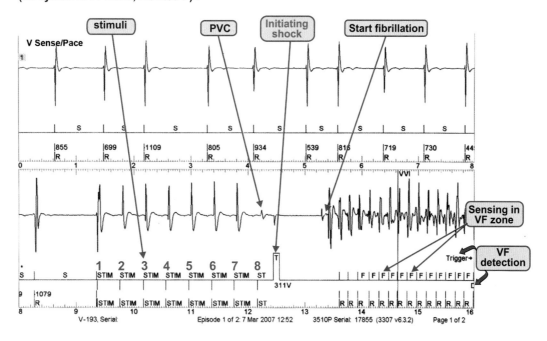

After reconfirmation (marked R) a shock of 490 V terminated VF. The ICD released the programmed shock because VF was reconfirmed (requiring at least 6 appropriate intervals).

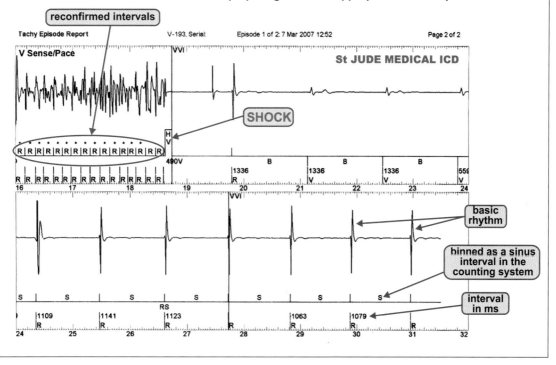

Figure 13.30

ATRIAL FIBRILLATION & STABILITY DISCRIMINATION
CASE 24 - part 1

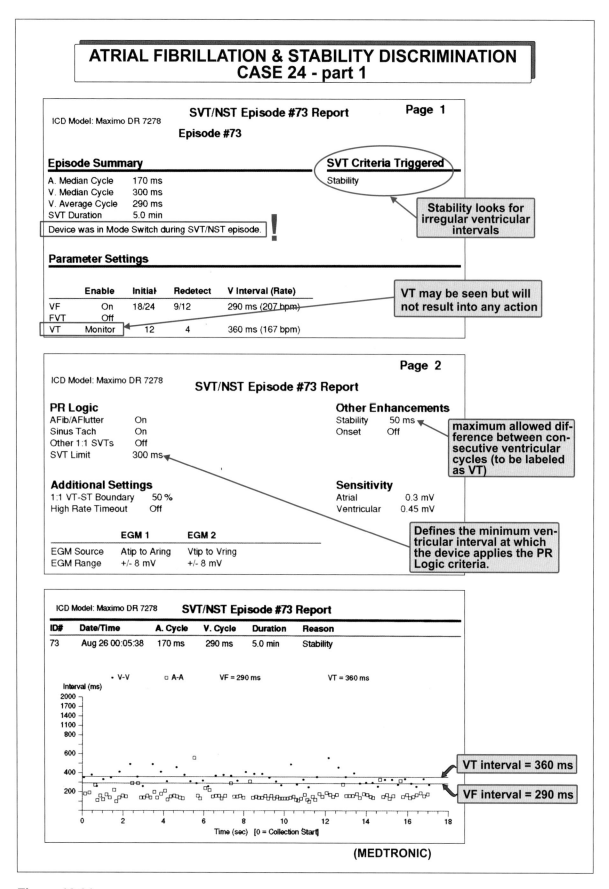

SVT/NST Episode #73 Report   Page 1

ICD Model: Maximo DR 7278

Episode #73

Episode Summary   **SVT Criteria Triggered**

A. Median Cycle   170 ms   Stability
V. Median Cycle   300 ms
V. Average Cycle   290 ms   *Stability looks for irregular ventricular intervals*
SVT Duration   5.0 min
Device was in Mode Switch during SVT/NST episode. **!**

Parameter Settings

	Enable	Initial	Redetect	V Interval (Rate)
VF	On	18/24	9/12	290 ms (207 bpm)
FVT	Off			
VT	Monitor	12	4	360 ms (167 bpm)

VT may be seen but will not result into any action

Page 2

ICD Model: Maximo DR 7278

SVT/NST Episode #73 Report

PR Logic   **Other Enhancements**
AFib/AFlutter   On   Stability   50 ms
Sinus Tach   On   Onset   Off
Other 1:1 SVTs   Off
SVT Limit   300 ms   *maximum allowed difference between consecutive ventricular cycles (to be labeled as VT)*

Additional Settings   **Sensitivity**
1:1 VT-ST Boundary   50 %   Atrial   0.3 mV
High Rate Timeout   Off   Ventricular   0.45 mV

	EGM 1	EGM 2
EGM Source	Atip to Aring	Vtip to Vring
EGM Range	+/- 8 mV	+/- 8 mV

Defines the minimum ventricular interval at which the device applies the PR Logic criteria.

ICD Model: Maximo DR 7278   **SVT/NST Episode #73 Report**

ID#	Date/Time	A. Cycle	V. Cycle	Duration	Reason
73	Aug 26 00:05:38	170 ms	290 ms	5.0 min	Stability

• V-V   □ A-A   VF = 290 ms   VT = 360 ms

Interval (ms)
2000
1700
1400
1100
800
600
400
200

0   2   4   6   8   10   12   14   16   18
Time (sec) [0 = Collection Start]

VT interval = 360 ms
VF interval = 290 ms

(MEDTRONIC)

Figure 13.31

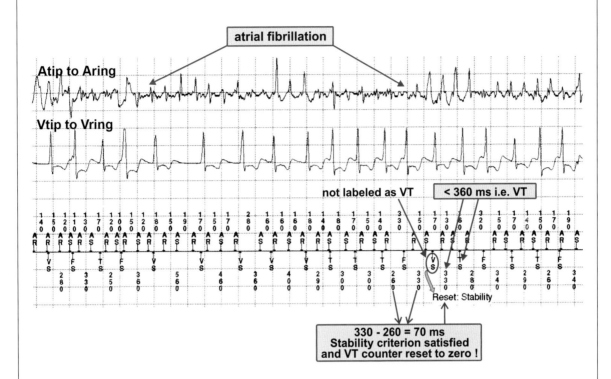

ATRIAL FIBRILLATION & STABILITY DISCRIMINATION
CASE 24 - part 2

atrial fibrillation

Atip to Aring

Vtip to Vring

not labeled as VT   **< 360 ms i.e. VT**

Reset: Stability

**330 - 260 = 70 ms
Stability criterion satisfied
and VT counter reset to zero !**

COMMENT :

The device was in mode switch during the SVT/NST episode. The device was programmed for a VT zone (monitoring only) between 167 and 207 bpm (intervals from 360 to 290 ms). The detection enhancement criterion only functions in the VT zone.

The interval-stability criterion examines the regularity of R-R intervals to discriminate AF with a rapid ventricular response from VT. An interval is labeled as unstable if the difference between it and any of the three previous intervals is longer than the programmed stability interval (here 50 ms). A cycle interpreted as unstable ends with a VS marker even if the cycle is shorter than the programmed VT interval.

Although shorter than 360 ms, the interval ending with the circled marker (VS) is not interpreted as VT since its difference with the preceding interval is 70 ms. The VS marker resets the VT counter to zero. Then the stability again requires 3 preceding cycles to look at. Thus, the 330 ms cycle after the circled VS is labeled TS as three cycles for comparison and activation of the stability search have not yet occured. In other words the VT count must be 3 before "stability" kicks in.

(MEDTRONIC)

Figure 13.32

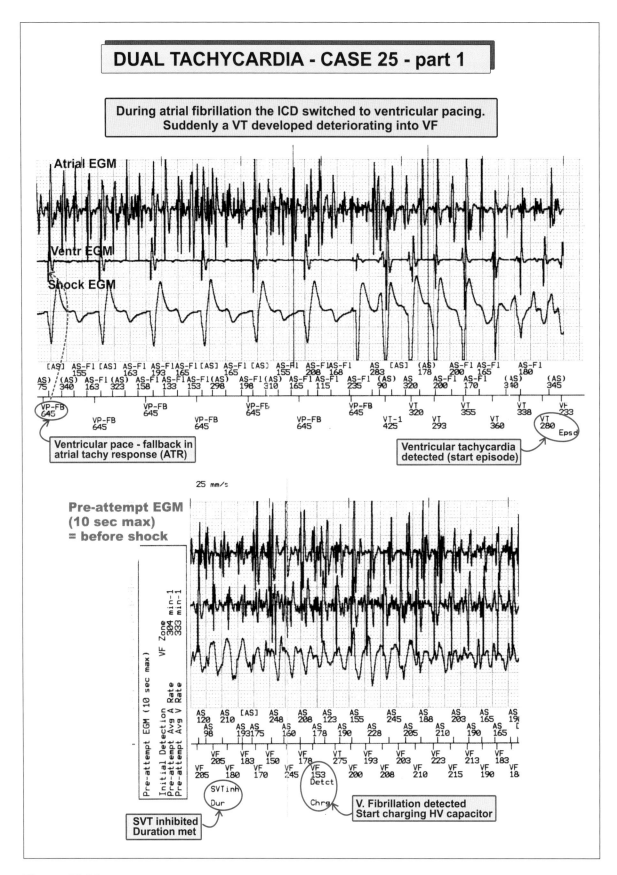

Figure 13.33

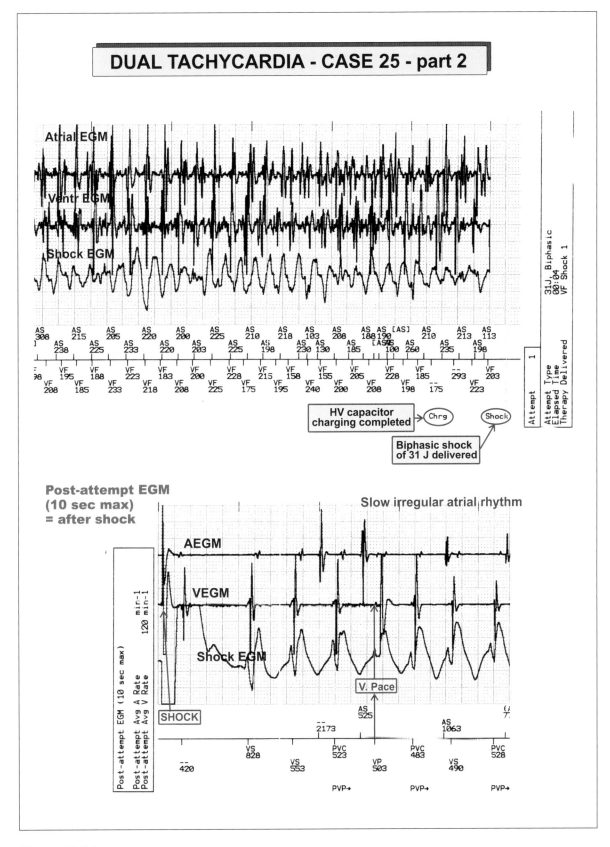

Figure 13.34

T WAVE OVERSENSING - CASE 26

Inappropriate detection of VF due to T wave oversensing during sinus tachycardia.
No shock was delivered because T wave oversensing was intermittent.
T wave oversensing disappeared after reprogramming the ventricular sensitivity to
the least sensitive setting of 1.2 mV (increasing the risk of undersensing a VF).
The problem was eventually solved by the implantation of a new pacing/sensing lead.
This solution is rarely needed for the treatment of T wave oversensing often correctible by programmability.

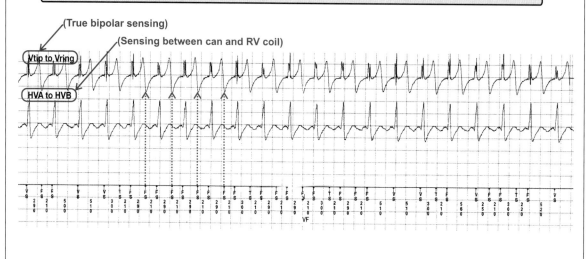

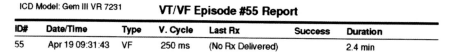

ICD Model: Gem III VR 7231   **VT/VF Episode #55 Report**

ID#	Date/Time	Type	V. Cycle	Last Rx	Success	Duration
55	Apr 19 09:31:43	VF	250 ms	(No Rx Delivered)		2.4 min

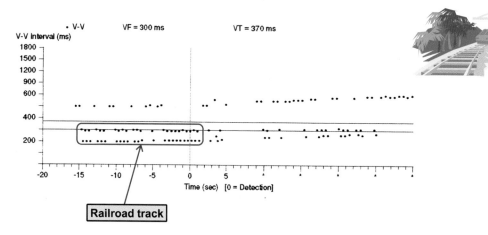

Railroad track

Consistent oversensing of T waves results in a typical "railroad track" appearance
on the interval plot.

Figure 13.35

SILENT LEAD MALFUNCTION - CASE 27

In this patient, lead malfunction was clinically silent and unsuspected during a long period of fol-low-up. Yet, it became manifest only after a test shock (during ICD replacement) when oversensing of false signals associated with noise on the shocking electrogram were recorded.

Ventricular fibrillation was induced during the replacement procedure by a 5 J shock on T wave. Ventricular fibrillation was adequately detected (FD) and was terminated by a 20 J shock. Post shock there was oversensing (FS) of false signals at a sensitivity of 0.15 mV and 0.3 mV. Undersensing of VF (not shown) occurred at a sensitivity of 1.2 mV.

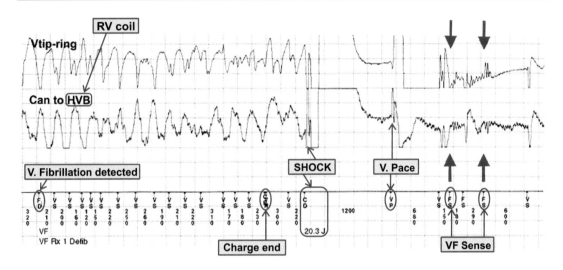

Note the corresponding smaller noise signals in the shocking electrodes, suggestive of additional RV coil malfunction.
The appearance of noise after a shock may be a specific sign of coaxial polyurethane(PU) ICD lead failure and may be due to degradation of the PU insulation by metal ion migration.

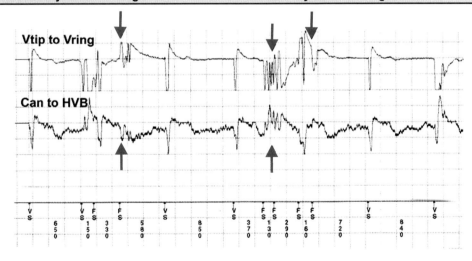

ICD lead problems may become evident only after a high voltage shock. Therefore, leads known for suboptimal survivability should be tested every 1-2 years with a maximal defibrillation shock.

Figure 13.36

ATRIAL FLUTTER - CASE 28

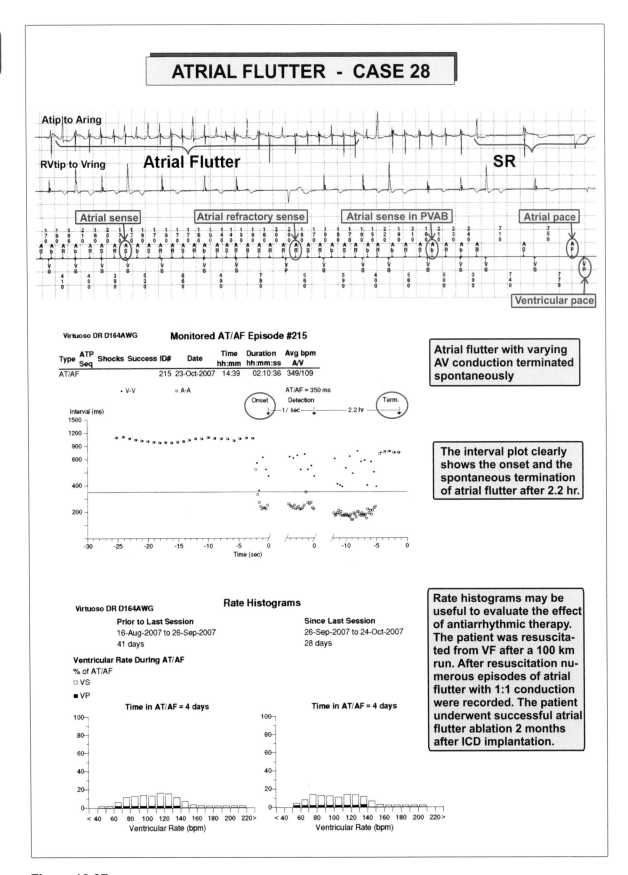

Atip to Aring

RVtip to Vring — Atrial Flutter — SR

| Atrial sense | Atrial refractory sense | Atrial sense in PVAB | Atrial pace |

Ventricular pace

Virtuoso DR D164AWG   **Monitored AT/AF Episode #215**

Type	ATP Seq	Shocks	Success	ID#	Date	Time hh:mm	Duration hh:mm:ss	Avg bpm A/V
AT/AF				215	23-Oct-2007	14:39	02:10:36	349/109

• V-V   □ A-A   AT/AF = 350 ms

Onset — Detection —1/sec— — 2.2 hr — Term.

Interval (ms)

Atrial flutter with varying AV conduction terminated spontaneously

The interval plot clearly shows the onset and the spontaneous termination of atrial flutter after 2.2 hr.

Rate Histograms

Virtuoso DR D164AWG

Prior to Last Session
16-Aug-2007 to 26-Sep-2007
41 days

Since Last Session
26-Sep-2007 to 24-Oct-2007
28 days

Ventricular Rate During AT/AF
% of AT/AF
□ VS
■ VP

Time in AT/AF = 4 days   Time in AT/AF = 4 days

Ventricular Rate (bpm)

Rate histograms may be useful to evaluate the effect of antiarrhythmic therapy. The patient was resuscitated from VF after a 100 km run. After resuscitation numerous episodes of atrial flutter with 1:1 conduction were recorded. The patient underwent successful atrial flutter ablation 2 months after ICD implantation.

Figure 13.37

AV CROSSTALK WITH VENTRICULAR INHIBITION IN A DUAL CHAMBER ICD - CASE 29

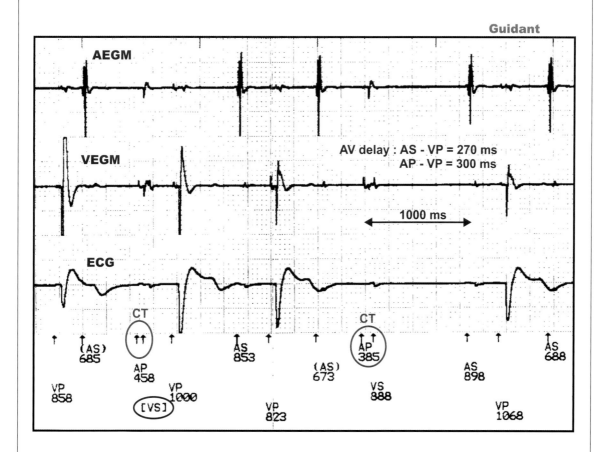

Guidant

AEGM

VEGM

AV delay : AS - VP = 270 ms
AP - VP = 300 ms

1000 ms

ECG

COMMENT :

Pacing is an integral part of ICD function. The pacing component of an ICD may therefore exhibit the same complications as conventional pacemakers. The ventricular channel detected the atrial stimulus, an abnormality known as AV crosstalk (CT). In the first CT activity, the ICD detected the atrial stimulus within the postatrial ventricular blanking period and no ventricular inhibition occurred. The marker depicted the situation as "[VS]". In the second CT activity, the ventricular channel sensed the atrial stimulus depicted by a "VS" marker beyond the postatrial ventricular blanking period (a blanking period designed to prevent CT), and the ventricular output was inhibited. A pause occurred because the patient was in complete AV block. The markers "(AS)" denote atrial sensing in the relatively long postventricular atrial refractory period. Treatment should include increasing the duration of the postatrial ventricular blanking period and decreasing the atrial output. Decreasing ventricular sensitivity may not be an option in an ICD but if reprogrammed, the device should be tested with VF induction to document correct ventricular sensing with an appropriate safety margin for sensing.

Figure 13.38

LONG QT SYNDROME and T WAVE OVERSENSING AT IMPLANTATION - CASE 30

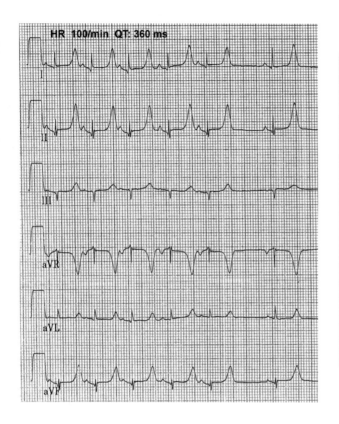

A 3-year-old girl suffered an out-of-hospital cardiac arrest during playing. The patient was defibrillated in time with full recovery.
The ECG showed a long QT syndrome. Family history is negative for long QT syndrome and sudden cardiac death.

A single chamber ICD was implanted abdominally with epicardial pacing/sensing leads.
Prior to induction of VF, real-time recording showed a long QT interval with intermittent sensing of the T wave.

VF could not be induced at implantation with shock on T at 340 ms (10 J, 1 J), nor with shock at 360 ms (1 J). Finally VF was induced by a 50 Hz burst. VF was terminated by a shock of 20 J.

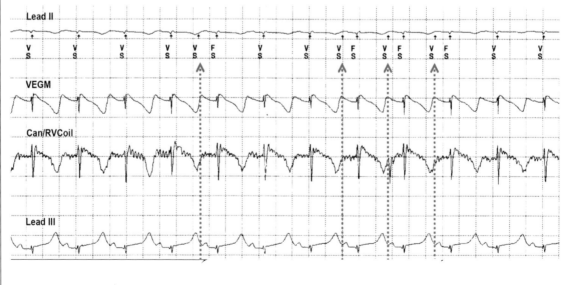

Figure 13.39

LONG QT SYNDROME and T WAVE OVERSENSING AT IMPLANT - CASE 30 - part 2

T wave sensing disappeared after reprogramming RV sensitivity from 0.3 to 0.9 mV. Detection of VF was appropriate at 0.9 mV.

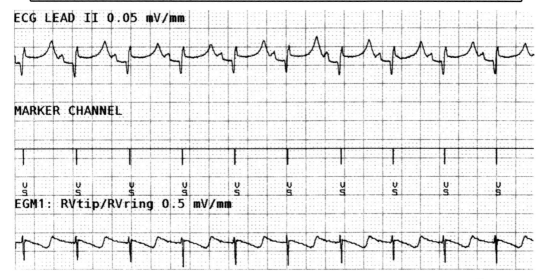

No problems were seen during tachypacing at a RV sensitivity set at 0.9 mV. Pacing was not performed at 0.3 mV.

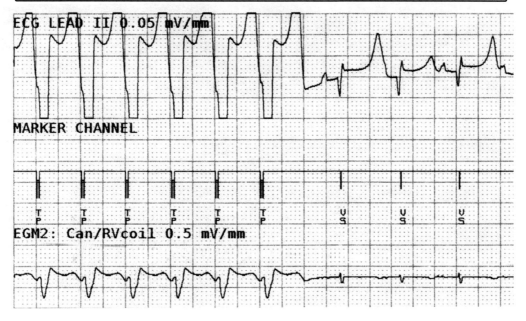

Figure 13.40

P WAVE OVERSENSING - CASE 31

P wave oversensing on the ventricular channel resulted in intermittent double counting (RR) and detection in the VF zone (F).

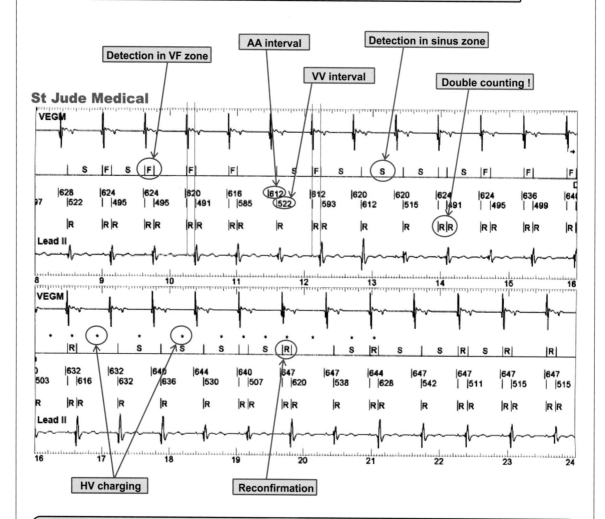

Oversensing of the P wave by the ventricular channel was due to displacement of the lead too close to the tricuspid valve. Repositioning of the lead solved the problem.
This ICD does not require consecutive intervals or a percentage (e.g. 75%) of short intervals for detection. In this case after VF detection (using an averaging algorithm), charging begins. During charging the device verifies continuation of the tachyarrhythmia. For a shock to be delivered, it must count 6 short (F) intervals (not necessarily consecutive) during charging to establish a sustained arrhythmia requiring therapy. When this requirement is satisfied, then at the end of charging, the device looks for another non-sinus interval to synchronize the shock. Return to sinus is declared (and shock aborted) at any time by counting 5 sinus intervals (as programmed) without intervening F intervals. In this tracing, six F intervals were counted during charging. At the end of charging, the ICD will seek another non-sinus interval (not shown) to synchronize the shock. If this interval failed to occur and the device saw 5 sinus intervals, the shock would be aborted.

Figure 13.41

CAPACITOR CHARGING DURING ANTITACHYCARDIA PACING - CASE 32

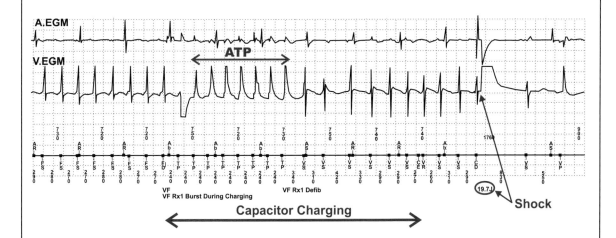

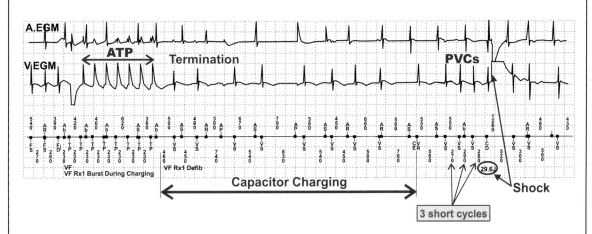

COMMENT :

Top : ATP followed by a shock.
Bottom : ATP terminates VT; Occasional VPCs in the confirmation period after the capacitor charging ends, cause delivery of a shock.
Tho device counts the confirmation intervals (VT interval + 60 ms) beginning with the first interval beyond completion of charging. The device cancels the shock if 4 of 5 cycles are longer than the confirmation interval. The VPCs created 3 short cycles in the confirmation resulting in the delivery of a shock before the episode termination criteria were met.
(Medtronic)

Figure 13.42

BIVENTRICULAR ATP MORE EFFECTIVE THAN RIGHT VENTRICULAR ATP - CASE 33

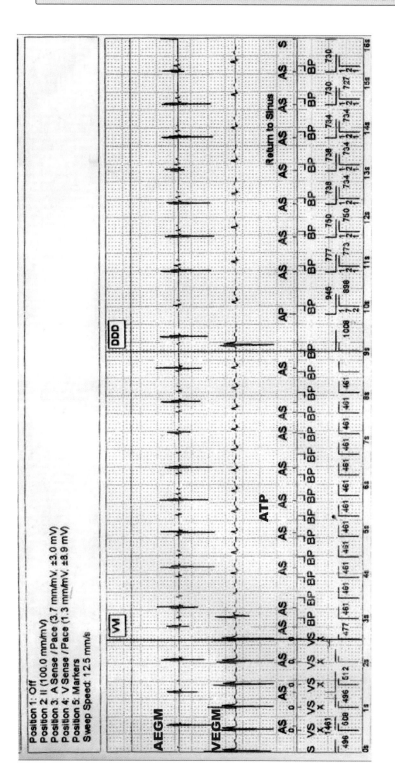

A biventricular ICD was implanted in a patient with poor LV function and heart failure due to non-ischemic cardiomyopathy. The patient had never experienced VT previously. A few hours after implantation, the patient developed many attacks of relatively slow VT. RV ATP was mostly ineffective but biventricular ATP was able to terminate most episodes with only one burst. These observations are consistent with studies that have shown that biventricular ATP is generally more effective than RV ATP presumably because the LV pacing site is closer to the VT reentrant circuit. VT was eventually controlled with large doses of beta-blockers. Speed: 12.5 mm/sec.

Figure 13.43

T WAVE OVERSENSING DURING SLOW VT - CASE 34

Oversensing of the T wave only during slow VT at a rate of 120 bpm.
The ICD detected slow VT as VF because of T wave sensing (double counting).
Therefore the ICD delivered a 25 J shock that terminated VT.

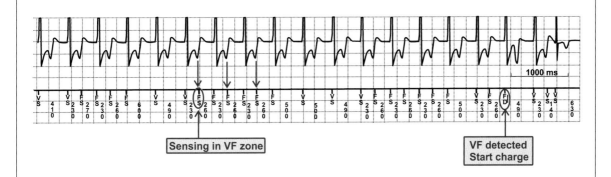

Sensing in VF zone

VF detected
Start charge

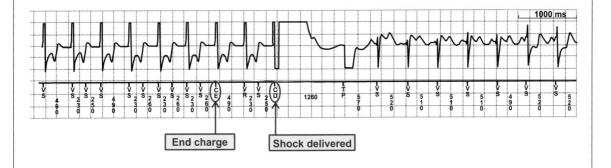

End charge

Shock delivered

Figure 13.44

COMBINED COUNT DURING AF AND INAPPROPRIATE SHOCK
CASE 35

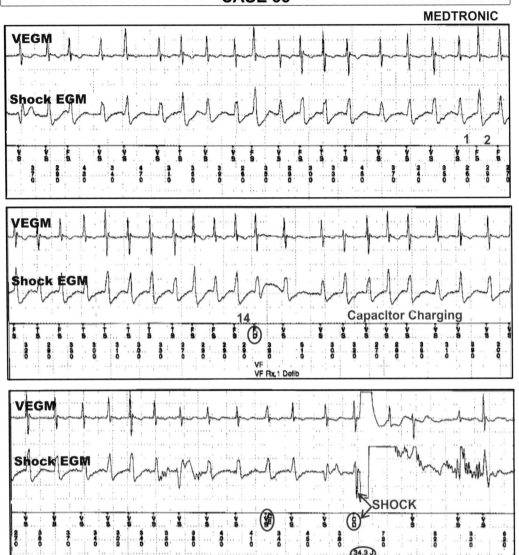

COMMENT :

The ICD was programmed as follows: VT at 176 bpm (340 ms) for 16 beats and VF at 200 bpm (300 ms) for 12/16 beats. The device counted VF and VT events separately according to design. Counting of VF and VT cycles started at the interval labeled 1 and ended at interval 14. When the VF counter reached 6, the combined count function was activated. The number of combined VF and VT beats to count for detection was calculated by the ICD by multiplying 12 (number of VF beats to detect) by 7/6 to provide the combined beats to detect at 14 as shown. The ICD reviewed the last 8 intervals of the 14 cycle sequence. Because one or more the last 8 intervals were classified as VF the ICD initiated VF therapy by charging the capacitor. During charging the ICD failed to abort the shock because 4 of 5 of the intervals were not longer than the confirmation interval equal to the VT interval + 60 ms = 400ms. The recording illustrates how a very fast ventricular response in atrial fibrillation can be associated with an almost regular rhythm and be responsible for inappropriate shock delivery

Figure 13.45

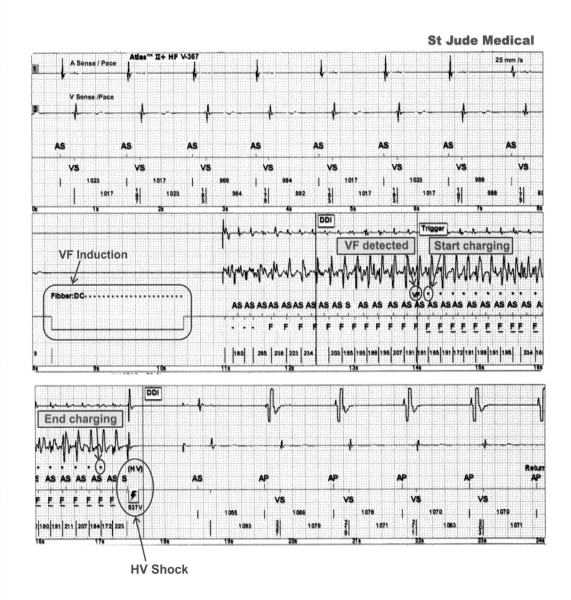

VF INDUCTION BY DC FIBBER - CASE 36

St Jude Medical

Figure 13.46

Note : When the word *"fibber"* is used alone, it is general in meaning and describes all types of fibrillation inductions (pacing burst, shock on T, DC pulse).
"DC Fibber" is a feature of St Jude Medical ICDs by which a single direct current (DC) pulse is delivered through the high-voltage electrodes.

REVERSED COIL CONNECTIONS IN A DUAL COIL INTEGRATED DEFIBRILLATION LEAD - CASE 37

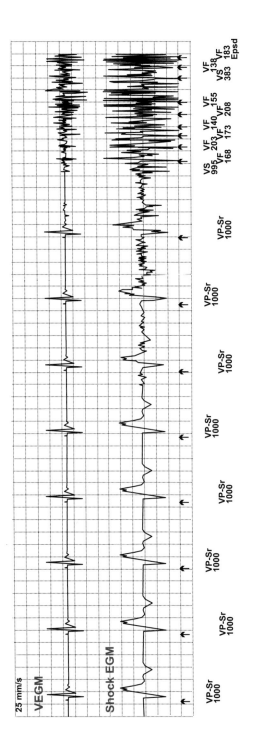

The DF-1 pins were put into the incorrect connectors. The rate sensing function was therefore connected to the active can. There was noise (myopotentials) in both the rate sensing and the shock electrograms. This problem may cause sensing of thoracic pectoral myopotentials and atrial activity with resultant ICD inhibition and/or inappropriate therapy (shocks).

Figure 13.47

INAPPROPRIATE THERAPY FOR SVT - CASE 38

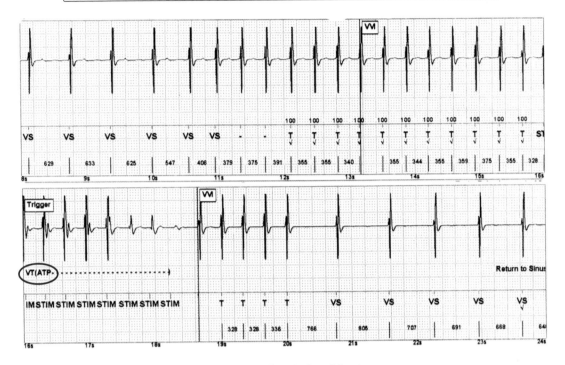

Atlas™+ VR V-193

Tachy Episode (Archive)

Tachy Episode 10 of 12	Date/Time: 3 May 2007 15:11	Type: VT (Therapy Delivered)	Episode Duration: 0:12

Diagnosis: VT

Time to Diagnosis: 4.00 sec CL 355 ms/169 min⁻¹

VT Diagnosis Criteria:	Any

Morphology.
Programmed: On, ≥ 60% is a match,
≥ 5 of 8 matches indicate SVT
Template Updated: 7 Mar 2006 02:40

Measured:
Min Match Score: 100%
Max Non-Match Score: N/A
No. Template Matches: 8 of 8 (SVT Indicated)!

Interval Stability.
Programmed: On w/SIH, ≥ 80 ms or
SIH Count ≥ 2 indicates SVT

Measured:
Stability Delta: 35 ms
SIH Count: 0 (VT Indicated)

Sudden Onset:
Programmed: On, <100 ms indicates SVT
Measured Max Delta: 270 ms (VT Indicated)

Alerts: 1

SVT discriminators disagree !

Therapy:	Results:
ATP	Below Rate Detection (CL 720 ms)

ATP Therapy Details: VT
Successful BCL: 312 ms
Burst 1: 312, 312, 312, 312, 312, 312, 312 ms

The patient developed an SVT at a rate of 169 bpm (QRS complexes were identical to those in sinus rhythm !). The template match was 100%, indicating SVT.
The "sudden onset" was programmed "ON" with a programmed maximum delta < 100 ms. The measured maximum delta was 270 ms, indicating VT according to the design of the ICD algorithm. Similarly the "stability" discriminator also indicated VT.
As the diagnosis criteria were programmed on "ANY", the device delivered inappropriate therapy. This case illustrates the importance of judicious programming of the dicriminators and the fact that activating too many of them can backfire. Both VT and SVT can develop suddenly and exhibit stability. Thus, these two discriminators may confuse the situation because the ICD interpreted both as representing VT. These discriminators cancelled the important data from the "morphology" discriminator because the system was programmed to make the diagnosis of VT should "ANY" of the 3 discriminators indicate VT.

Figure 13.48

VT/SVT DISCRIMINATION BY THE V > A RULE
CASE 39

VT at a rate of 148 bpm was terminated by ATP (8 stimuli at a cycle length of 344 ms) based upon rate branch (V > A) and morphology. Discrimination was programmed "IF ANY".

AV dissociation with the ventricular rate (V) faster than the atrial rate (A) is the hallmark of VT. Thus, a dual chamber ICD makes the diagnosis of VT simply and only on the basis of when V > A. All Discriminators are bypassed. In this case, although the *morphology* discriminator indicated "no match" (VT), this information was not used for the diagnosis. Discriminators are useful when A = V or A > V, but not when V > A as in this example.

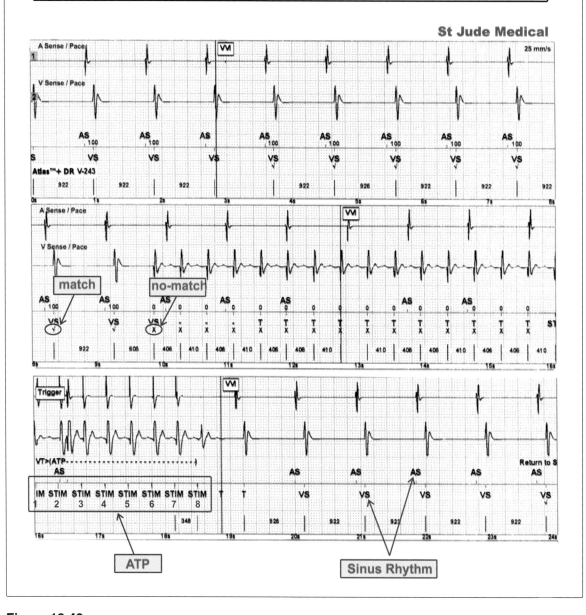

Figure 13.49

VT ACCELERATION WITH INTERMITTENT DOUBLE R WAVE COUNTING INDUCED BY ATP - CASE 40

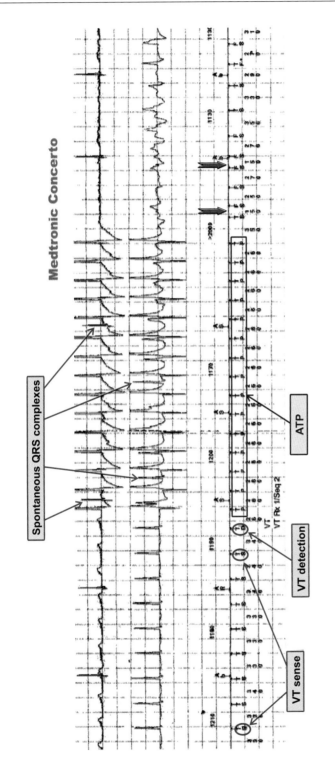

The ICD detected VT and delivered rather prolonged burst pacing. The spontatenous QRS complex can be seen as a distinct deflection through the burst indicating lack of capture. If capture occurred it must have been late into the burst. The burst induced a faster VT with varying and wider VEGM morphology. This caused intermittent double counting of the R wave (arrows). The Ab marker indicates a signal within the postventricular atrial blanking period where it is used by the PR Logic algorithm but not by the antibradycardia function. In previous models this event was depicted by an AR marker.

Figure 13.50

DIAPHRAGMATIC MYOPOTENTIAL INTERFERENCE - CASE 41

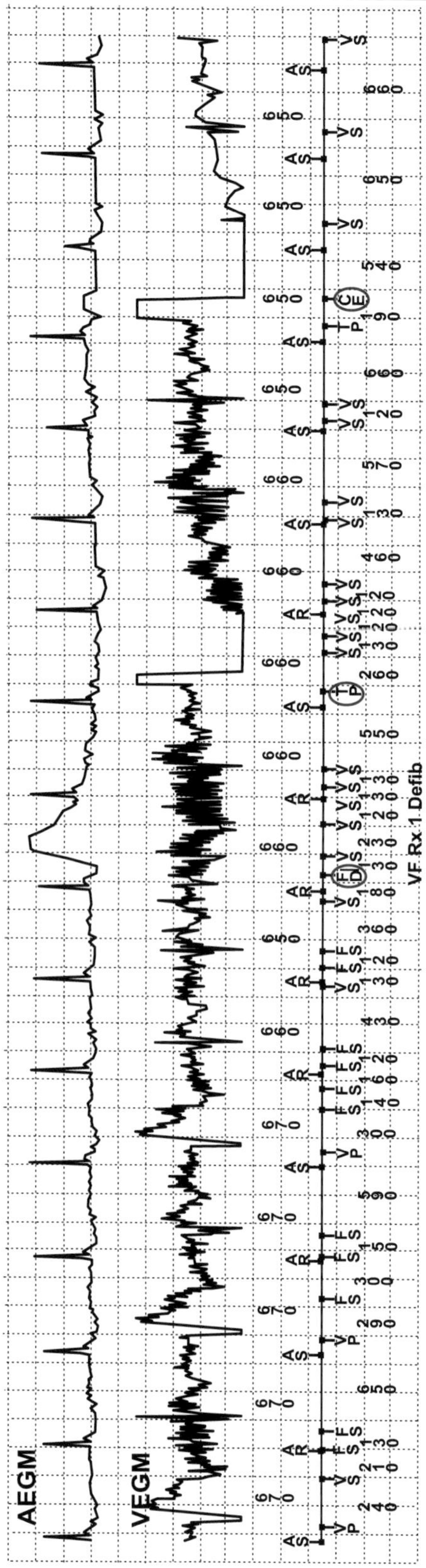

During coughing, myopotentials were sensed by the integrated bipolar ventricular lead. The extraneous signals were interpreted as VF by the ICD and a shock was delivered. Note the characteristic interference on the ventricular sensing channel.

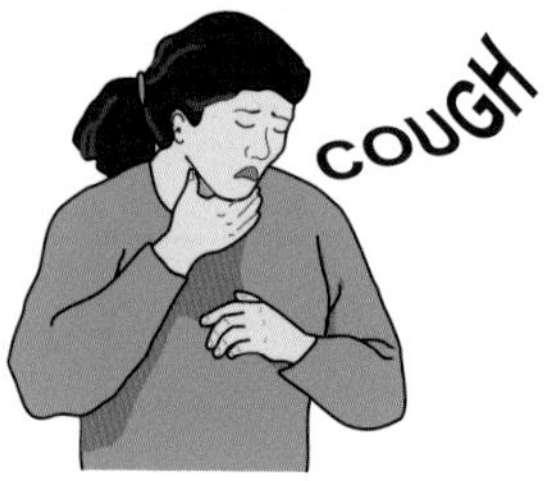

COUGH

Figure 13.51

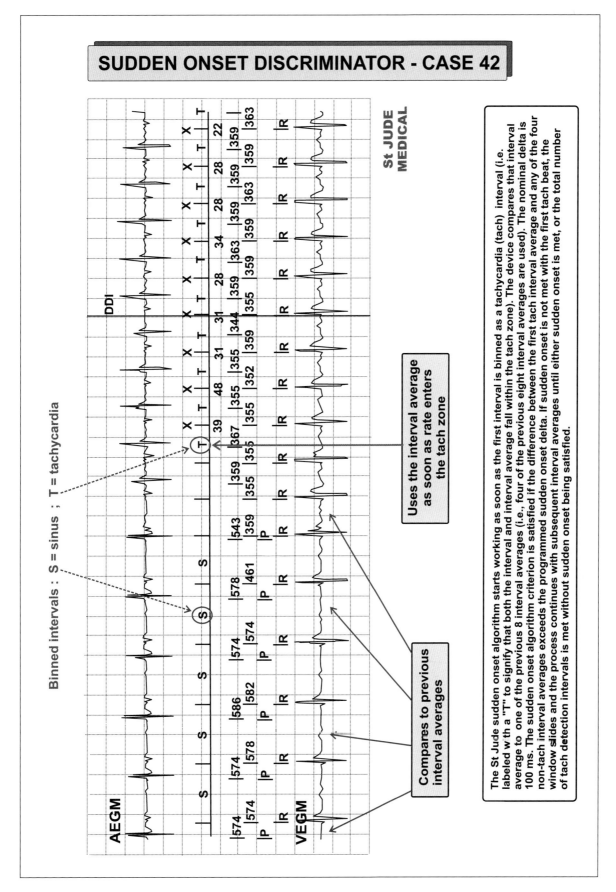

Figure 13.52

SUDDEN ONSET DISCRIMINATOR - CASE 42

The St Jude sudden onset algorithm starts working as soon as the first interval is binned as a tachycardia (tach) interval (i.e. labeled with a "T" to signify that both the interval and interval average fall within the tach zone). The device compares that interval average to one of the previous 8 interval averages (i.e., four of the previous eight interval averages are used). The nominal delta is 100 ms. The sudden onset algorithm criterion is satisfied if the difference between the first tach interval average and any of the four non-tach interval averages exceeds the programmed sudden onset delta. If sudden onset is not met with the first tach beat, the window slides and the process continues with subsequent interval averages until either sudden onset is met, or the total number of tach detection intervals is met without sudden onset being satisfied.

Figure 13.52

INTERMITTENT LEAD MALFUNCTION WITH OVERSENSING - CASE 43

Two years after ICD implantation, the patient experienced several inappropriate shocks. The sensing ventricular lead recorded irregularly occurring artifacts (false signals) typical of lead malfunction from either an intermittent fracture or insulation defect. The device responded to the noise by binning F intervals and detected VF after counting 12 F intervals not necessarily consecutive. The capacitor began charging at the trigger point. The shock was aborted because the ICD detected 5 S (sinus) intervals without interspersed F events. Consequently with return to sinus, the shock was aborted.

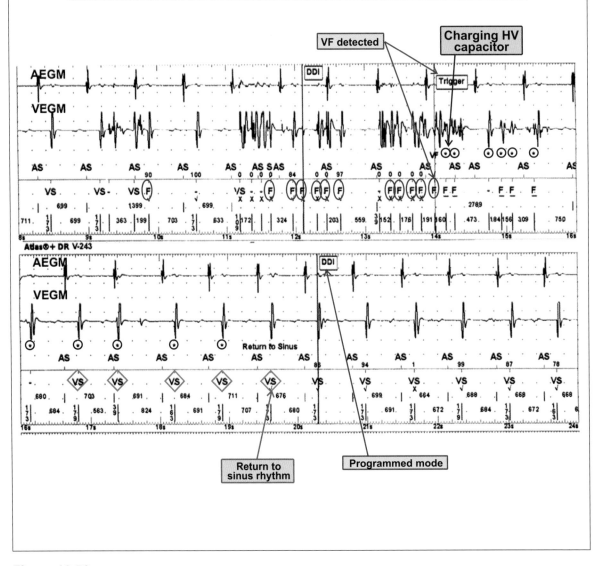

Figure 13.53

SHOCK TO VT WITH 1:1 CONDUCTION CAUSING ACCELERATION - CASE 44

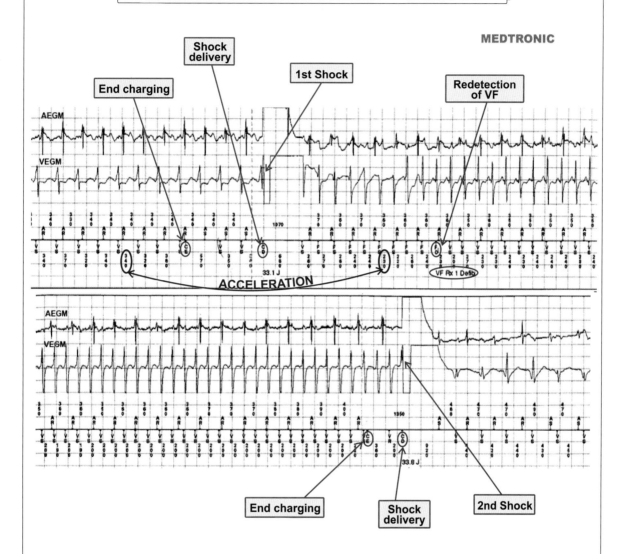

A shock to VT with 1:1 retrograde VA conduction causing acceleration.
VT with 1:1 retrograde VA conduction was treated with a shock which caused acceleration.
The faster VT then stabilized into ventricular flutter with a cycle length of 200 ms. Atrial
activity became dissociated from ventricular activity because of the fast ventricular rate. A
second shock restored sinus rhythm.

Figure 13.54

DOUBLE COUNTING OF THE R WAVE - CASE 45

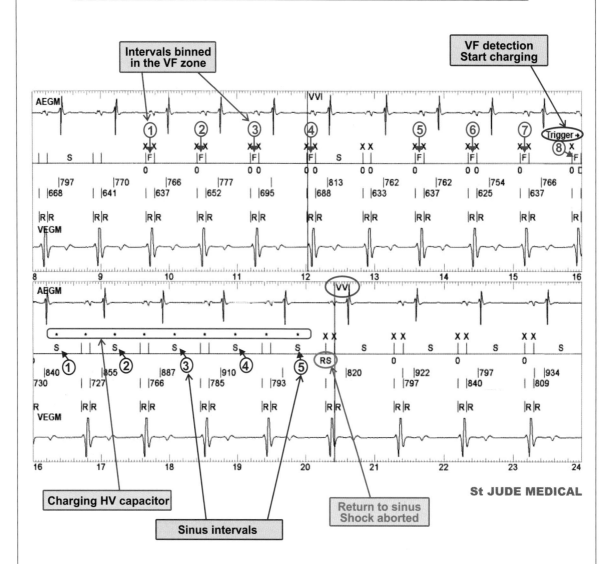

Figure 13.55

The ICD counted 8 F intervals (averaged intervals according to the St Jude binning system) and VF was detected. Note that these F intervals need not be consecutive. The unlabeled events were not binned. Charging began after VF detection. However the shock was aborted because the ICD detected 5 S (sinus events) without intervening F cycles. RS depicts return to sinus. The basic rhythm was probably a ventricular rhythm with retrograde VA conduction. Sinus rhythm with an exceedingly long PR interval and AV conduction would be highly unlikely.

IRREGULAR VT DETECTED BY ICD - CASE 46

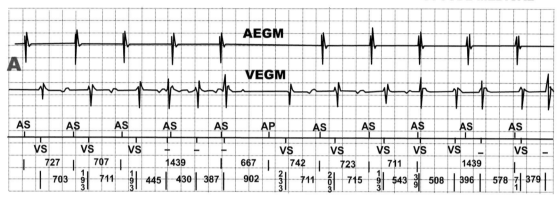

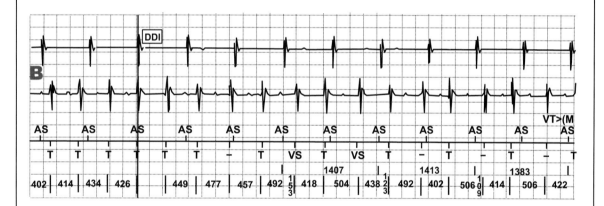

Comment :

VT is obviously irregular and associated with AV dissociation. This device does not detect VT by counting consecutive short intervals or a fixed % of short intervals (x out of y). The averaging algorithm of this ICD counts the number of T cycles (binned when the current interval and average interval are similar) which need not to be consecutive. The ICD detects VT at the end of the tracing. Programming a stability discriminator might have prevented VT detection.

Figure 13.56

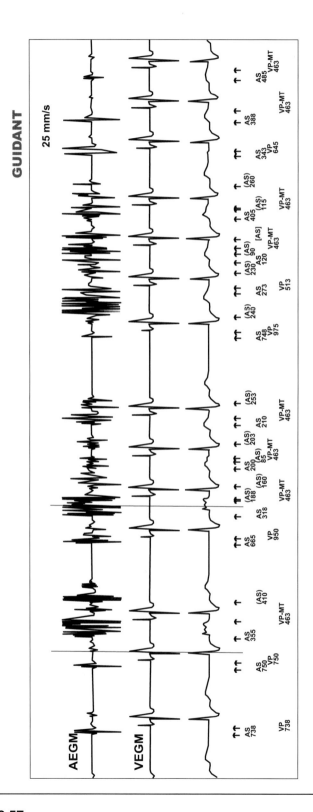

ATRIAL LEAD FRACTURE - CASE 47

GUIDANT
25 mm/s

AEGM

VEGM

Dual chamber ICD with interference (false signals) in the atrial electrogram generated by an intermittent fracture of the atrial lead. The device sensed the atrial signals whereupon it triggered a corresponding ventricular output. At times, sensing of atrial interferences pushes the ventricular pacing rate to the programmed upper rate.

Figure 13.57

T WAVE OVERSENSING - CASE 48
COMMITTED ICD SHOCK UPON VF REDETECTION

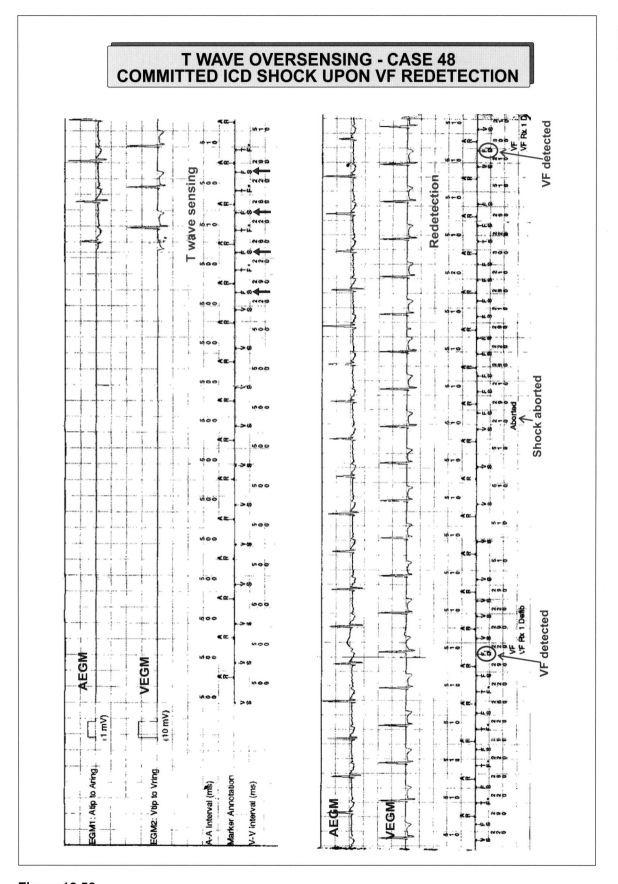

Figure 13.58

T WAVE OVERSENSING - CASE 48 cont'd
COMMITTED ICD SHOCK UPON VF REDETECTION

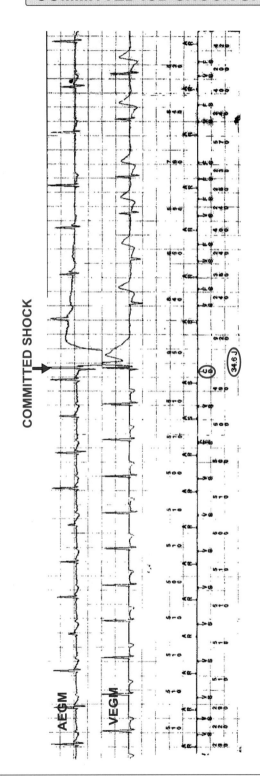

COMMITTED SHOCK

AEGM

VEGM

34.6 J

COMMENT :

T wave oversensing by an ICD was interpreted as VF and the capacitor began to charge. However, during charging ("second look" phase) the ICD detected 4 of 5 intervals longer than the confirmation interval (VT cycle + 60 ms). The shock was therefore aborted. Return to sinus requires the detection of 8 consecutive intervals longer than the programmed VT interval. T wave oversensing recurred and did not permit these critical intervals to occur. Consequently VF redetection took place but this time the capacitor charged to its full programmed value and an committed shock was delivered despite the transient disappearance of T wave oversensing. If the ICD detects VT/VF and the shock is aborted, redetection will induce a committed shock. This response was designed to ensure VT/VF therapy in the case of intermittent undersensing.

Figure 13.59

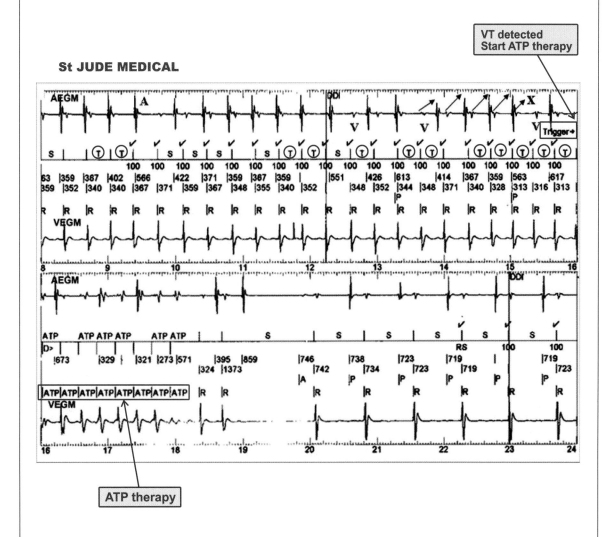

VT WITH RETROGRADE VA CONDUCTION SHOWING WENCKEBACH BLOCK - CASE 49

VT detected
Start ATP therapy

St JUDE MEDICAL

ATP therapy

VT with gradual prolongation of retrograde conduction in the form of a Wenckebach phenomenon which culminated in a beat with blocked VA conduction. ATP terminated the VT.
The ICD detected VT after 12 non-consecutive T cycles without the occurrence of a sequence of 5 S (sinus) cyles free of T intervals in the progression. These 5 S cycles would have indicated return to sinus.

Figure 13.60

COMMITTED ICD RESPONSE TO UNSUSTAINED VT
CASE 50

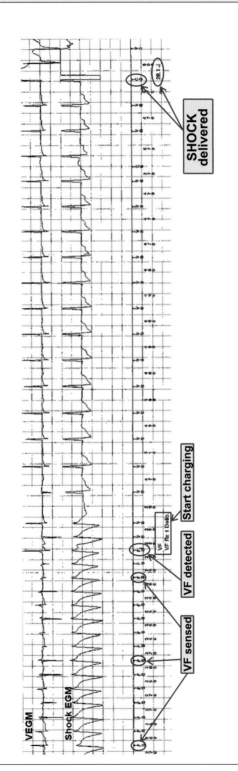

VEGM

Shock EGM

VF sensed

VF detected

Start charging

SHOCK delivered

Prior to this recording, an episode of unsustained VT was detected as VF by the ICD (not shown). The HV capacitor began to charge but the VT terminated spontaneously. The shock was therefore aborted (uncommitted shock). The second episode of unsustained VT (detected as VF) shown in this tracing restarted soon afterwards but the ICD response was different. The HV capacitor began to charge again as expected. The VT terminated spontaneously again, yet the shock was not aborted and the ICD behaved like a committed device by delivering the shock during sinus rhythm. This response should not be interpreted as ICD malfunction ! If an ICD detects VT/VF and the shock is aborted, redetection will induce a committed shock. This response was designed to ensure VT/VF therapy in case of intermittent undersensing.

Figure 13.61

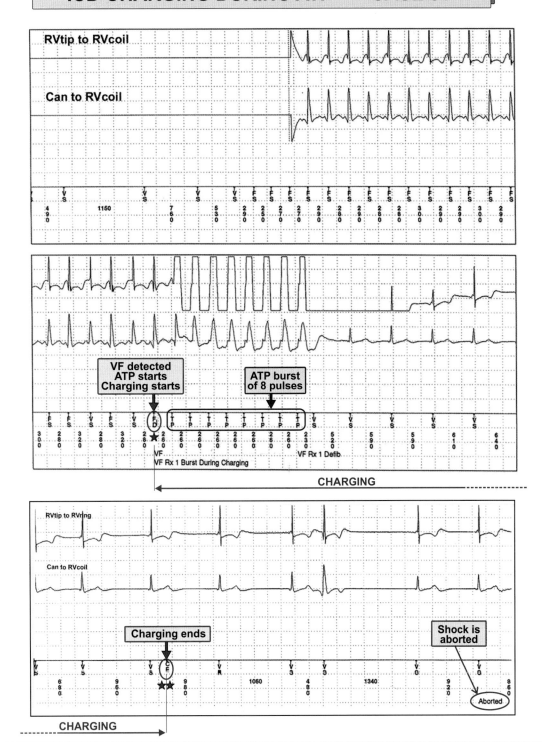

ICD CHARGING DURING ATP   -   CASE 51

The ICD detected VF (*) and released ATP. HV capacitor charging started coincidentally with ATP initiation. ATP terminated VT and maximum charging was completed (**) relatively soon after cessation of ATP. The shock was aborted because ATP restored sinus rhythm. The new ICDs permit simultaneous ATP and charging for first VF detection as a programmable option. This was designed because a fast organized VT can sometimes be terminated by ATP though detected as VF by a device. This example demonstrates the benefit of this design to avoid shocks.

Figure 13.62

INTERMITTENT PRE-VENTRICULAR AND POST-VENTRICULAR ATRIAL FAR-FIELD SENSING OF THE R WAVE - CASE 52

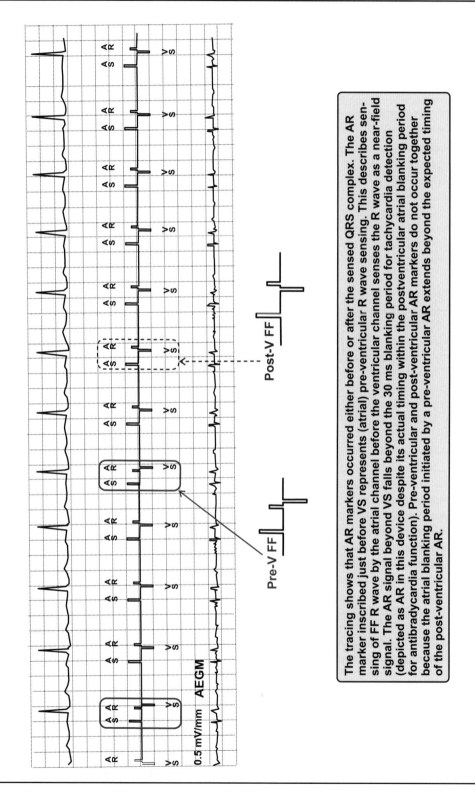

The tracing shows that AR markers occurred either before or after the sensed QRS complex. The AR marker inscribed just before VS represents (atrial) pre-ventricular R wave sensing. This describes sensing of FF R wave by the atrial channel before the ventricular channel senses the R wave as a near-field signal. The AR signal beyond VS falls beyond the 30 ms blanking period for tachycardia detection (depicted as AR in this device despite its actual timing within the postventricular atrial blanking period for antibradycardia function). Pre-ventricular and post-ventricular AR markers do not occur together because the atrial blanking period initiated by a pre-ventricular AR extends beyond the expected timing of the post-ventricular AR.

Figure 13.63

ATRIAL SENSING OF FAR-FIELD R WAVE - CASE 53

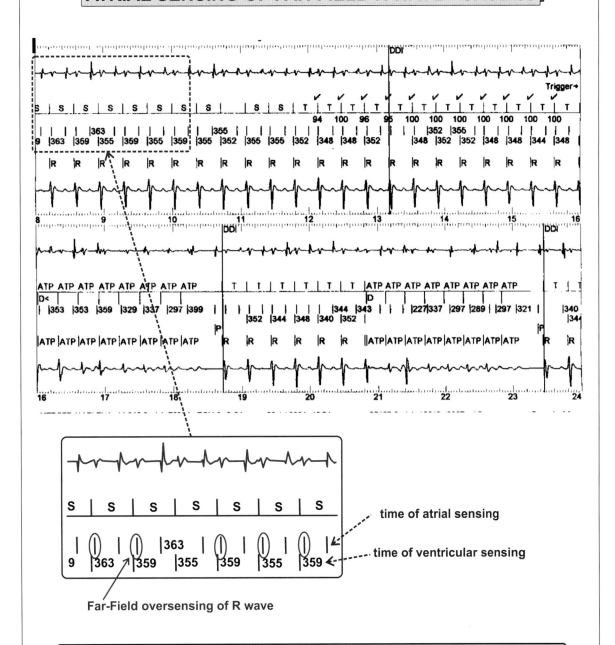

time of atrial sensing

time of ventricular sensing

Far-Field oversensing of R wave

The atrial channel sensed almost all the R waves as FF signals. The morphology dicriminator was programmed on "Monitor". The basic rhythm was either atrial tachycardia or sinus tachycardia. The device interpreted the tachycardia as VT and delivered ATP which was unsuccessful. The device made the diagnosis of FF oversensing and discounted the additional atrial signals during tachycardia.

Figure 13.64

VT WITH RETROGRADE WENCKEBACH - CASE 54

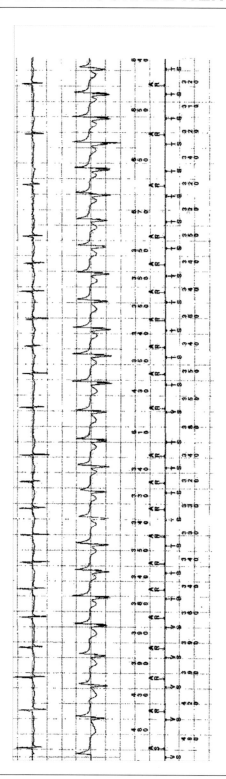

COMMENT :

VT exhibited gradual acceleration into the VT zone. There is retrograde VA conduction with a gradual increase in the VA conduction time culminating in retrograde VA conduction block. This represents a Wenckebach form of retrograde VA conduction. The missing P wave from blocked VA conduction excludes SVT and clinches the diagnosis of VT. The gradual increase in the VT rate means that if an onset discriminator had been programmed, the device might have interpreted the arrhythmia as sinus tachycardia.

Figure 13.65

UNSUCCESSFUL ATP FOLLOWED BY SUCCESSFUL ATP - Part 1
CASE 55

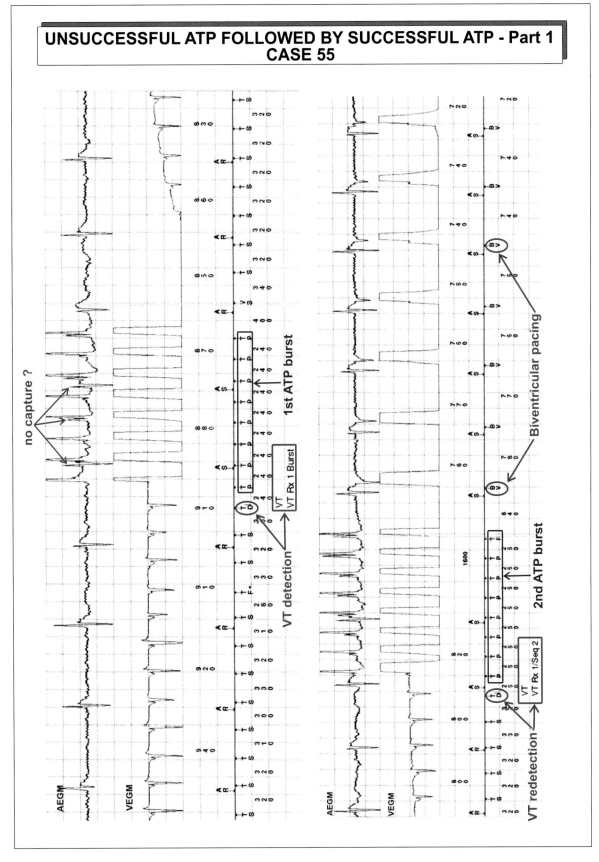

Figure 13.66

UNSUCCESSFUL ATP FOLLOWED BY SUCCESSFUL ATP - Part 2
CASE 55

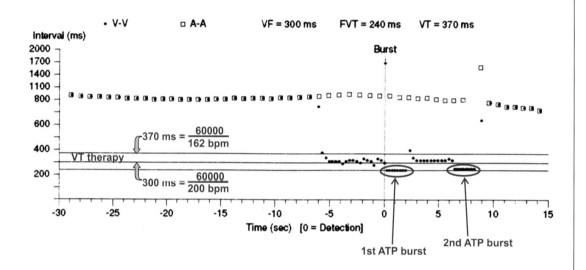

ICD Model: InSync Sentry 7298   **VT/VF Episode #57 Report**

ID#	Date/Time	Type	V. Cycle	Last Rx	Success	Duration
57	Dec 23 19:22:34	VT	300 ms	VT Rx 1	Yes	14 sec

> The patient received an ICD-CRT device for heart failure and recurrent VT.
> Programmed VT therapy : (162-200 bpm) 3 x burst pacing followed by 5 x 35 J shocks.
> The first burst sequence did not stop the tachycardia.
> The seond burst terminated the tachycardia after which biventricular pacing resumed.

Figure 13.67

FAR-FIELD R WAVE SENSING DETECTED AS AF/AT - CASE 56

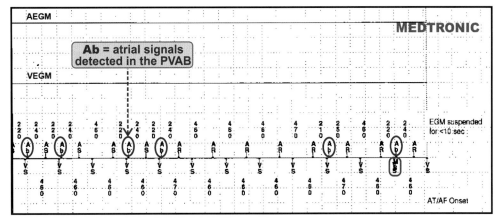

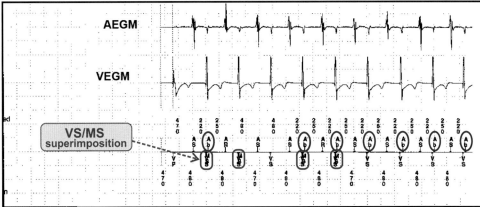

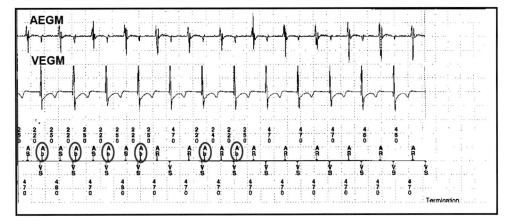

COMMENT :
The sinus rate was fast and the PR interval relatively long. This combination in association with FF R wave atrial sensing tends to produce nearly equal intervals between detected atrial events. The ICD interprets this arrangement as AF/AT. The dense markers represent the superimposition of VS and MS markers. The device detects the Ab (in the postventricular blanking period) signals used only by the PR Logic for the diagnosis of atrial tachyarrhythmias.

Abbreviations : AR = atrial sense during refractory period; FF = far-field; MS = mode switching; PR Logic = discrimination algorithm used in Medtronic ICDs;

Figure 13.68

DETECTION OF TACHYCARDIA WITH COMBINED COUNT
CASE 57

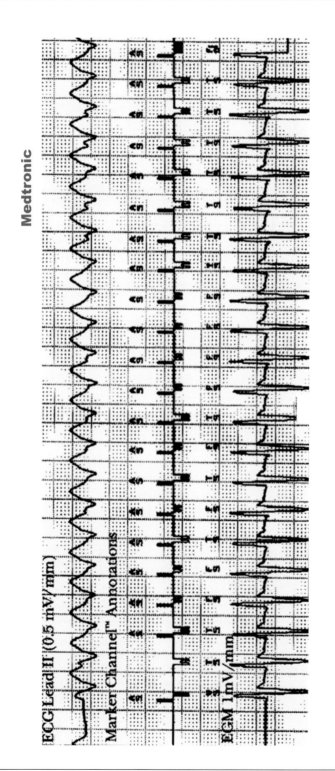

Medtronic

Because the device counts VT and VF events separately, a rhythm with variable cycle length can cause VT and VF counts to increment separately. The device can automatically perform a combined count to prevent therapy delay. If the VF counter reaches 6, the device activates the combined count function. The combined beats to count (initial or redetect) are multiplied by 7/6. If VF to detect is 18/24, the combined beats to detect becomes 18 x 7/6 = 21. Then the ICD reviews the last 8 intervals.

1. If any of the intervals were VF, VF therapy is applied
2. Fast VT therapy is applied if none of the last 8 intervals was counted as VF, but one or more cycles were detected in the fast VT zone
3. VT therapy is applied if all 8 intervals are outside the VF and the fast VT zones

Figure 13.69

DOUBLE TACHYCARDIA IDENTIFIED BY ICD - CASE 58

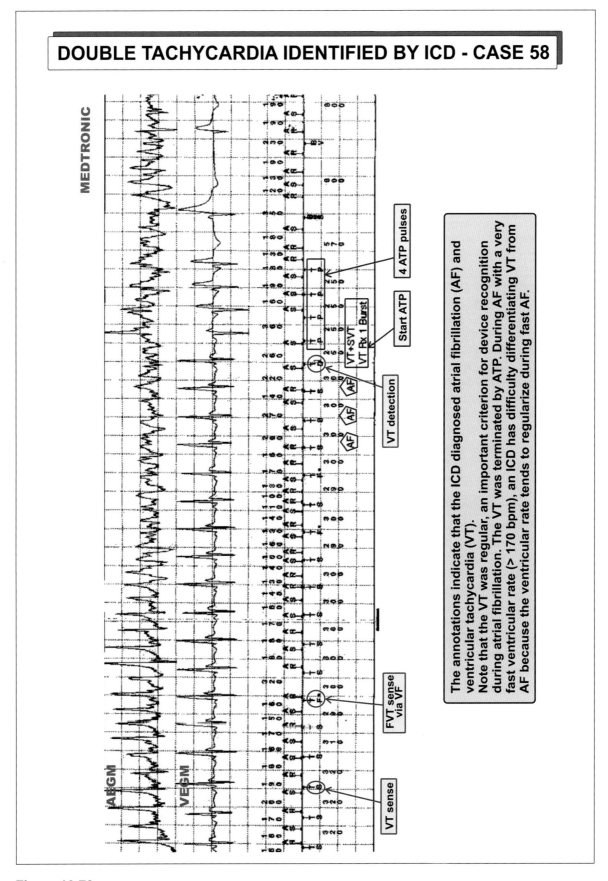

The annotations indicate that the ICD diagnosed atrial fibrillation (AF) and ventricular tachycardia (VT).

Note that the VT was regular, an important criterion for device recognition during atrial fibrillation. The VT was terminated by ATP. During AF with a very fast ventricular rate (> 170 bpm), an ICD has difficulty differentiating VT from AF because the ventricular rate tends to regularize during fast AF.

Figure 13.70

RESPONSE OF ONSET DISCRIMINATOR - CASE 59

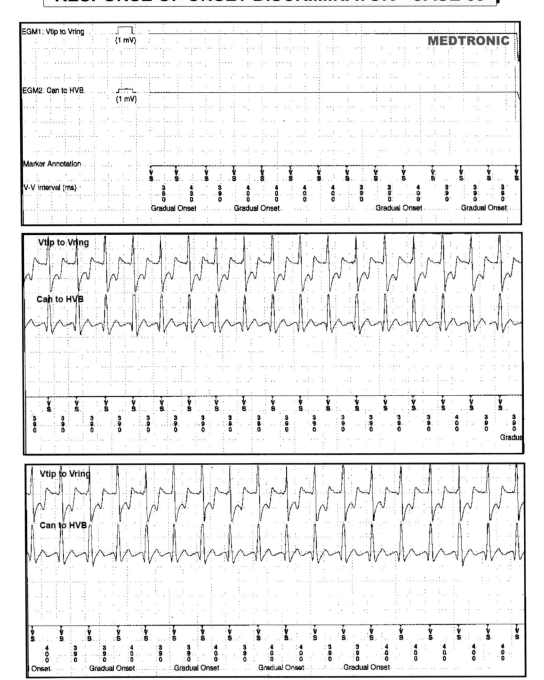

The ICD was programmed to detect VT at 400 ms. The onset criterion was programmed "ON". The onset algorithm evaluates acceleration of the ventricular rate to prevent the detection of sinus tachycardia as VT based on the concept that sinus tachycardia exhibits a gradual increase in rate and the initiation of VT does not. When the device detects a gradual increase of the ventricular rate in the VT zone, it stops counting VT events (labeled as VS in the VT zone). The onset criterion was programmed to 81% in this case. The device compares the average of the 4 most recent ventricular intervals (Re) with the average of the 4 previous intervals (Pr). The ratio Re/Pr is multiplied by 100. If the value is less than the onset criterion, the ICD detects a rapid rate. In this case the value was > 81% because of the very gradual increase in the ventricular rate. Therefore the ICD stopped counting intervals < 400 ms as VT. The onset criterion must be programmed cautiously as the sensitivity for VT detection decreases when the percentage decreases.

Figure 13.71

AIR ESCAPE by Vtip SEAL PLUG - CASE 60

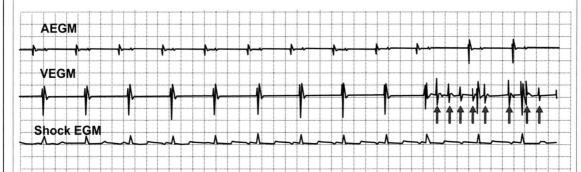

AEGM

VEGM

Shock EGM

Noise recorded on the sensing lead was most probably due to mechanical forces on the contact in the header caused by escaping air. This may be seen for a couple of days after implantation and eventually air will be expelled until the pressure equalizes between the header and the lead.
Intrusion of body fluid into the set screw area of the header is very likely.

NOISE FROM CONTACT OF TWO VENTRICULAR LEADS
CASE 61

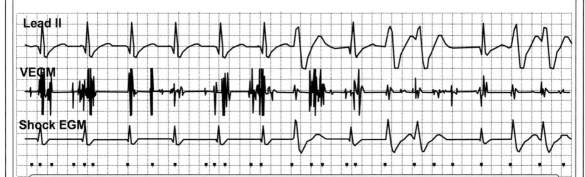

Lead II

VEGM

Shock EGM

Lead-on-lead contact cause noise coincident with cardiac contraction which approxi mated the leads to make contact. The nois amplitude can sometimes be modulated by respiration.

Figure 13.72

REVERSAL OF SHOCKING LEADS IN HEADER - CASE 62

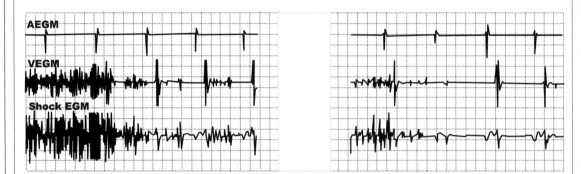

A bipolar integrated dual coil defibrillation RV lead was implanted. Several inappropriate shocks occurred soon after implantation. Recordings revealed obvious noise in the sensing VEGM and the shock EGM. The noise was easily reproduced by arm movement. The distal coil had been connected to the device header into the port designed for the proximal coil and vice versa. This creates a "proximal coil" capable of sensing pectoral myopotentials. Note the absence of interference in the atrial EGM. In this device the can is an active electrode situated in the pocket and connected directly to the proximal shocking coil-connector inside the device.

ATRIAL LEAD ABRADING INTO RV LEAD - CASE 63

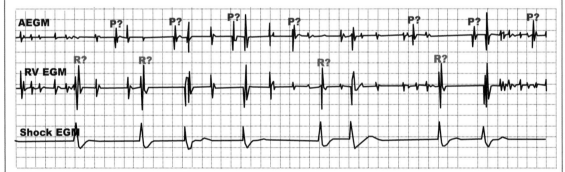

COMMENT :

Contact of the insulation-defective atrial and ventricular leads generated noise concurrently in both channels. The similar timing of these signals in both channels is typical for transient potentials due to intermittent contact (ON/OFF) between the atrial and ventricular conductors. Isolated signals (apart from the false signals) in either the atrial or ventricular channel in all likelihood represent P waves in the AEGM and R waves in the VEGM.

Figure 13.73

NOISE DUE TO ELECTROCAUTERY - CASE 64

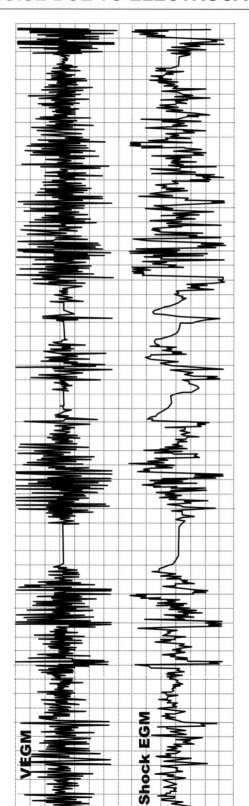

VEGM

Shock EGM

COMMENT :

Typical noise recorded during electrocautery. The noise involved the AEGM (not shown), VEGM and Shock EGM. The interference can be interpreted as VF by an ICD with resultant delivery of a shock. Hence the importance of turning off the tachy function with magnet application during surgery when electrocautery is used.

Figure 13.74

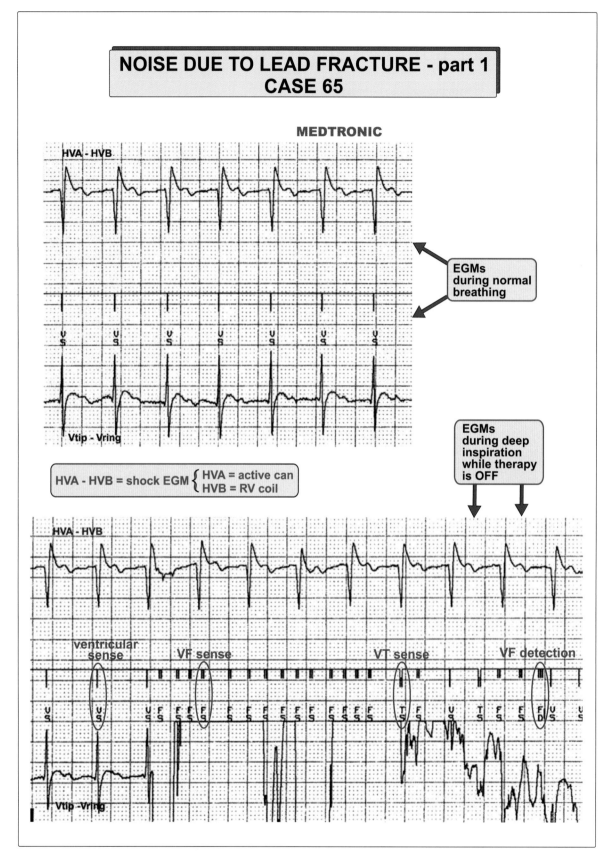

**NOISE DUE TO LEAD FRACTURE - part 1
CASE 65**

MEDTRONIC

HVA - HVB

EGMs
during normal
breathing

Vtip - Vring

HVA - HVB = shock EGM { HVA = active can
HVB = RV coil

EGMs
during deep
inspiration
while therapy
is OFF

HVA - HVB

ventricular
sense   VF sense   VT sense   VF detection

Vtip -Vring

Figure 13.75

NOISE DUE TO LEAD FRACTURE - part 2
CASE 65

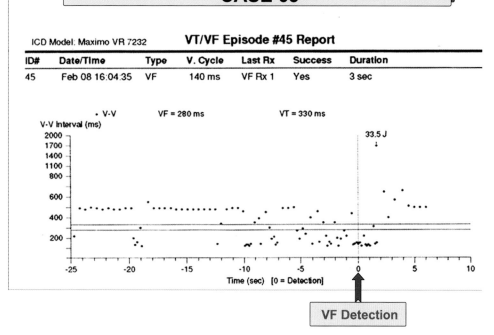

ICD Model: Maximo VR 7232   **VT/VF Episode #45 Report**

ID#	Date/Time	Type	V. Cycle	Last Rx	Success	Duration
45	Feb 08 16:04:35	VF	140 ms	VF Rx 1	Yes	3 sec

VF = 280 ms   VT = 330 ms

33.5 J

V-V Interval (ms)

Time (sec) [0 = Detection]

VF Detection

Status Report

ICD Model: Maximo VR 7232

Battery Voltage

(ERI=2.62 V)
Feb 08, 2007 16:13:26
Voltage   2.89 V

Last Capacitor Formation

Feb 08, 2007 15:45:52
Charge Time   3.66 sec
Energy   12.1 - 35.0 J

Last Charge

Feb 08, 2007 16:04:36
Charge Time   1.32 sec
Energy   25.5 - 35.0 J

Sensing Integrity Counter

(if >300 counts, check for sensing issues)
Since Feb 06, 2007 18:05:45
120-130 ms V-V intervals   1859

high number of short V-V intervals

Lead Impedance

Feb 08, 2007 03:00:05
V. Pacing   496 ohms
V. Defib   33 ohms
SVC (HVX) Defib   46 ohms

EGM Amplitude

Feb 08, 2007 03:00:12
R-Wave Amplitude   8.1 mV

Last High Voltage Therapy

Feb 08, 2007 16:04:37
Measured Impedance   32 ohms
Delivered Energy   33.5 J
Waveform   Biphasic
Pathway   AX>B

Device Status

Charge Circuit is OK.

Malfunction of ICD sensing lead was unmasked by deep respiration. During normal respiration the baseline VEGM appeared normal. Deep respiration precipitated a shower of ventricular signals considered non-physiologic because of their short V-V intervals. The prominent baseline disturbance ruled out diaphragmatic myopotential oversensing. The false signals induced VT and VF detection by the ICD and resulted in the delivery of an inappropriate shock. The findings were consistent with lead malfunction probably related to a lead insulation defect. Despite the recorded abnormalities, lead and shock impedances remained normal. The sensing integrity counter registered a high number of short V-V intervals highly suggestive of a lead problem. This case illustrates that the earliest manifestation of a lead problem may be reflected in the short V-V interval count at a time when lead impedances still remain within the normal range.

Figure 13.76

Cardiac tachyarrhythmias are subdivided into supraventricular and ventricular arrhythmias (Fig. 1.01).

1.1 Mechanism of tachycardias

There are three basic mechanisms of arrhythmias common to both atrial and ventricular arrhythmias: automaticity, afterdepolarizations and reentry.

1. *Automaticity* describes the spontaneous development of a new site of depolarization (ectopic focus) in non-nodal tissue.
2. *Afterdepolarizations* consist of secondary depolarizations arising *during* repolarization (early afterdepolarization: EAD) but also just *after* complete repolarization of the cellular membrane: delayed afterdepolarization (DAD). Afterdepolarizations may reach the threshold level and generate an action potential giving rise to tachycardia.
3. *Reentry* occurs when an impulse depolarizes the myocardium and then perpetuates activation in an anatomic or functional loop producing repetitive beats or sustained tachycardias. Reentrant circuits require three functional or structural conditions:
   (a) an impulse conducted through two pathways with different conduction velocities and refractoriness;
   (b) pathways joined proximally and distally to form a continuous loop;
   (c) unidirectional block in one pathway to initiate the process.

Slow conduction in the loop allows the previously blocked pathway time to recover excitability. A critically timed impulse conducts anterogradely through the only open pathway and returns retrogradely via the other pathway responsible for unidirectional block. If the anterograde pathway has recovered from refractoriness, the returning impulse can then reactivate the earlier site and start a self-perpetuating reentrant tachycardia (Fig. 1.02).

1.2 Supraventricular tachyarrhythmias

The maintenance of supraventricular tachyarrhythmias (SVT) involves structures above the division of the His bundle. Supraventricular tachyarrhythmias comprise atrial tachycardia (AT), atrial flutter (AFL), atrial fibrillation (AF) and atrioventricular (AV) junctional tachycardias. Atrioventricular junctional tachycardias include AV nodal reentrant tachycardia (AVNRT) and AV reentrant (orthodromic reciprocating) tachycardia (AVRT/ORT) incorporating one or more accessory AV pathways in a reentry circuit.

1.2.1 AV nodal reentrant tachycardia

Atrioventricular nodal reentrant tachycardia (AVNRT) involves an AV nodal reentry circuit that consists of two atrionodal connections or pathways and a component of atrial myocardium joining them.

The common type of AVNRT (slow–fast) involves two functionally and anatomically separate atrionodal pathways with different refractory periods. The fast conducting pathway possesses a long refractory period and the slow pathway a short refractory period. During sinus rhythm, anterograde conduction proceeds simultaneously over both AV nodal pathways but retrograde invasion of the impulse coming from the fast pathway blocks anterograde conduction over the slow pathway. The tachycardia typically starts with a premature atrial beat with critical timing that finds the fast pathway refractory but open conduction over the nonrefractory slow pathway (with a long PR-interval). Upon reaching the lower common pathway of the reentry circuit, the wavefront returns retrogradely to the atria via the fast pathway. The process establishes a reentrant SVT using the slow pathway as the anterograde limb and the fast pathway as the retrograde limb (Fig. 1.03). Atrial and ventricular activation occur nearly simultaneously. During the common slow–fast AVNRT, retrograde P-waves hide within the QRS complex or emerge at the end of the QRS complex producing terminal "pseudo s waves" in the inferior leads or more frequently "pseudo r waves" in lead V_1. Rarely the P-wave precedes the beginning of the QRS complex, resulting in "pseudo-q waves" in the inferior leads.

The reverse form of AVNRT (fast–slow AVNRT) is rare. It engages the fast pathway as the anterograde limb and the slow pathway as the retrograde limb of the reentry circuit.

1.2.2 Orthodromic reciprocating tachycardia

Orthodromic reciprocating tachycardia (ORT) often occurs in patients with an obvious accessory pathway (atrium to ventricle as in the Wolff–Parkinson–White syndrome). However, some patients show no evidence of preexcitation during sinus rhythm because the accessory pathway can only conduct in the retrograde direction from ventricle to atrium. In this situation, an ORT utilizes the accessory pathway as the retrograde limb and the AV node as the anterograde limb of a reentry circuit (Fig. 1.04). Orthodromic reciprocating tachycardia usually starts with either an atrial or ventricular premature beat. When the accessory pathway conducts rapidly, the retrograde P-wave is inscribed at approximately 140 ms (range 80–160 ms) after the QRS complex with an RP interval shorter than the PR interval. The QRS complex is identical to that during sinus rhythm unless rate-related bundle branch aberrancy supervenes.

1.2.3 Atrial tachycardia

Atrial tachycardia can originate from anywhere in the atria. The mechanisms are unclear but may be related either to localized atrial reentry or a focus of enhanced automaticity. The atrial rate generally runs between 150 and 200 b.p.m. but occasionally as fast as 300 b.p.m. During atrial tachycardia the P-wave precedes the QRS complex. The morphology of the P-wave depends on the site of origin and differs from the sinus P-wave. The ventricular rate depends on AV nodal transmission. The AV relationship can be 1:1, or governed by second-degree AV block, which may itself also be variable (Fig. 1.05). The QRS complex remains the same as during sinus rhythm.

1.2.4 Atrial flutter

Atrial flutter (AFL) is sustained by a macro-reentrant atrial tachycardia usually located in the right atrium. During the common "typical" counterclockwise (CCW) right AFL the activation wavefront proceeds in a caudo-cranial direction along the interatrial septum. Then it returns cranio-caudally down the right atrial free wall towards the cavo-tricuspid isthmus (the area between the inferior vena cava and tricuspid valve) where there is marked slowing of conduction. During the less common "reverse typical" type of right AFL the macroreentry circuit rotates in a clockwise (CW) direction, down the interatrial septum and up the right atrial free wall (Fig. 1.06).

In typical CCW AFL, atrial activity (F-waves) inscribes a characteristic "saw-tooth" configuration with a dominant negative deflection in the inferior leads. In the uncommon CW AFL the inferior leads register positive flutter waves. The atrial rate approximates 300 b.p.m., and the AV ratio is usually 2:1 or greater depending on the status of AV nodal conduction. The AV ratio may change irregularly. Atrial flutter can also occur in the left atrium, especially after pulmonary vein isolation (ablation) for the treatment of atrial fibrillation.

A 1:1 AV ratio is exceptional. It may result from the proarrhythmic effect of class IC antiarrhythmic drugs that reduce atrial conduction velocity. The marked slowing of the atrial rate (190–240 b.p.m.) (Fig. 1.07) permits the development of 1:1 "slow" AFL with rate-related bundle branch block – a situation often misdiagnosed as ventricular tachycardia (VT).

1.2.5 Atrial fibrillation

The electrophysiologic basis of atrial fibrillation remains obscure. Two major hypotheses prevail:
1. "Multiple wavelets."
2. A single or a small number of high-frequency sources ("rotors" or "drivers") of stable micro-reentry ("mother wave") primarily located at the left atrium/pulmonary vein junction. Passive fibrillatory conduction gives rise to "daughter waves" (Fig. 1.08).

During atrial fibrillation the fibrillatory waves (f-waves) exhibit a rate of 350–500/min. Only part of the many atrial impulses actually travel at irregular intervals through the AV nodal filter to the ventricles. The electrocardiogram (ECG) shows an irregular ventricular response. The ventricular rate becomes regular and not fast, only in combination with complete AV block. In the presence of a fast ventricular response (> 170 b.p.m.), the ventricular rate tends to regularize, and an implantable cardioverter defibrillator (ICD) may therefore face difficulty in discriminating atrial fibrillation from ventricular tachycardia.

1.3 Ventricular arrhythmias

Ventricular tachycardia (VT) and ventricular fibrillation (VF) are the major causes of sudden cardiac death in patients with structural heart disease. Ventricular fibrillation (VF) and/or ventricular tachycardia (VT) can also occur far less commonly in patients with structurally normal hearts. Sudden cardiac death is defined as death from an unsuspected circulatory arrest, usually due to an arrhythmia occurring within an hour of the onset of symptoms and when medical intervention such as defibrillation reverses the event.

1.3.1 Ventricular tachycardia

Ventricular tachycardia is defined as three or more consecutive premature ventricular complexes with a QRS duration > 120 ms at a rate between 100 and 300 b.p.m. The QRS complexes are not preceded by atrial deflections. The VT may be monomorphic or polymorphic. *Monomorphic VT* consists of a stable (organized) single QRS morphology often with a left bundle or right bundle block pattern. *Polymorphic* or *multiformic VT* exhibits an irregularly changing QRS configuration with variable cycle lengths between 600 and 180 ms. Torsades de pointes is a form of polymorphic VT associated with a long QT interval and characterized by twisting of the peaks of the QRS complexes.

Ventricular tachycardia may be *sustained* (duration > 30 s) and/or require termination due to hemodynamic compromise in less than 30 s) or *non-sustained* (three or more beats but less than < 30 s).

Special types of VT include:
1. Bidirectional VT, which displays beat-to-beat alternans of the QRS complexes.
2. Bundle branch reentrant VT, which occurs usually in the setting of cardiomyopathy and involves reentry in the His–Purkinje system traveling from one bundle branch to the other. The common type is associated with left bundle branch block morphology. Diagnosis is important because the common form can be easily eliminated by ablation of the right bundle branch.

1.3.2 Ventricular flutter

This type of VT runs usually close to 300 b.p.m. At fast rates, VT is so rapid that one cannot distinguish the QRS complexes from the T-wave. In other words there is no isoelectric interval between successive QRS complexes. This tachycardia is regular with cycle length variability of 30 ms or less.

1.3.3 Ventricular fibrillation

Ventricular fibrillation produces a completely disorganized tachyarrhythmia usually faster than 300/min with chaotic, random, asynchronous electrical activity of the ventricles. There are no discrete QRS complexes. Ventricular fibrillation shows marked variability of QRS cycle length, morphology and amplitude. For ICD work, VF may be defined as a polymorphic rhythm with a cycle length < 250 ms associated with no blood pressure. Spontaneous VF is often preceded by organized monomorphic VT. At its onset, VF registers a coarse electrical pattern. As the heart becomes less viable the fibrillation becomes fine and then as an agonal event all electrical activity ceases (flat line).

1.4 Causes of wide QRS tachycardia

There are various causes of tachycardia with a wide QRS complex (Fig. 1.11):
1. Ventricular tachycardia, by far the most common cause, constitutes more than 90% of wide QRS tachycardias in the emergency department. A history of prior myocardial infarction or congestive heart failure yields a positive predictive accuracy of > 95% for VT.
2. Supraventricular tachycardia (including sinus tachycardia, atrial tachycardia, AFL, AF, AVRT and AVNRT) with preexisting or rate-related bundle branch block or QRS widening due to class IC drugs or hyperkalemia.
3. Antidromic AVRT with anterograde conduction over an accessory pathway and retrograde conduction over the AV node or another accessory path.
4. Supraventricular tachycardia with anterograde conduction over an accessory pathway. Atrial fibrillation in the Wolff–Parkinson–White syndrome creates a fast and irregular tachyarrhythmia with a wide QRS complex.
5. Antidromic AVRT involving a Mahaim fiber (atriofascicular connection from the right atrium to the right bundle branch) with decremental conduction similar to the AV node. A Mahaim reentrant tachycardia uses the connection as the anterograde limb and the AV node as the retrograde limb of the reentry circuit. The ECG during tachycardia shows left bundle branch morphology because the anterograde limb inserts into or near the right bundle branch.
6. Bundle branch reentry tachycardia. The QRS morphology during sustained tachycardia exhibits a typical left bundle branch pattern (rarely right bundle branch block). Bundle branch reentry tachycardia should be considered in patients with nonischemic dilated cardiomyopathy and evidence of His–Purkinje conduction disease, manifested by a prolonged PR interval and/or QRS duration. This tachycardia depends on block in one bundle (long refractory period), and slow retrograde conduction along the other bundle (Fig. 1.14). Patients commonly present with syncope or sudden cardiac death with tachycardia rates often 200–300 b.p.m. During tachycardia, a His (H) bundle potential precedes each QRS complex and variations in VV interval are preceded by similar changes in H–H intervals. Recognition is important because catheter

ablation of the right bundle branch (in the common form) can easily eliminate the tachycardia. However, depending on the severity of underlying left ventricular (LV) function, patients with bundle branch reentry VT may also benefit from primary sudden death prevention with an ICD.

1.5 Electrocardiographic diagnosis of ventricular tachycardia

Despite numerous established criteria for the differentiation of ventricular from supraventricular tachycardia (SVT) with aberrant conduction, the differential diagnosis of a wide QRS complex tachycardia (QRS > 120 ms) remains a challenge.

Stepwise approach (Fig. 1.12)

Step 1: Absence of RS complexes in any of the precordial leads

The absence of RS complexes in any precordial lead strongly suggests VT. If RS complexes are present proceed to step 2.

Step 2: Duration of RS interval in the precordial leads

An interval of the R-wave onset to the S-nadir > 100 ms favors VT.

Step 3: Atrioventricular dissociation, capture or fusion beats

The presence of *AV dissociation*, i.e. independent atrial and ventricular activity, during a wide QRS tachycardia is diagnostic of VT. It occurs in about half the VT cases; in the other half there is retrograde VA conduction. With 1:1 retrograde VA conduction, the AV/VA relationship cannot differentiate VT from SVT. The presence of second-degree VA conduction block indicates VT.

During relatively slow VT, part of or all the ventricles may be activated by a supraventricular impulse (e.g. sinus beat) conducted through the AV junction. This phenomenon results in *"capture beats"* (with supraventricular QRS configuration) reflecting complete ventricular activation from the impulse coming from AV node. *"Fusion beats"* (intermediate QRS morphology) occur when both the ectopic ventricular impulse and a supraventricular beat activate the ventricle to a varying degree. These phenomena are diagnostic of VT.

Step 4: QRS morphologies in V1 and V6

Ventricular tachycardias may present either with a right (RBBB) or left bundle branch block (LBBB) pattern (Fig. 1.13).

SVTs with RBBB usually display a triphasic pattern in V_1 and V_6. Lead V_1 shows an rSR' pattern, lead V_6 shows a narrow q wave and the R/S ratio is typically > 1.

VTs with RBBB show a monophasic or biphasic QRS complex in lead V_1. The presence of a deep S wave with an R/S ratio < 1 or QS or QR pattern in lead V_6 supports the diagnosis of VT.

SVTs with LBBB show a narrow r wave (< 30 ms) in lead V_1 with a fast downstroke of the S wave. The interval from the onset of the QRS to the nadir of the S wave measures < 60 ms.

VTs with LBBB show in lead V_1 a broad R wave (≥ 30 ms) and a slow descent from the beginning of the QRS to the nadir of the S wave (> 60 ms). A prominent Q wave in lead V_6 is diagnostic for VT.

QRS duration

VT is the most probable diagnosis when QRS duration is > 140 ms in patients with a RBBB configuration and > 160 ms in LBBB in the absence of antiarrhythmic drug therapy.

QRS axis in the frontal plane

A frontal plane QRS axis between − 90° and ± 180° (right superior axis) suggests VT. Thus, mostly negative QRS complexes in leads I, II and III are useful criteria for identifying VT.

Concordant negative ECG patterns in the precordial leads

If all precordial leads generate predominantly negative QRS deflections, VT is the likely diagnosis. If all precordial leads are mostly positive, the differential diagnosis consists of VT and an antidromic tachycardia using a left-sided accessory pathway anterogradely.

The indications for ICD implantation have expanded over the past few years. In addition to secondary prevention for patients with prior life-threatening events, ICDs are now implanted for primary prevention in patients without a prior event but at high risk for sudden death (see appendix and Fig. 2.01).

The American College of Cardiology (ACC) and the American Heart Association (AHA) together with the Heart Rhythm Society (HRS) have issued guidelines on ICD indications (Fig. 2.02; see Appendix). These guidelines represent the consensus of medical opinion as to the use of ICDs. Guidelines use a class system (class I to III) for indications and rank the weight of evidence in levels (level A to C).

The guidelines describe indications as class I as a condition for which there is evidence and/or general agreement that ICD implantation is useful and effective (Fig. 2.03). Class II indications are conditions for which there is conflicting evidence concerning usefulness or efficacy; in class IIa (Fig. 2.04) the weight of opinion favors ICD implantation, whereas in class IIb the evidence generally opposes use of an ICD. Class III includes several patient populations for whom the consensus of medical opinion holds that ICD implantation is not useful or effective and in some cases may be harmful (Fig. 2.05).

The evidence that supports a recommendation is ranked as level A if the data were derived from multiple randomized clinical trials involving a large number of individuals. The evidence is ranked as level B when the data are derived from a limited number of trials involving a smaller number of patients or from well-designed data analyses of nonrandomized studies or observational registries. Evidence is ranked as level C when the consensus opinion of experts was the primary source of recommendation. This does not necessarily mean that a recommendation based on level C evidence is worse than one based on level A evidence. Especially in patient cohorts with rare diseases, randomized trials will be difficult to conduct and possibly never be done.

Reversible ventricular tachyarrhythmias

An ICD should not be considered if ventricular tachyarrhythmias are transient and reversible. Such causes include hypokalemia, hypomagnesemia and proarrhythmic effects of class III drugs (all of which can cause torsades de pointes even in a structurally normal heart), and digitalis toxicity. A long list of cardiac and noncardiac drugs can cause QT prolongation and torsades de pointes. Ventricular fibrillation occurring in the first 48 hours after an acute coronary syndrome and myocardial infarction is associated with an increase in hospital mortality but not with increased long-term mortality. Patients with polymorphic VT (with a normal QT interval) should be considered for urgent coronary angiography to determine a possible ischemic cause. If severe coronary artery disease is complicated by ventricular tachyarrhythmias, there is a good likelihood that revascularization will reduce or eliminate the arrhythmias. In this situation if left ventricular ejection is normal or near normal, the indication for an ICD is debatable.

Single or dual chamber ICD

Dual chamber ICDs are indicated in patients who have conventional indications for dual chamber pacing such as chronotropic incompetence, sick sinus syndrome or abnormalities in AV conduction. However, many practitioners favor the use of dual chamber ICDs in many other patients because atrial monitoring provides useful data for the diagnosis of various tachyarrhythmias.

2.1 The cardiac action potential and malfunction of ion channels

2.1.1 The cardiac action potential

Resting membrane potential

Cardiac cells are covered with a semipermeable membrane (sarcolemma) that maintains steep gradients of ions between the intracellular and extracellular environment, an arrangement responsible for the membrane potential. Pumping of sodium ions out of the cell and potassium ions into the cell maintains the resting membrane potential.

At rest, during diastole when no electrical charge flows, the interior of the cell is negatively charged and the outside is positively charged so that the sarcolemma is polarized. The ionic movements accompanying the wave of electrical excitation, a process called depolarization, reverses this polarization state.

The juxtaposition of the depolarized and polarized cells allows current to flow so that current spreads further and other adjacent cells become depolarized.

During a cardiac cycle the membrane potential changes from the polarized state (resting membrane potential) to depolarization, then repolarization, and back to the polarized state.

The cardiac action potential is governed by the complex interaction between depolarizing inward currents (making the interior of the cell more positive) and repolarizing outward currents (making the interior of the cell more negative). These phenomena are caused mainly by transmembrane movements of sodium, calcium and potassium ions (Fig. 2.06).

The sequence of electrical changes during the cardiac action potential is divided into five arbitrary phases: phase 0, the upstroke phase of rapid depolarization; phase 1, the phase of initial rapid repolarization; phase 2, the plateau phase; phase 3, the final repolarization; and phase 4, in cells with pacemaker activity, spontaneous depolarization of the membrane generates a new action potential.

Phase 0: Rapid depolarization

During the rapid phase of initial depolarization (phase 0) the action potential opens the sodium channels when the voltage reaches -70 to -60 mV, which is the threshold of activation. Upon depolarization, sodium ions enter the cell very rapidly during the first milliseconds of depolarization (inward Na^+ current) and the cell membrane potential turns positive ($+30$ mV).

Phase 1: Initial fast repolarization

Cessation of depolarization gives way to a period of fast repolarization (Fig. 2.07) before the pattern levels off to form the plateau phase. This rapid repolarization produces the "dart–dome" configuration of the action potential in myocardial and Purkinje cells. The repolarization process stems mainly from the combination of the fast inactivation of sodium channels and a transient outward potassium current i_{to}.

Phase 2: Plateau phase

The plateau phase is due to a "fine balance" between the depolarizing late inward calcium (i_{CaL}) and late sodium current (i_{NaL}) and repolarizing outward potassium current (i_{K1}).

Phase 3: Final repolarization

The final repolarization comes mostly from the combined action of the repolarizing outward rapid i_{Kr} and slow i_{Ks} potassium currents and the depolarizing late inward currents i_{NaL} and i_{CaL}.

Phase 4: Diastolic depolarization

Finally, the cell reenters the polarized state. In the sinoatrial and atrioventricular nodes spontaneous depolarization can occur normally and initiate a propagated impulse.

2.1.2 Malfunction of ion channels

Gene mutations may cause either a *gain or loss of function* of the important ionic channels governing the repolarization process and hence action potential duration. Normal repolarization represents the result of a fine balance between repolarizing and depolarizing currents (Fig. 2.07). An imbalance will result in abnormalities of action potential duration that may cause arrhythmias. This concept underlies the long QT, short QT and Brugada syndromes.

When the repolarizing currents (i_{Kr} and i_{Ks}) are stronger than the depolarizing currents (i_{NaL} and i_{CaL}), the action potential duration and the QT interval shorten. Conversely, the action potential duration and the QT interval lengthen when the repolarizing currents (i_{Kr} and i_{Ks}) become smaller and the depolarizing currents (i_{NaL} and i_{CaL}) larger.

2.2 ICD therapy in specific diseases

2.2.1 The long QT syndrome

The QT interval extends from the beginning of the QRS complex to the end of the T-wave. It represents the sum of cardiac depolarization and repolarization times, and basically corresponds to the duration of the action potential. Because the QT interval shortens with tachycardia and lengthens with bradycardia, it is corrected for heart rate using Bazett's formula (divide the QT interval by the square root of the RR interval) (Fig. 2.06). The corrected QT interval (QTc) normally measures 400 ± 40 ms.

The long QT syndrome (LQTS) is the phenotypic description of a group of disorders characterized by a prolonged QT interval in the electrocardiogram (Fig. 2.08). The LQTS may be acquired or genetic.

Acquired LQTS may be due to QT-prolonging drug therapy (such as antiarrhythmic drugs, certain antihistamines, macrolide antibiotics, antipsychotic and antidepressant medications) or electrolyte disturbances (hypokalemia, hypomagnesemia). Bradycardia can potentiate the risk of drug-induced LQTS.

The LQTS carries an increased risk of life-threatening ventricular arrhythmias known as torsades de pointes (TdP). Patients with a QTc > 500 ms carry a higher risk of syncope, cardiac arrest or sudden death.

Torsades de pointes is a dangerous arrhythmia describing a form of polymorphic VT with cycling of the QRS axis through 180° (Fig. 2.09). The peaks of the QRS complexes display an undulating pattern and appear to "twist" around the isoelectric line; hence the name torsades de pointes, or "twisting of the points". The ventricular rate usually ranges from 200 to 250 b.p.m. TdP is usually short-lived and often terminates spontaneously but may give rise to syncope. Most patients experience multiple episodes of TdP that may recur in rapid succession, potentially degenerating into VF with sudden death.

TdP may be accounted for by early afterdepolarizations (EADs), which are single or multiple oscillations of the membrane potential occurring during phase 2 or 3 of the action potential. Bradycardia potentiates EADs, which also emerge often after a compensatory pause related to a premature ventricular complex.

Seven causal genes have been identified in patients with genetic LQTS; five are associated with potassium channels, one with ankyrin B (*ANK2* gene) and one with the sodium channel. The distinct genetic types are designated LQT 1 through 7. The LQT syndromes LQT1, LQT2 and LQT3 account for more than 90% of cases of congenital LQTS, with LQT1 and LQT2 being more common than LQT3 (Fig. 2.08).

The LQT1 syndrome is caused by mutations in the *KCNQ1* gene resulting in a loss of function of the slowly acting component i_{Ks} of the repolarizing outward potassium current. The LQT2 syndrome is caused by mutations in the *KCNH2* (*HERG*) gene resulting in a loss of function of the rapidly acting component i_{Kr} of the repolarizing outward potassium current. The LQT3 syndrome is caused by mutations in the cardiac sodium channel gene resulting in a gain of function of the late sodium current i_{NaL}.

Three clinical phenotypes have been described in congenital LQTS according to the type of inheritance and the presence or absence of sensorineural hearing loss. The more common autosomal dominant form, the *Romano–Ward syndrome*, has a purely cardiac phenotype. The autosomal recessive form, the *Jervell and Lange-Nielsen syndrome*, is associated with LQTS and deafness. The Jervell and Lange-Nielsen

syndrome thus far has only been described in LQT1 and LQT5, both of which affect i_{Ks}.

The uncommon clinical phenotype called Andersen–Tawil syndrome (previously classified as LQT7) is an autosomal dominant disorder characterized by the clinical triad of periodic paralysis, facial/skeletal dysmorphism and ventricular arrhythmias. The syndrome is caused by a mutation of the *KCNJ2* gene encoding the repolarizing outward potassium current (i_{KI}). The reduced i_{KI} current is responsible for the prolonged terminal phase of the cardiac action potential, delayed afterdepolarizations (DADs) and arrhythmias. Electrocardiographic manifestations include mild QTc prolongation and prominent U-waves. Ventricular ectopy is common and includes polymorphic VT, bidirectional VT and TdP. Sudden death may occur.

A relationship exists between genotype and morphology of the T-wave. Patients with LQT1 show a broad-based T-wave of high amplitude. The electrocardiographic hallmark for patients with LQT2 consists of notched "bifid" low-amplitude T-waves. Patients with LQT3 show a long isoelectric ST segment and a late-onset, peaked asymmetrical T-wave. However, ECG patterns may be overlapping.

A relation was found between specific genotypes and the conditions that trigger cardiac events in LQTS (Fig. 2.10). Patients with LQT1 have a propensity to develop arrhythmias during physical exercise, especially swimming. In contrast, LQT2 and LQT3 patients have only a modest probability of cardiac events during exercise. Auditory stimuli act as a specific trigger for LQT2 patients, whereas LQT3 patients are at greatest risk when at rest or during sleep.

All patients with LQTS, even if asymptomatic, should be treated with beta-blockers. They are effective in LQT1 but less effective in LQT2 and LQT3. Patients with LQT1 have a low incidence of cardiac events with beta-blocker therapy, whereas patients with LQT2 and LQT3 have a higher risk of cardiac events even on beta-blocker therapy. An ICD should be seriously considered in asymptomatic patients with LQT2 with a QTc > 500 ms and in all LQT3 patients. Beta-blockers should be continued after ICD implantation.

2.2.2 Brugada syndrome

The Brugada syndrome (BS) is characterized by:
1. ST-segment elevation in the right precordial ECG leads V_1 to V_3 resembling a right bundle branch block pattern;
2. a high incidence of sudden death at rest or during sleep, and a structurally normal heart (Fig. 2.11).

The disease is genetically determined, with an autosomal dominant pattern in 50% of familial cases. The genetic abnormalities causing BS have been linked to mutations in the ion-channel gene *SCN5A*, which encodes the cardiac sodium channel. Mutations in this channel result in loss of function of the channels or rapid recovery from inactivation enhancing the repolarization process with resultant abbreviation of the action potential duration. Arrhythmias are based on phase 2 reentry.

Three ECG repolarization patterns in the right precordial leads (V_1–V_3) are recognized.

Type 1, called the "coved-type" (upward convexity), is diagnostic of Brugada syndrome. It inscribes coved ST-segment elevation ≥ 2 mm (0.2 mV) followed by a negative T-wave so there is no isoelectric segment. The QT interval is normal.

Type 2, called the "saddle-type", is characterized by a saddleback appearance with a high-takeoff ST-segment elevation (≥ 2 mm) followed by a gradually descending ST segment (remaining ≥ 1 mm above baseline) and positive or biphasic T-waves.

Type 3 shows either coved or saddleback morphology, with an ST-segment elevation of < 1 mm.

The ECG manifestations of the BS may be transient or concealed but can be unmasked primarily by sodium channel blockers (i.e. flecainide, procainamide, ajmaline) but also during a febrile state or with vagotonic agents. Beta-adrenergic stimulation (isuprel or exercise) normalizes the ECG pattern whereas it is exaggerated by beta-blockers. Type 2 and type 3 patterns are considered significant if there is a conversion to a type 1 pattern, either spontaneously or during administration of class I A/C antiarrhythmic drugs (flecainide, etc.). Placement of the right precordial leads in a superior position (two intercostal spaces above normal) can increase the sensitivity of the ECG for detecting the Brugada phenotype in some patients, both in the presence or absence of a drug challenge.

Currently, an ICD is the only proven effective treatment for the disease. Recommendations for ICD implantation are summarized in Fig. 2.12. Quinidine is the only drug that may be useful.

Symptomatic patients displaying the type 1 Brugada ECG (either spontaneously or after sodium channel blockade) who present with aborted sudden death should receive an ICD without a preliminary electrophysiologic study. Similar patients presenting with syncope, seizure, or nocturnal agonal respiration also should undergo ICD implantation after noncardiac causes are carefully ruled out. An electrophysiologic study is recommended in symptomatic patients only for the assessment of supraventricular arrhythmias.

Asymptomatic patients displaying a type 1 Brugada ECG (either spontaneously or after sodium channel blockade) should undergo an electrophysiologic study if there is a suspected family history of sudden cardiac death from Brugada syndrome. With a negative family history for sudden cardiac death, an electrophysiologic study is justified if the type 1 ECG pattern occurs spontaneously. The patient should then receive an ICD for inducible VT/VF. Asymptomatic patients with no family history who develop a type 1 ECG pattern only after sodium channel blockade should be closely followed.

2.2.3 The short QT syndrome

Patients with the short QT syndrome (QT interval < 300 ms) present with malignant ventricular tachyarrhythmias at a young age, a history of familial sudden death and a structurally normal heart (Fig. 2.13). The QRS complex is normal, and the ST segment virtually nonexistent. The short QT syndrome originates from a gain in function of the i_{Kr} and i_{Ks} potassium channels, increasing the speed of repolarization so that the action potential duration shortens considerably. The gain of function is caused by mutations of the *KCNQ1* gene (responsible for i_{Ks}) and/or the *KCNH2* gene (responsible for i_{Kr}). Currently, ICD implantation provides the only therapeutic option and prophylactic implantation should be strongly considered, although it is not really feasible in very young children. Quinidine may be helpful in prolonging the QT interval.

2.2.4 Hypertrophic cardiomyopathy

Hypertrophic cardiomyopathy (HCM) is an inherited myocardial disorder (Fig. 2.16) linked to a variety of gene mutations encoding protein components of the cardiac sarcomere. Hypertrophic cardiomyopathy carries the risk of ventricular tachyarrhythmias and sudden death, especially in young patients. Drug therapy includes beta-blockers and amiodarone. Alcohol septal ablation or septal myectomy do not lower the risk of sudden death. Patients with a prior cardiac arrest or sustained VT/VF should obviously receive an ICD for secondary prevention in view of the recurrence risk. The precise identification of patients who should be targeted for primary prevention with an ICD remains challenging.

Risk stratification requires a detailed personal and family history, physical examination including provocative maneuvers, 12-lead ECG, and two-dimensional echocardiography with assessment of resting and provoked left ventricular outflow gradients, 24-h ambulatory ECG monitoring, and exercise testing. Massive left ventricular hypertrophy (interventricular septal thickness > 30 mm) is a powerful independent marker for sudden death, even in the absence of demonstrable ventricular arrhythmias.

Implantation of an ICD for primary prevention of sudden death in HCM patients depends on the risk profile, and is considered in the presence of two or more risk factors, although some authorities recommend an ICD in the setting of only one risk factor (Fig. 2.17).

2.2.5 Arrhythmogenic right ventricular dysplasia

Arrhythmogenic right ventricular dysplasia (ARVD) is characterized by varying degrees of patchy replacement of the right ventricular myocardium with fatty or fibrous-fatty tissue that underlies the substrate for reentrant circuits responsible for ventricular tachyarrhythmias (Fig. 2.02). The lesions affect the right ventricular inflow, apex and infundibulum more frequently. The left ventricle may rarely also be affected. The condition is frequently transmitted in an autosomal dominant manner, with disease-causing mutations identified in genes encoding the cell adhesion proteins plakoglobin and desmoplakin.

T-wave inversion in leads V_1 to V_3, and a prolonged S-wave upstroke (> 55 ms) in leads V_1 to V_3 are the most common ECG findings. The myocardial process can cause delayed activation in the right ventricle, manifested in some cases as a potential in the terminal portion of the QRS in V_1–V_3 leads defined as an "epsilon wave". More frequently the signal-averaged ECG (SAECG) detects fragmented electrical activity.

Patients with ARVD mostly suffer from palpitations due to frequent premature ventricular complexes (1000/24 h on Holter monitoring) or syncope associated with episodes of sustained or nonsustained VT with a LBBB pattern originating in the right ventricle. Patients with a history of syncope or frequent VT should receive an ICD.

The role of ICD therapy in the primary prevention of sudden death remains unclear to date in the light of only preliminary data.

2.2.6 Cathecholaminergic polymorphic ventricular tachycardia

Cathecholaminergic polymorphic ventricular tachycardia (CPVT) is a genetically determined disorder associated with syncope and sudden death (Fig. 2.15). Features include:
1. a direct relationship between adrenergic activation at the onset of ventricular tachyarrhythmias;
2. a typical pattern of bidirectional VT with an unremarkable resting electrocardiogram (with the exception of mild sinus tachycardia);
3. a structurally normal heart.

Physical exercise or acute emotional stress provides specific triggers for arrhythmia. The disturbance is caused by genetic mutations of the cardiac ryanodine receptor RyR2 and calsequestrin proteins responsible for the regulation of calcium in the heart. The mutations cause an overload of calcium in the heart causing delayed afterdepolarizations (DADs). Delayed afterdepolarizations are spontaneous diastolic depolarizations that can initiate action potentials and arrhythmias. Beta-blockers are the cornerstone of therapy but an ICD is also recommended in most patients.

2.2.7 Lamin A/C gene mutation

Dilated cardiomyopathy with conduction defects has been associated with mutations in the *LMNA* gene encoding the inner nuclear membrane protein lamin A/C. Atrial fibrillation, sinus node dysfunction, AV conduction defects, heart failure and sudden cardiac death due to ventricular tachyarrhythmias are common in patients with lamin A/C gene mutations. Because sudden cardiac death may occur even before the development of severe left ventricular systolic dysfunction, prophylactic implantation of an ICD rather than permanent pacing should be considered at an early stage of this entity.

3 ICD hardware

The ICD system consists of a pulse generator and one or more leads or patches capable of sensing, pacing and defibrillation (Fig. 0.01). The ICD generator houses the battery (the power source), one or two high-voltage capacitors (reservoir of electrical charge) and the electronic circuitry responsible for timing, tachyarrhythmia detection, therapy delivery, bradyarrhythmia pacing, diagnostics and telemetry.

3.1 ICD can and header

The ICD generator casing (called the "can") is a hermetically sealed metal housing made of either stainless steel or titanium. Titanium is the preferred material because of its strength, biocompatibility or nonreactivity in body fluids, and low density. The metal housing protects the battery and the electronic circuitry from the corrosive effects of body fluids and external electromagnetic interference (EMI). However, the can may also serve as an active shocking (high-voltage) electrode in current ICD models.

After mounting the battery and the electronic components, the two halves of the metal housing are welded together using a laser or TIG (tungsten inert gas welding). Before completing the seal, the unit is filled with helium. After final sealing, the hermetic seal is tested at ultra-high vacuum by a helium leak tester. The header generally consists of clear PMMA (polymethylmethacrylate resin or acrylic glass) so that the connections with the leads can be visually confirmed during implantation or troubleshooting. When there are more ports in the header than leads to be used, the inactive port is sealed with a silicone plug.

3.2 Battery

The lithium-iodine battery used in pacemakers was designed to deliver a low current for a long time (typically 10 µA for 5 years or more). However, in addition to this small current, the battery of an ICD must provide very high current pulses to charge the capacitor for defibrillation (typical current is 2 A

for at least 10 s). Therefore, an ICD battery must possess high energy density, high current delivery capability and low self-discharge (i.e. low loss of charge due to internal leakages). The battery in most ICDs is the lithium/silver–vanadium oxide cell, or SVO battery).

3.2.1 Active components

The active cathode material is silver vanadium oxide ($Ag_2V_4O_{11}$). The active material forms a mixture together with a Teflon binder and conductive carbon. The reduction of vanadium (in steps from V^{5+} to V^{3+}) and silver (from Ag^+ to Ag^0) absorbs electrons from the external circuit. The anode is pure lithium metal pressed onto a nickel current collector. The oxidation of lithium delivers electrons to the external circuit. One mole of $Ag_2V_4O_{11}$ can react with seven moles of Li. Conventional Li/SVO batteries are called cathode-limited because the capacity of the cathode must not exceed the capacity of the anode (lithium). The term cathode-limited was used for the original SVO battery design and implies that depletion occurs when the cathode material is depleted (Fig. 3.01).

The surface area of both cathode and anode must be sufficiently large to provide the current delivery to meet the shock requirements. Therefore, a folded construction or a flattened coil permits both sides of the electrodes to be active (Fig. 3.02).

3.2.2 Battery indicators

The SVO battery generates an open circuit voltage or "electromotive force" of 3.2 V at full charge (i.e. at the beginning of life, or BOL). The progressive chemical reactions inside the unmodified battery generate a specific discharge curve with two regions of nearly constant voltage: one at 3.2 V and another at 2.6 V. These regions are joined by a segment of sloping voltage. The voltage also slopes downward after the 2.6-V plateau. Generator replacement is recommended when a specific indicator of battery depletion, termed the elective replacement indicator (ERI), is reached. The battery voltage normally triggers the ERI point. Consequently the ERI voltage must be set slightly below the 2.6-V plateau to achieve higher longevity. At the ERI point, generator replacement can be scheduled usually within 2–3 months but preferably sooner. A late indicator, designated as end of life (EOL) reflects a lower voltage of approximately 2.2 V and indicates the need for urgent generator replacement.

3.2.3 Battery voltage during capacitor charging

Note that the loaded voltage of a battery is always less than the open circuit voltage. The equivalent series resistance (ESR) of a SVO battery is about 0.3 Ω. During charging of the high-voltage (HV) capacitor, a current drain of up to 2 A may be needed, yielding (according to Ohm's law: $R \times I = V$) an internal voltage drop of $0.3\ \Omega \times 2\ A = 0.6\ V$. Thus, during charging of the HV capacitor, the loaded voltage of the battery may drop below the ERI voltage. However, the device does not measure this low loaded voltage and therefore does not activate the ERI point during the short capacitor charging time. The status of the battery voltage and the ERI indicator are exclusively based on the open circuit voltage (also called the monitoring voltage or unloaded voltage) when there is no capacitor charging. There is always, of course, a very small current drain in terms of some microamperes for the microprocessor, memory, etc. Due to differences in this overhead current drain, the ERI voltage varies from manufacturer to manufacturer even though they use the same type of power source.

Some ICDs use two SVO batteries in series and hence have a BOL voltage of 6.4 V.

3.2.4 Capacitor charging time

The internal resistance (ESR) of the battery decreases slightly during the 3.2-V plateau, then increases steadily until depletion. The combination of a decreasing voltage and increasing internal resistance influences the charging time of the HV capacitor. The charging time may double from about 5–7 s to about 15 s. In view of the importance of rapid capacitor charging, some ICDs incorporate the charging time in the ERI warning (i.e. the device declares ERI with a low battery voltage or excessively long capacitor charging time).

3.2.5 Dual battery sources

Some devices use a dual energy source: a Li/SVO battery for defibrillation shocks requiring a high current delivery capacity, and a separate Li/iodine battery for monitoring functions and electronics. The dual source solution may result in a smaller overall battery volume because the classic Li/iodine battery possesses a greater energy density.

3.2.6 Voltage delay and internal battery impedance

When the battery has reached its 2.6-V plateau, a "chemical buildup" around the cathode may occur when a high charging current has not been delivered during a couple of months. The buildup increases the ESR and lengthens the charging time. This phenomenon is called "voltage delay" because it may delay the delivery of the shock. Because the chemical buildup disappears after a new charging cycle of the capacitor, it is recommended to "reform" the capacitor every 3 months when the 2.6-V plateau is reached (Fig. 3.04). The capacitor reforming recommended by the manufacturers partly reflects this battery requirement.

3.2.7 New battery technology

A new battery invented by Medtronic (Minneapolis, MN, USA) is anode-limited and has the advantage of maintaining a higher voltage throughout the life of the battery. The constituents are rebalanced with a lesser amount of lithium, and the altered composition of the battery eliminates the second voltage plateau of cathode-limited batteries. There is no dual-plateau depletion curve as in cathode-limited batteries. The battery discharge is substantially completed as the open circuit battery voltage drops to about 2.6 V. With the new battery, the depletion curve is roughly linear after the first plateau, with the elective replacement indicator (ERI) set at about 2.62 V. The advantage of the higher voltage in anode-limited batteries is a greater "push" for charging capacitors. There is also less need for relatively frequent capacitor reforming (in contrast to ICDs with a cathode-limited battery) when the battery voltage approaches the ERI point. In this respect, Medtronic specifies capacitor reforming (see below) every 6 months. Frequent capacitor reforming reduces battery life.

3.3 Capacitors and capacitor charging

The high-voltage (HV) capacitor is an important component of the ICD. Understanding ICD function requires some knowledge of capacitors and their charging capability. Most ICDs are equipped with two HV capacitors, both able to withstand, say, 400 V. When fully charged, the capacitors are connected in series and together they deliver a pulse to the heart of $2 \times 400\ V = 800\ V$.

3.3.1 Amplification of battery voltage

As the ICD battery generates only a low voltage (3.2 V, or 6.4 V with two batteries), it cannot quickly deliver the charge (shock) required to defibrillate the heart. Therefore, a charger (or DC–DC converter) transforms this low voltage to a high voltage (up to 750–800 V). The HV charge for defibrillation then builds up gradually over several seconds and is temporarily stored in a HV capacitor, from which delivery to the heart takes place in only a few (6–10) milliseconds. This process is analogous to a bucket being continuously and slowly filled with water from a garden hose (low volume per second, or a small current). The bucket is then tipped over followed by rapid dumping of the water (high volume per second, or a very large current). The volume in the bucket represents the total charge stored in the capacitor (Fig. 3.04).

3.3.2 Basic properties of capacitors

A capacitor stores electrical charge. Specifically, it is a temporary storage compartment for charge or energy. A simple capacitor consists of two conductors, called plates or electrodes (e.g. parallel metallic plates), separated by an insulator, called the dielectric. Upon connecting a voltage source to a capacitor, the free electrons in the plates are redistributed: electrons are removed from one plate and pumped into the other plate. This forms an electrical component containing one positively charged plate and one negatively charged plate together with a voltage (potential difference) between the plates. After removal of the voltage source, the capacitor retains the charge.

Capacitance is the ability of a capacitor to store electrical charge. The capacitance is large when a small voltage can store a large charge into a capacitor. Mathematically, the capacitance (C) may be expressed as the ratio between charge and voltage: $C = Q/V$ (Fig. 3.05). The basic unit of capacitance is the farad (symbol F). A capacitor has a capacitance of 1 F when 1 coulomb (1 C) of charge is stored as 1 volt (1 V) is applied to the plates of a capacitor. However, for practical purposes, the farad unit is far too large. Electronic devices usually require much smaller subunits: the microfarad (µF) is a million times smaller than the farad, and the nanofarad (nF) is a billion times smaller than the farad (Fig. 3.06).

Before connecting an external voltage source (e.g. a battery) to a capacitor, both of its plates contain the same quantity of positive and negative charges: it is electrically neutral and the voltage between the plates is zero. Immediately after connecting the voltage source, many electrons are pumped from one plate to the other and initially a large current flows through the external circuit (i.e. external to the capacitor). However, the buildup of charge on the plates creates a voltage between them that opposes the source voltage. Consequently, the current through the external circuit (which started at a high value) gradually decreases while the voltage between the capacitor plates gradually increases starting from zero. Finally, the capacitor voltage becomes equal to the source voltage and the current (flow of electrons) ceases (Fig. 3.07).

The current flow is limited by the external circuit. There is no current flow through the capacitor itself because the dielectric works as an insulator (if the insulator is not perfect a small leakage may occur; that is why the charge cannot be stored indefinitely in a practical capacitor). The current through the external circuit must comply with Ohm's law. This means that the resistance in the feeding circuit limits the magnitude of the current. Thus, a smaller current Ic secondary to a larger circuit resistance R, will prolong the time required fully to charge the capacitor (Fig. 3.08).

3.3.3 Time constant of capacitors

Mathematically, the current decrease Ic and the voltage rise Vc are both exponential; that is, their rate of change is governed by the time constant $\tau = RC$. The time constant τ represents the time for the voltage across the capacitor plates or the current through the external circuit to change by a factor of 63.2%. It is also the product of the charged capacitor (C) and the resistance in the charging circuit (R). During each time interval equal to RC, the difference between the source voltage (Vs) and the actual voltage between the capacitor plates (Vc) is further reduced by 63.2% (i.e. 63.2% of Vs – Vc) (Fig. 3.09).

Obviously, capacitor charging proceeds more slowly when the time constant becomes larger, that is, with a larger capacitor or a greater resistance connected in series. For all practical purposes, it is generally accepted that a capacitor is fully charged after a time equal to $5 \times \tau$ or 5RC.

3.3.4 Capacitor discharge

Discharging a capacitor – the inverse of charging – is governed by the same simple electrical laws. Once again, the curves are exponential and ruled by a time constant. The current in the external circuit now flows in the opposite direction and the resistance in the discharging circuit may be different from that of the charging circuit. If the resistance (R_2) in the discharging circuit exceeds that of the charging circuit (R_1) capacitor charging is quicker than discharging (Fig. 3.10).

The formation of the output pulse of an elementary pacemaker is an illustration of these simple principles. The output capacitor C_o (connected to the lead) slowly charges from the battery toward the voltage V_s. The current through the heart is very small, mostly limited by the large resistance R_{ch} (the pacing resistance itself, R_p, is rather small). It follows that the charging current does not affect the heart. When a switch S is closed by a timing mechanism, the capacitor suddenly starts discharging, causing the rapid delivery of a large charge bolus to the heart. The discharging current is large as it is only restricted by the smaller pacing resistance R_p. Hence the discharging current stimulates the heart. The discharging time is kept within strict limits by the same timing mechanism and when the switch S is opened again the capacitor C_o restarts charging (Fig. 3.11).

The very short duration of a pacemaker pulse causes a very small "droop" (i.e. the voltage difference between the leading edge and the trailing edge). Therefore, this pulse is known descriptively as a constant voltage type. In contrast, the high-voltage pulse (shock) of an ICD is different.

The shock resistance during discharge of the HV capacitor is minimal and the duration of the shock is much longer than a pacemaker pulse. It follows that the exponential decay or decline of the capacitor voltage is much more pronounced. The difference between the leading and the trailing edges is called the "tilt" (Fig. 3.12).

3.3.5 Capacitor voltage tilt

Tilt defines the percentage of the initial voltage on the HV capacitor lost during the shock. In mathematical terms, tilt = $(V_L - V_T)/V_L$ where V_L is the voltage at the start and V_T the voltage at the end of the waveform or shock. For a given shock duration, the tilt varies as a function of the shock resistance R; the smaller the resistance, the larger the tilt. Conversely, for a fixed tilt, the duration of the shock depends upon the shock resistance R; the larger the resistance, the larger the duration to obtain the same tilt. In other words, the capacitor is not completely discharged even with a maximal shock, so that a residual charge remains immediately after therapy. Some ICDs permit programming of the tilt, which represents an indirect way of programming pulse width. Tilt, therefore, depends on lead impedance, the capacitance, and the duration of the waveform. The optimal tilt for defibrillation ranges from 40% to 65%. In other words, in order for an ICD to deliver a programmed amount of energy (in joules) with a fixed tilt system, it has to vary the pulse width. Programming the pulse width rather than the tilt (available in St. Jude Medical devices; St. Jude Medical, St. Paul, MN, USA) may occasionally be helpful in reducing the energy requirements for defibrillation. In such a case, the device adjusts the tilt to provide the programmed energy. Advice from the manufacturer is vital when programming pulse duration in a difficult situation.

Most contemporary ICDs deliver biphasic high-voltage shocks. The same high-voltage capacitor generates both phases, and a switch with multiple positions changes the polarity of the waveform to the heart. Of course the shock resistance, mainly determined by the heart, remains the same for both phases and the tilt varies because the durations of the two phases are different (Fig. 3.13).

3.3.6 Potential energy

In order to charge a capacitor, electrons move from one plate to the other, a process requiring work. The battery must deliver "energy". The capacitor stores this energy as potential energy in the electric field between its plates (potential energy means the capacity for work upon capacitor discharge). The potential energy (W) associated with the stored charge is given by: $W = 0.5 \times CV^2$ where C is the capacitance and V the voltage between the plates. Note that the stored energy increases as the square of the voltage. Doubling the voltage will increase the energy by a factor of 4 (Fig. 3.14).

3.3.7 Energy vs voltage

ICD devices should be characterized by: (i) voltage; (ii) capacitance; (iii) tilt or pulse duration (if not programmable); and (iv) internal resistance. All other parameters can be derived from them by simple calculations. Yet energy is always expressed in joules (J; i.e. the mechanical unit of work). The joule is also used for programming ICDs based on historical reasons. Classic external defibrillators did not use shock truncation. The voltage on the HV capacitor always drooped to zero at the end of the shock and hence only the maximum voltage could be properly stated. Expressing a voltage–time relation was impossible (because shock duration was unknown). However, the stored energy was easily calculated if the capacitance of the HV capacitor was known ($0.5 \times CV^2$). Because old habits are hard to change, ICD programming is still done in terms of joules rather than volts (Fig. 3.16). The energies used during defibrillation are large. Such large energies can produce lesions in the heart tissue, and huge high-voltage shocks should only be used when strictly needed (Fig. 3.15).

3.3.8 Capacitor reformation

A capacitor appears superficially to be a simple component: the larger the surface area (A) of the plates and the smaller the distance (d) between them, the larger the capacitance ($C \propto kA/d$). However, the HV capacitors used in ICDs require a unique combination of properties: high voltage (up to 850 V), high capacitance (up to 200 µF), small size (less than 25 cm^3) and small weight (Fig. 3.17). These requirements confine the possible dielectrics to aluminum oxide in electrolytic capacitors (although efforts are being made to develop alternative dielectric materials).

Capacitor reformation is a maintenance process required periodically over the life of the capacitor and requires charging the capacitor completely. Capacitors can be reformed manually or automatically by the ICD at programmed intervals. If done manually, allow at least 10 min for charge dissipation. When aluminum electrolytic capacitors remain unused for an extended period of time, the oxide coating on the anode foil can decompose, resulting in an increase in static leakage current. This process is called "deformation" and can usually be reversed by the application of a reformation current for a sufficient length of time to redeposit aluminum oxide onto the foil. Deformation lengthens the charge time because some of the energy from the battery is used to re-form the oxide coating rather than charge the capacitor. The amount of additional energy needed to charge the capacitor depends on the length of time since the last time the capacitor was charged. To control this degradation (or deforming of the dielectric) and to limit the charging time to an acceptable duration, the capacitor has to be "reformed" regularly. This means fully charging the capacitor. This can be accomplished manually but all devices perform this task at regular intervals. The charge on the capacitor is then dissipated internally without patient awareness.

Ultimately, aluminum electrolytic capacitor charge times are primarily dependent on two factors:
1. the time when the capacitor was last reformed;
2. the viability (voltage) of the battery that is pushing charge onto the capacitor.

A prolonged charging time might be due to a lowered battery voltage close to the ERI (Figs 3.04 and 3.18).

More frequent charging results in reduced charge times; this occurs with the passage of time and is not harmful to the capacitor. However, too frequent (auto)reformation results in reduced projected longevity.

3.4 The high-voltage charging circuit

Defibrillation requires a high voltage to deliver a high-energy shock in less than 10 ms. The 3.2-V SVO battery source cannot deliver such a high voltage and therefore the ICD uses a "charger" or DC–DC converter for this purpose (Fig. 3.19).

The central part of the charger is a transformer that can transform a small alternating voltage (AC) into a large one. Because the battery only delivers a direct voltage (DC), a switch is placed between the battery and the transformer to convert DC into AC. At the output of the transformer a rectifying diode reconverts the AC to DC for the HV capacitor.

The switching occurs at a high frequency (e.g. 50 kHz) precluding mechanical switches (Fig. 3.20). The actual switching is done by a MOSFET transistor (metal oxide semiconductor field effect transistor).

A basic transformer has two coils of wire wound on a ferromagnetic core (ferrite). The first coil, identified as the "primary winding", functions as the input of the transformer. The second coil, known as the "secondary winding", functions as the output. The varying electrical current through the primary winding creates an alternating magnetic field, which in turn induces a voltage in the secondary winding. The voltage on both coils is proportional to their number of turns. By putting a large number of turns in the secondary winding, a huge secondary voltage may be obtained (Fig. 3.21).

A semiconductor diode only conducts in one direction and rectifies the alternating voltage (Vs) from the secondary winding of the transformer. A small amount of charge is added to the high-voltage capacitor C each time the voltage Vs becomes larger than the voltage Vc on the capacitor. When the secondary voltage Vs decreases below the capacitor voltage Vc the diode stops conducting and no charge can leak away from the capacitor (Fig. 3.22).

Capacitor charging time

Charge time is linearly related to the voltage and therefore energy being delivered. The charge time of the HV capacitor therefore depends upon the programmed energy. Programming an unnecessarily high energy (i.e. a higher voltage) requires a longer charging time and hence delays therapy (see Fig. 4.14). This is why the first shock for VF is sometimes programmed to a safe value (discussed later) below the maximal output of the ICD. This reduces capacitor charging time so that the ICD delivers an earlier shock.

3.5 ICD leads

The lead conducts electrical impulses from the ICD to the patient. An intracardiac ICD lead is composed of two, three or four conductors and electrodes, insulating coating, two or more connector pins and a fixation mechanism. The electrode is the active portion of the lead in direct contact with tissue.

The defibrillation electrodes have a relatively large surface area and are positioned to maximize the density of current flow through the ventricular myocardium. The ICD leads with their electrodes have three essential functions:
1. sensing intracardiac signals;
2. delivering pacing pulses for bradycardia and tachycardia;
3. delivering HV shocks.

3.5.1 ICD lead design

The first ICD lead systems used two epicardial patches. For sensing, two epicardial screw-in leads were also implanted. This method necessitates thoracotomy and is now used only in exceptional cases (Figs 3.23 and 3.24).

Contemporary transvenous leads provide defibrillation, pacing and sensing functions. The technology used for sensing and pacing resembles that of pacemakers. However, high-energy shocks require specialized leads capable of conducting the large current to the heart and withstanding a high voltage.

3.5.2 Types of transvenous leads

Transvenous defibrillator leads contain either one or two shocking coils. Both types use a distal coil close to the lead tip for right ventricle (RV) positioning. A dual-coil lead also incorporates a proximal coil located in the superior vena cava or subclavian vein. Both single-coil and dual-coil defibrillation leads come with active or passive fixation.

A subcutaneous or submuscular patch or subcutaneous array can be implanted in patients with a high defibrillation threshold. Contemporary transvenous leads, electrically active cans and the use of biphasic shocks have largely eliminated the unacceptably high defibrillation thresholds seen in the past.

ICD leads use only a bipolar configuration for sensing. There are, however, two types of bipolar configuration: "integrated bipolar" and "true bipolar". For pacing and sensing an integrated bipolar configuration connects the lead tip and the distal defibrillation coil whereas a true bipolar configuration utilizes the tip and an additional ring electrode. True bipolar leads provide the best sensing and pacing performance and are less susceptible to sensing far-field signals and diaphragmatic myopotentials. Integrated bipolar leads might be more favorable for defibrillation as the distal coil can be mounted closer to the tip and hence closer to the RV myocardium. New leads using a short tip-to-ring spacing (8 mm or less) bring the shocking coil nearer to the RV wall.

3.5.3 Lead construction

ICD leads can be coaxial or multiluminal. The coaxial design consists of a coiled conductor with an enveloping insulation layer between each of the conductors. Typically the tip conductor is central, with the ring conductor and the defibrillation conductor more peripheral. Lead implantation requires the insertion of a stylet through a channel within the innermost conductor. Coaxial leads are restricted to three conductors (single-coil leads) to avoid an excessively large and stiff product (Fig. 3.25).

The multiluminal design houses coiled and straight conductors running in parallel through a single insulating body. Each conductor is sheathed with an additional insulating layer. In a multiluminal lead, more conductors fit into an overall smaller body with probable lower electrical resistance of the HV shocking conductors.

Defibrillation conductors must resist corrosion and fatigue, and perform with the flexibility of traditional pacemaker lead conductors. Moreover, they must have a very low electrical resistance to minimize voltage loss. Peak current in a traditional pacemaker lead does not exceed 15 mA, but the current through a defibrillation conductor may attain 40 A (Ohm's law: $800\,V/20\,\Omega$). So-called "composite wires" achieve the required low resistance. These sophisticated wires combine the great conductivity of silver with the mechanical strength of titanium or stainless steel (such as MP35N, an alloy of Ni, Co, Cr and Mo). The wires are further formed into coils or twisted into small-diameter cables to improve flexibility and fatigue resistance. Coiling enhances fatigue life and flexibility, but increases the wire length and thus the electrical resistance.

3.5.4 Lead connections

Each defibrillator lead connects to the ICD with a total of two or three pins: one IS-1 (International Standard 3.2-mm connector) connection for pacing and sensing and one or two DF-1 (standard 3.2-mm connector) connections for defibrillation according to the number of coils (according to the ISO-11318 standard to ensure interchangeability). Dual-chamber ICDs require a separate bipolar atrial lead with an IS-1 connection (Fig. 3.26).

A new International Standard for a four-pole pacemaker and defibrillator connector system is currently being developed by manufacturers of cardiac rhythm management devices, with industry experts working together in the connector task force under ISO/IEC (International Organization for Standardization/International Electrotechnical Commission) Joint Working Group and the AAMI CRMD (Association for the Advancement of Medical Instrumentation Cardiac Rhythm Management Devices) Committee. Active industry participants currently include: Biotronik (Berlin, Germany), Guidant (Boston Scientific, St. Paul, MN, USA), Medtronic and St. Jude Medical (Fig. 3.27).

3.5.5 Lead insulation

Lead insulation influences lead reliability. The most commonly used insulation materials are silicone, polyurethane and fluoropolymers (polytetrafluoroethylene [PTFE], e.g. Teflon; or ethylene tetrafluoroethylene [ETFE], such as Etzel).

Polyurethane is biocompatible and has a high tensile strength making small lead diameters possible. The fundamental disadvantage of polyurethane insulation involves environmental stress cracking and metal ion oxidation, which affect reliability. Pre-treating polyurethane by heating it in inert gas greatly reduces the risk of environmental stress cracking.

Silicone rubber insulation is highly biocompatible, inert and biostable, but has a high friction coefficient. Its softness makes it prone to damage during implantation and carries the risk of abrasion.

Fluoropolymer insulation is highly biocompatible, allows a small lead diameter but stiffness limits its uses (maximal thickness 0.08 mm). Fluoropolymers have the greatest dielectric strength, making them the favorite material for HV lead insulation.

Contemporary leads possess a body of silicone supplemented by an outer layer of pretreated polyurethane to reduce the friction coefficient and scar formation. The lack of contact of the polyurethane with the metal conductors prevents metal ion oxidation. The HV conductors connected to the shocking electrodes are coated with an extra layer of a fluoropolymer.

3.6 The ICD programmer

Assuming proper programmer selection, most programmers will automatically identify the type of implanted device upon telemetric connection between the ICD and the programmer. Interrogation yields a vast amount of information for review. This includes pacing function, detection/delivery of tachyarrhythmia therapies and stored intracardiac electrograms with annotated markers.

4.1 Shocking vectors

Downsizing of ICD pulse generators has allowed routine pectoral implantation, and the use of the outer casing as the second or third defibrillation electrode. The latter system is known as "active can" or "hot can". The ICD should be implanted on the left pectoral side for optimal function of the active can (Figs 4.01 and 4.02).

For a single-coil lead system, shocks are delivered between the right ventricular (RV) coile (usually the anode or the positive pole) and the active can (cathode or negative pole). If this configuration does not produce an adequate defibrillation threshold, a separate SVC coil may be added or a dual-coil lead can be used instead. In this configuration both coils and the ICD participate in the shock vector. In some ICDs the active can be programmed out of the shock pathway. In rare cases the defibrillation threshold remains unacceptably high even with an appropriately positioned dual-coil system. In such instances, the proximal coil should be taken out of the defibrillation circuit or a subcutaneous array or patch can be added (Figs 3.24 and 4.22). At each step of the testing protocol, with unsuccessful defibrillation, the polarity of the shock pulse can be inverted and testing repeated although substantial improvement in the defibrillation threshold (DFT) is unusual.

4.2 Defibrillation testing

For ventricular defibrillation the shock must alter the transmembrane potential throughout the myocardium in such a way that it eliminates the fibrillation wavefronts without inducing new wavefronts capable of VF reinitiation.

During implantation one must test the ability of the ICD to convert VF successfully. Therefore testing requires VF induction (Fig. 4.06). One must be absolutely certain that VF and not fast VT is being induced for testing. The method of VF induction depends upon the manufacturer, and the capabilities of the device and programmer. The desired method is selected on the programmer screen and the programmer then transmits the command to the ICD.

There are several methods for VF induction, with little difference in their effectiveness.

1. *Shock-on-T-wave*. Pace the RV at a cycle length of 400 ms for eight beats and determine the coupling interval to the peak of the T-wave. Deliver a low-energy shock of 1 J at the top of the T-wave (usually at a coupling interval of approximately 310 ms) to initiate VF (Fig. 4.07).
2. *High-frequency ventricular burst pacing*. Induce VF by the delivery of a 1–2-s stimulation train of 50 Hz (Fig. 4.08).
3. Application of a relatively prolonged *DC (direct current) voltage*.

4.3 Defibrillation waveforms

The electrical shocks delivered by an ICD originate from capacitor discharge to the heart via the high-energy electrodes. The resultant waveform exhibits a voltage declining exponentially (Fig. 3.13). The waveform terminates prematurely (truncated) before full capacitor discharge. Truncation avoids the refibrillatory (proarrhythmic) effects induced by the low-voltage tail of complete capacitor discharge. Moreover, an excessively long shock waveform wastes much energy because the maximum membrane voltage captures the largest number of cells, that is, long before complete discharge of the HV capacitor (Fig. 4.09). The rate of voltage decay (tilt) is inversely proportional to both the (shocking) impedance of the lead system and the total capacitance in the ICD (Fig. 3.12).

Early models used a monophasic waveform that was truncated at 35% of the leading edge voltage. This is referred as a 65% tilt monophasic shock. In this waveform, all energy was delivered during *one and the same phase of the pulse* (i.e. the polarity was not reversed during the pulse). Contemporary ICDs incorporate biphasic waveforms because biphasic defibrillation is significantly superior to monophasic defibrillation, requiring less energy and causing less damage with greater success rates. A biphasic shock is split into two phases of opposite polarity. After an initial pulse (phase 1), a second pulse with the opposite polarity (phase 2) is delivered after 2 or 3 ms (Fig. 4.10). In other words, the waveform reverses direction in mid-shock instead of traveling in one direction only. Phase 1 depolarizes and/or extends the refractory period of most ventricular cells like a monophasic shock. Phase 2 acts as a powerful catalyst to reduce significantly the electrical requirements of the first phase. Phase 2 removes the charge ("burping") of cells that were not "captured" (where capture is used in the broad sense of extending refractory periods). This burping reduces the number of borderline stimulated cells that would otherwise exhibit delayed activation capable of desynchronizing the heart. Moreover, phase 2 removes charge from cells that were too close to the HV electrodes and hence were injured by excessive fields (at least temporarily).

The duration of each phase of a biphasic waveform depends on the manufacturer and may be programmable. The initial voltage of the second phase is the same as the residual voltage on the capacitor after truncation of phase 1. In other words the trailing edge of phase 1 always equals the leading edge of phase 2 (Figs 4.11 and 4.12).

Pulse voltage and pulse width are not programmable in ICDs as in pacemakers. Defibrillation is most efficient at a certain voltage and pulse duration. As energy is an indirect parameter, a larger quantity may not necessarily provide the optimal voltage–pulse duration relationship for effective defibrillation. It is acceptable for ICDs to use energy as "dosage" provided that lead impedance, capacitance values and pulse duration do not change.

Because the defibrillation pulses are always truncated, the voltage over the HV capacitor never reaches zero volts. Therefore, there is always energy remaining in the capacitor at the end of the shock. The difference between the stored or available energy at the start of the discharge and the energy remaining at the end of the discharge is the energy delivered to the heart. Obviously, the delivered energy is always smaller than the available energy (Fig. 4.13).

It should be noted that the charging time increases linearly with the stored or available energy (Fig. 4.14). The larger the stored energy (i.e. more joules), the longer the charging time (more milliseconds). Therefore, some physicians program the first shock as low as safely possible to ensure a more rapid shock delivery to the patient.

4.4 Defibrillation threshold

Induction of VF at ICD implantation aims to assess:
1. Electrical integrity of the connections between the lead system and the device.
2. Reliable sensing, detection, and redetection of VF. Testing usually starts by programming a ventricular sensitivity of 1.2 mV. If the device senses VF satisfactorily, the ventricular sensitivity is usually programmed permanently to 0.3 mV.
3. Efficacy of programmed shock strength. The efficacy of antitachycardia pacing is no longer routinely tested.

The defibrillation threshold (DFT) defines the lowest energy level that achieves successful defibrillation. However, the DFT does not represent a constant value because defibrillation requirements vary as a result of many factors. Therefore, there exists no true threshold at which defibrillation will always be successful. Instead, the likelihood of defibrillation at any energy level is a probability of success. Patient-specific defibrillation testing aims at estimating an energy output with an extremely high probability (> 99%) of successful defibrillation (Figs 4.15–4.18). Determination of a complete defibrillation probability-of-success curve for an individual patient is impractical and unsafe because it requires numerous fibrillation–defibrillation episodes. Table 4.1 outlines the factors influencing the DFT.

4.4.1 Methodology

The RV coil should be the anode. Programming the RV coil as the cathode does not improve defibrillation efficacy. There are many methods to estimate defibrillation efficacy, but two are commonly used (Fig. 4.19). In both methods the first shock is set at least 10 J less than the maximal output of the device (e.g. 30 − 10 = 20 J using a 10-J safety margin). In one method, the same successful defibrillation shock is repeated at 20 J as in the above example (*single-energy success protocol*). This method, using two equivalent shocks, does not assess the DFT but ensures an adequate 10-J safety margin. Alternatively, progressively lower-intensity shocks are delivered (*step-down protocol*) until a shock fails. The lowest successful shock energy level defines the DFT. By convention, programming a safety margin of 10 J above the DFT is widely accepted and generally provides reliable defibrillation. Although a 10-J margin is considered the traditional "standard of care", this number was derived before the introduction of more efficient defibrillation technology. There is evidence that a lower value may be acceptable with contemporary ICD systems. The interval between test shocks should be 5 min. Finally, two external defibrillators should be available for rescue shocks.

4.4.2 Single-shock protocol

The efficacy of modern ICDs using a pectoral implant with an active can and biphasic shock waveforms

Table 4.1. Factors influencing the defibrillation threshold

Generator-dependent factors	Active can and its site (right- or left-sided pectoral implant)
	Shock waveform – monophasic or biphasic (tilt and pulse duration) and polarity
	Lead system, number of electrodes, surface area
	Subcutaneous electrodes or array
Patient-related factors	LV mass, dilatation
	Body size and position
	Metabolic causes (hypercapnea and acidosis with deep sedation without intubation)
	Implantation site right or left
	Underlying heart disease, ischemia, presence of heart failure, hypertrophic cardiomyopathy
	Cocaine use
	Pneumothorax, left pleural effusion, pericardial effusion
Antiarrhythmic agents	Amiodarone, etc.
Ventricular fibrillation	Duration of VF
	Defibrillation protocol
	Prolonged procedure with multiple VF induction and defibrillation
	Type of anesthesia

now permits successful ICD implantation with a "safety margin" of at least 10 J in over 95% of cases (Fig. 4.21). A single VF induction at implantation using one defibrillation success at 14 J is attractive because it simplifies the implantation procedure and might reduce procedure times and complications. Such an approach depends on the DFT and is feasible in about 80% of patients. The long-term safety and efficacy of single-shock defibrillation testing has not been evaluated prospectively. In one retrospective analysis a single shock at 14 J, as the criterion for implantation, resulted in a similar success as 31-J shocks for the termination of spontaneous or induced VF episodes. The criterion of a single successful shock at 14 J is also comparable to a more traditional clinical approach of two successful shocks at 21 J for a 31-J maximal output device. These data suggest that single-shock testing appears to be a reasonable compromise to minimize testing, but a larger safety margin of 15–20 J is needed to ensure a high probability of defibrillation success. Further prospective studies to validate this approach are warranted.

Other data from DFT testing

1. Appropriate sensing and detection of VF. If sensing at the apex is inadequate, leads should be placed in the RV outflow tract or septum. Alternatively, a separate rate-sensing lead may be positioned in a different RV location.
2. The shocking impedance is within the acceptable range.
3. The charge time is acceptable.

4.4.3 High DFT

With present technology, the failure of transvenous ICD implantation because of a high DFT is rare (1–2%). Pneumothorax should be included in the differential diagnosis when unexpected high DFTs are found during ICD implantation or predischarge testing. No clinical, echocardiographic, or radiological variable is a strong predictor of high DFT (Fig. 4.22). The diagnosis of a high DFT mandates identification and correction of acutely reversible causes such as myocardial depression, pharmacological effect or left pleural effusion. A subcutaneous patch electrode or electrode array is the most effective of the commonly used methods for reducing DFTs (Table 4.2). The procedure requires deep sedation or general anesthesia during lead insertion and carries the potential long-term risks of infection, erosion and chronic pain. Patients with a history of habitual cocaine use may be at increased risk of a

---

Table 4.2. Management of high defibrillation threshold (DFT)

- Reevaluate lead position (is it truly at the RV apex?)
- Check high-voltage impedance and all the connections
- Exclude proximal coil if low in the right atrium. Position in high SVC or innominate (brachiocephalic) vein or use separate coil to innominate or left subclavian vein
- Always program right ventricular polarity to anode
- Correct reversible causes: acidosis, hypercapnia, hypoxia, ischemia, fragments of old electrodes, etc.
- Right-sided implant: exclude active can
- Alter transvenous shock vector
- Change waveform: reprogram pulse duration if available
- Implant subcutaneous electrode or electrode array
- Use a high-output generator
- Epicardial implantation

---

high DFT during ICD implantation so that larger output generators or subcutaneous arrays might be required.

4.4.4 Upper limit of vulnerability testing

Determination of the upper limit of vulnerability (ULV) provides another method to estimate the DFT while minimizing or even eliminating the need for VF induction (Fig. 4.20). The concept behind ULV stems from the observation that there exists a shock strength above which VF will no longer be induced with a shock delivered near the peak of the T-wave (the vulnerable period of repolarization). Testing for the ULV provides a direct measure of a point high on the defibrillation probability-of-success curve.

Programming first ICD shocks based on patient-specific measurements of ULV rather than routine programming to maximum output shortens charge time and may reduce the probability of syncope as ICDs age and charge time increases. Disadvantages of this testing method include the inability to evaluate correct VF sensing and lack of testing of the subsequent decision-algorithm for the delivery of VF therapy.

Table 4.3. Contraindications to DFT testing

Absolute	Intracavitary thrombus
	Atrial fibrillation without systemic anticoagulation
	Severe aortic stenosis
	Severe coronary artery disease with ischemia or unstable angina
	Suboptimal anticoagulation with a prosthetic valve
	Hemodynamic instability treated with intravenous inotropic agents
	Inadequate sedation and anesthesia
Relative	?Left ventricular mural thrombus with adequate anticoagulation
	Marked obesity that may prevent external defibrillation if needed
	Severe coronary artery disease
	Recent coronary stent
	Recent stroke or transient ischemic attack
	Hemodynamic instability (systolic blood pressure ≤ 85 mmHg) requiring treatment
	Very severe left ventricular dysfunction
	Likelihood that a newly placed coronary venous lead might become displaced

4.4.5 Is defibrillation testing always warranted?

The need for DFT testing is an important issue surrounded by a lot of recent controversy, now that current device technology utilizing biphasic waveforms and high-output devices has enabled successful implantation in most patients. The risks of DFT testing are related to VF inductions and shocks: intractable VF, cerebral hypoperfusion (a potential cause of transient ischemic attack [TIA]) and myocardial ischemia with post-shock electromechanical dissociation. Death is rare. The risks of shocks include anesthesia-related complications, myocardial depression, atrial fibrillation and arterial thromboembolism mainly from conversion of atrial fibrillation by the ventricular shock or from an LV thrombus.

Severe aortic stenosis, unstable angina, and risk-associated anesthesia constitute absolute contraindications to DFT testing (Table 4.3). Contraindications to DFT testing also include: atrial fibrillation with poor anticoagulation control, especially if transesophageal echocardiography reveals thrombus in the left atrial appendage; LV mural thrombus; re-cent coronary stenting or severe unrevascularized coronary artery disease; recent stroke or TIA, and hemodynamic instability. In the case of intracardiac thrombi, DFT testing should be postponed until all thrombi have disappeared during anticoagulant therapy (Fig. 4.21).

In view of the high reliability and low DFTs of contemporary ICDs, DFT testing can be deferred for 1–2 months with little risk in patients for whom DFT evaluation is considered to pose a high risk. Some workers believe that DFT testing can be postponed indefinitely.

4.4.6 Follow-up DFT testing

With contemporary devices, the use of DFT testing before hospital discharge is questionable. The biphasic DFT remains stable over time. Consequently there is no need for DFT testing at regular intervals (such as once a year) as was done in the past with devices generating monophasic waveforms. Follow-up DFT testing is necessary in patients with a change in antiarrhythmic drug therapy or sensitivity, in the setting of a marginal DFT at implantation, and when a shock fails to terminate VT or VF.

5 Sensing and detection of ventricular tachycardia/fibrillation

5.1 Sensing

An ICD senses or sees the intracardiac electrogram (EGM) by recording the potential difference (voltage) between the positive and negative electrodes (Fig. 5.01). Although pacemakers use either unipolar or bipolar sensing, ICDs only use bipolar sensing. In contrast to the term "sensing", "detection" refers to the diagnosis and appropriate response of an ICD to certain tachyarrhythmias. Sensing and the sensing circuit in an ICD differ from those in a pacemaker. The ICD contains only ventricular blanking periods. No ventricular refractory periods exist (Fig. 5.02).

ICDs use the *near-field ventricular EGM* for rate sensing; that is, for true bipolar leads the local bipolar electrogram is registered between the tip and ring electrodes, and for integrated leads the bipolar electrogram is recorded between the tip electrode and the distal defibrillation coil in the RV (Fig. 5.03). Electrode configuration has been shown to have little effect on the amplitude or slew rate of the intracardiac EGM, but it does have an effect on the duration of the sensed electrogram. Furthermore, a true bipolar lead detects the ventricular EGM slightly later than an integrated lead.

5.1.1 Signal amplitude

R-wave signals (ventricular EGMs) presented to a typical pacemaker system generally fall between 5 and 25 mV. By contrast, an ICD needs to detect VF wavelets sometimes as small as 0.1 mV. Sensing of VF and VT by ICDs must be reliable because the amplitude of the ventricular signals during VF fluctuates markedly and diminishes to approximately 25% of the ventricular EGM amplitude during sinus rhythm (Fig. 5.04). If the amplitude of the ventricular EGM during sinus rhythm at implantation is greater or equal to 5 mV (with a slew rate > 1 V/s, which is commonly not measured), nominal settings with a maximum sensitivity near 0.3 mV usually provide adequate VF sensing. More sensitive settings (numerically lower than 0.3 mV) increase the risk of oversensing T-waves or myopotentials, whereas less sensitive settings (numerically > 0.3 mV) increase

the risk of undersensing VF. The aim is to minimize both undersensing during VF and oversensing during regular rhythms. To achieve this goal, ICDs use a feedback mechanism based on R-wave amplitude to adjust the sensing threshold dynamically.

5.1.2 Sensitivity

An ICD cannot function with the fixed sensitivity of pacemakers because it has to deal with wide variations of EGM size. All contemporary ICDs function with automatic dynamic sensitivity in the form of either an automatic gain control or autoadjusting sensitivity to ensure reliable sensing of VF EGMs of low and variable amplitude while simultaneously avoiding T-wave oversensing. These algorithms automatically increase amplifier sensitivity over time after a paced or sensed event until the maximum sensitivity is reached or the next sensed/paced event occurs. In other words, the longer the ICD goes without sensing a signal, the more sensitive it becomes until it reaches a plateau determined by the highest sensitivity. Then, upon sensing, the sensitivity returns to a lower (less sensitive) level determined by the amplitude of the sensed R-wave or to a fixed sensitivity in case of a paced event. After a pacing pulse the starting point of the sensitivity decay curve is different from that after sensing (Fig. 5.05). Devices perform the automatic adjustment of sensitivity in different ways. The sensitivity may be adapted exponentially (Medtronic: Fig. 5.06), or in small steps (Fig. 5.07) or linearly (Fig. 5.08). To avoid T-wave sensing, the decay of the sensitivity curve can be delayed in some ICDs (St. Jude Medical: Fig. 5.09). This programmable time interval is called "decay delay".

In dual-chamber ICDs, far-field oversensing of R-waves by the atrial channel can be circumvented by prolonging the postventricular atrial blanking period (Fig. 5.10).

With contemporary ICD technology, failure to sense VT or VF is rare with appropriate programming of sensitivity, but delayed sensing and arrhythmia detection may sometimes occur from "signal dropout" related to spontaneous changes in the ventricular EGM.

5.2 Detection

In contrast to sensing, detection is the process by which an ICD analyzes a number of sensed intracardiac signals and their timing, then classifies the rhythm and decides the need for therapy (Fig. 5.11). Detection of the ventricular EGM depends entirely on the quality of the intracardiac signal determined at implantation. The device detects and makes the diagnosis of ventricular arrhythmias mainly on the basis of two parameters: rate and duration of the tachycardia.

The minimum duration of tachycardia required for detection is programmable either in seconds or indirectly by setting the number of tachycardia intervals for detection (Fig. 5.12). The ICD detects a tachycardia episode (device diagnosis leading to therapy) when the minimum rate and duration criteria are satisfied.

A high rate criterion is very sensitive but lacks specificity because the device will sense virtually all fast arrhythmias with a fast ventricular response. Specificity may be improved by using a number of discriminators (described later).

5.2.1 Detection zones

Because tolerance of VT often depends on heart rate, devices offer several detection zones, with independently programmable therapy for each zone. The zones define programmable rate cutoffs. An ICD may be programmed with as many as three detection zones: a single "VF zone" and two "VT zones" (Fig. 5.13).

The fastest tachycardia (VF) requires the most aggressive therapy with an immediate shock. Slower VTs can often be treated with painless antitachycardia pacing, eliminating the need for painful shocks. Further division of the VT zone into slow and fast VT permits application of different electrical treatments to VTs of different rates (Fig. 7.08).

5.2.2 How many zones?

A minimum of two zones should usually be programmed, even in patients with VF as the only clinical manifestation. Most VF episodes begin with a fast organized VT often terminable by antitachycardia pacing, which carries only a small risk of tachycardia acceleration or degeneration into VF.

The lower rate boundary for the slowest VT zone should be at least 40 ms longer than the expected VT cycle length to prevent underdetection. If therapy is not actively programmed for slow VT, the slow-rate zone may be programmed as a "monitor-only"

diagnostic zone with detection "on" and therapies "off".

5.2.3 Rate and detection algorithms

Rate and duration of arrhythmia determine the need for ICD treatment. Slow and short-lived arrhythmias do not require therapy. As a rule, faster rhythms require a shorter detection time. Slow and brief VTs do not require therapy. On the one hand, a short-duration parameter programmed for detection increases the likelihood that nonsustained VT or SVT may induce inappropriate capacitor charging with aborted or inappropriate shocks, a situation resulting in unnecessary battery depletion. On the other hand, waiting too long for an arrhythmia to end without an ICD intervention may increase the risk of syncope.

For VT detection (Fig. 5.12), but never for VF, some ICDs require that a programmable number of consecutive RR intervals (consecutive interval counting) be shorter than the tachycardia detection interval (TDI). The ICD delivers therapy upon reaching the programmable "number of consecutive intervals needed to detect" (NID). This approach is not feasible for VF detection because the amplitude and rate of the ventricular EGMs may fluctuate chaotically. Missing one beat during VF by counting consecutive intervals would reset the VF counter to the baseline (from which counting restarts from zero) thereby delaying detection and treatment. A more sensitive method for VF (VT) detection involves "x out of y counting" (Fig. 5.14). For diagnosis this algorithm requires only a percentage of intervals shorter than the VF (VT) detection interval, for example 75% or 12 events (shorter than the VF interval), in any order, in a sequence of 16 events. In patients with self-terminating device-detected VF, increasing the number of intervals to detect VF from 12/16 to 18/24 results in a clinically significant decrease in ICD detections and fewer unnecessary shocks with minimal incremental delay in VF detection.

The ICDs of one manufacturer (St. Jude Medical) classify intervals based both on the basis of the last (current) interval and the average of the last four intervals (Figs 5.15 and 5.16). If both the current and the average interval are in the same zone, the current interval is classified in that zone. If the two intervals fall in different VT or VF zones, the current interval is binned (used for counting) in the faster zone. If one interval falls in the sinus zone and the other in a VT or VF zone, the current interval is discarded or not binned (not used for diagnosis). This method may compensate for potential dips below the rate cutoff with the aim to prevent delayed detection and delivery of therapy.

One manufacturer (Medtronic) uses overlapping VT/VF zones. This provides antitachycardia pacing for rapid VTs actually in the VF zone that would otherwise receive a shock (Fig. 5.17). In this system, the diagnosis of fast VT (for antitachycardia pacing) requires constancy of a programmable number of consecutive intervals (such as the last 8 cycles). Any inconsistant interval (shorter than the programmed upper interval of fast VT detection) immediately triggers VF therapy. Appropriate settings for fast VT (FVT) detection depend on the patient's VT cycle lengths. If the patient presents with a clinical VT interval in the usual VF zone, FVT detection should be programmed as above via VF to ensure reliable VF detection. If the patient presents with two clinical VTs, both outside the usual VF zone, FVT detection via VT should be selected to offer separate therapy for each VT (Fig. 5.18).

Occasionally, the rhythm fluctuates between detection zones. Consequently some manufacturers permit simultaneous counting in two zones: VF and VT. In the *multizone configuration* from Guidant, timers run independently of each other. When the duration parameter in a higher zone (VF zone) has elapsed, it takes precedence (and therapy starts) over the programmed duration parameter of the lower zone (VT zone) (Fig. 5.19).

Combined count detection is an algorithm used by Medtronic devices to speed up the detection and redetection of tachyarrhythmias with ventricular intervals fluctuating between the boundaries of the VF and VT zones (Fig. 5.20). The combined count detection criterion compares the sum of the VF and VT event counts with the *combined number of intervals to detect* (CNID). If the CNID is met, the device reviews the intervals to determine if the episode should be treated as VF, fast-VT or a VT episode (Fig. 5.21).

6 SVT/VT discrimination

Inappropriate ICD therapy remains a major clinical challenge resulting in poorer quality of life, pain, psychological distress, shorter battery life and device proarrhythmia. ICDs have incorporated increasingly sophisticated algorithms to discriminate VT from SVT to reduce inappropriate shocks. Programming of discriminators should be tailored according to a patient's specific needs, type of heart disease and tendency for inappropriate therapy such as paroxysmal atrial fibrillation. Discrimination algorithms in single-chamber ICDs have historically been based on RR interval patterns (e.g. sudden RR onset is not characteristic of sinus tachycardia) and RR interval stability reflects the irregularity generated by atrial fibrillation. Ventricular EGM morphology algorithms for SVT discrimination were added to determine whether a tachycardia has changed EGM morphology in comparison with the usual rhythm.

6.1 Single-chamber SVT/VT discrimination enhancements

An ICD can erroneously interpret supraventricular tachyarrhythmias with a rapid ventricular response as VT or VF, resulting in inappropriate treatment, including shocks. The incidence of inappropriate shocks for SVT varies from 10% to 40%. Inappropriate ICD shocks are not only painful for patients, but also proarrhythmogenic and can reduce device longevity as a result of battery depletion. This problem of inappropriate shocks spurred the design of detection enhancements (SVT discriminators) in the VT zones of single-chamber ICDs to discriminate SVT from VT and withhold VT/VF therapy for ICD diagnosis of SVT (Figs 6.01 and 6.03). Although SVT discrimination has not eliminated inappropriate therapy, these algorithms may prevent inappropriate shocks in some patients.

Because faster rhythms are likely to cause hemodynamic intolerance, detection enhancements are not applied in the VF detection zone where a rapid delivery of therapy is essential.

6.1.1 Interval-stability criterion

The interval-stability criterion examines the regularity of RR intervals to discriminate atrial fibrillation (AF) with a rapid ventricular response from VT. The criterion depends on the analysis of cycle length variations and is continuously active during a tachycardia episode. AF conducted to the ventricles usually generates an irregular ventricular rhythm with unstable RR intervals, in contrast to monomorphic VTs. For most VTs the measured stability or the variation between RR intervals measures < 21 ms, as opposed to AF, which typically varies by 35–50 ms. The algorithm is highly effective for ruling out atrial fibrillation at slower rates. At faster rates, the ventricular rate during atrial fibrillation tends to become more regular and difficult to discriminate from VT (Fig. 6.04).

This discrimination enhancement may result in underdetection of irregular VT or polymorphic VT with periodic "dropout" of ventricular sensing. For this reason, stability should not be programmed "on" unless AF with a rapid ventricular response has been documented clinically.

6.1.2 Sudden-onset criterion

The sudden-onset criterion tries to distinguish sinus tachycardia from a relatively slow VT by examining the suddenness of tachycardia onset (Figs 6.05, 6.16 and 6.17). It is applied only once during a tachycardia episode. In general, the sinus rate increases gradually with RR intervals shortening by 2–3% per cycle, in contrast to VTs, which generally begin suddenly with a shortening of RR intervals by 10–20% at the onset. In this way, a device detects a sudden reduction in cycle length as VT but interprets a gradual rate increase as sinus tachycardia. The algorithms have a high specificity for rejecting sinus tachycardia but may prevent detection of VT that starts during SVT and VT that starts abruptly with an initial rate below the VT detection rate.

6.1.3 Morphology discrimination

Morphology discriminates VT from SVT on the basis of morphology-based algorithms that compare the differences between ventricular EGMs in a previously stored template of a normally conducted beat (in sinus rhythm or base supraventricular rhythm) with VT EGMs during a tachycardia episode. These features can increase the specificity of

VT detection. The computing power of ICDs permits sophisticated discriminators using morphology template matching and vector correlation. The microprocessor and its peripheral electronic components decompose the analog EGM signal into a series of samples, convert them into a digital format and store them temporarily into the random access memory (RAM) of the device (Fig. 6.06). During a learning phase, the ICD establishes a "template" composed of a number of normally conducted sinus beats or the supraventricular base rhythm. In most ICDs an automatic algorithm creates and updates templates from nonpaced slow rhythm and continuously checks the quality of the template used for arrhythmia discrimination. After careful alignment of the peak values of each of these EGM complexes, the corresponding samples are averaged to form a stored template (Fig. 6.07).

Morphology detection relies upon the *comparison* of each beat of the ventricular signal (ventricular electrogram, VEGM) of a suspected tachyarrhythmia with the stored sinus rhythm template. The actual comparison method depends on the ICD model and the manufacturer. The Marquis Medtronic ICD, for instance, breaks down the template and each beat of the suspected ventricular signal in some small rectangular waveforms called "Haar wavelets". A number of coefficients are calculated from the two sets of wavelets and the ICD compares these coefficients to find a match for SVT or otherwise for VT (Figs 6.08–6.10).

St. Jude Medical ICDs align the template and the suspected ventricular rhythm and calculate the area of difference between the peaks. Matching of the two sets is expressed as a percentage. If this percentage is larger than a preset percentage match, the ICD recognizes the tachycardia as VT (Fig. 6.11).

The vector-timing and correlation algorithm of the Vitality ICD (Guidant) stores templates of near-field and far-field EGMs during normal sinus rhythm and during tachycardia. It aligns the peaks of the near-field signals and calculates the dif-ferences between these peaks and those of the corresponding far-field signals.

Systems using peak alignment of ECGs introduce a potential difficulty when alignment is not straightforward (Fig. 6.12).

6.2 Dual-chamber SVT/VT discriminators

The additional information from the atrial channel in dual-chamber ICDs integrates the ventricular and the atrial electrograms for rhythm analysis. The comparison of atrial and ventricular activity enhances rhythm discrimination. The advantages of dual- over single-chamber discriminators have been difficult to establish. Despite the introduction of more advanced dual-chamber detection algorithms, a substantial number of patients still experience inappropriate therapy.

6.2.1 Atrial and ventricular rate counting

Comparison of atrial and ventricular rates with reliable identification of atrial EGMs provides a simple and powerful SVT/VT discriminator. The ICD faces a challenge in the presence of VT with atrial fibrillation or associated with 1:1 VA conduction (Figs 6.13–6.15, 6.18, 6.19, 1.09 and 1.10).

V-rate > A-rate

If the ventricular rate exceeds the atrial rate (i.e. V-rate > A-rate), the ICD classifies the tachycardia as VT. No other data are necessary. Fortunately V-rate > A-rate occurs in over 90% of VTs. Therefore additional criteria for device diagnosis may be necessary only in less than 10% of VTs.

Low-amplitude atrial signals, especially during atrial fibrillation, may be undersensed or simply blanked out by the device resulting in an erroneous determination that the ventricular rate exceeds the atrial rate. This causes the incorrect device diagnosis of SVT as VT. Conversely, atrial oversensing during VT, usually due to VA far-field sensing, may interfere with this criterion and prevent therapy for true VT.

V-rate = A-rate

When there is a 1:1 relationship between atria and ventricles, the ICD determines whether this is sinus tachycardia or SVT with a rapid ventricular response or VT with 1:1 retrograde VA conduction. In this situation the ICD can use sophisticated algorithms such as morphology to make the diagnosis. The device withholds therapy if it interprets the presence of a supraventricular rhythm (Fig. 1.09).

V-rate < A-rate

If the ventricular rate is slower than the atrial rate, the device interprets this situation as atrial flutter or SVT with multiblock so that the ICD automatically inhibits therapy (Fig. 6.20).

As patients with atrial fibrillation may develop a slow VT, an atrial/ventricular counting algorithm would classify the situation as SVT because the atrial rate exceeds the ventricular rate, and other SVT discriminators may be necessary for a proper device diagnosis. The best additional discriminator is morphology or stability.

6.2.2 Atrioventricular association

The AV association algorithm looks constantly at the atrial and ventricular EGMs to determine whether they are related or independent of each other. The AV association function also analyzes the constancy of the PR or RP interval (Figs 6.13 and 6.21).

Atrioventricular dissociation is a reliable diagnostic criterion for VT. However, changing PR intervals and varying ratios of AV block and atrial undersensing and oversensing can cause a device to miss AV association.

6.2.3 P:R pattern

The P:R pattern algorithm identifies consistent and complex timing relationships between atrial and ventricular EGMs during specific SVTs, such as sinus tachycardia and atrial flutter (Figs 6.24–6.28).

6.2.4 Chamber of origin

This algorithm only applies to tachycardias with 1:1 AV association. It discriminates sinus or atrial tachycardia with 1:1 AV conduction from VT with 1:1 VA conduction. Atrial tachycardia starts with a short PP interval, whereas VT begins with a short VV interval (Fig. 1.09). As this algorithm depends on accurate sensing of atrial and ventricular events it is susceptible to errors based on a single over-sensed or undersensed event.

6.2.5 Premature stimulation

The response of the opposite chamber to atrial or ventricular pacing is useful in the electrophysiology laboratory for diagnosing tachycardias with a 1:1 AV relationship. Premature stimulation discriminates VT from sudden-onset atrial tachycardia based on the response to a late premature stimulus in either the atrium or ventricle. A late premature stimulus advances activation in the other chamber only if the stimulus is delivered in the tachycardia chamber of origin. This feature has not been used so far in ICDs.

6.3 Sustained rate duration

Detecting VT as SVT can be harmful. For this reason ICDs contain a rate duration safety net (Fig. 6.01). To prevent excessive delay of therapy delivery in the case of possible sustained VT, the sustained-duration override (Boston Scientific-Guidant: Sustained-Duration Override [SRD]; Medtronic: High Rate Timeout; St. Jude Medical: Maximum Time to Diagnosis [MTD]) functions prevent SVT/VT discriminators from permanently withholding therapy truly aimed at VT as programmed (Figs 6.29 and 6.30). It delivers therapy if a tachycardia (VT or SVT) satisfies the VT rate criteria for a specified period of time (programmable), even if the discriminator had indicated and still indicates SVT. With this function, delivery of inappropriate ventricular therapy for SVT eventually occurs as long as the SVT cycle length remains shorter than the programmed tachycardia detection interval. This function must be used judiciously to avoid unnecessary shocks. The rationale of this backup function is based on the belief that VT will continue to satisfy the rate criterion for the programmed duration whereas the ventricular rate during transient sinus tachycardia or atrial fibrillation will decrease below the VT rate boundary. Using this function may perhaps be an admission that the SVT/VT discriminators are not entirely trusted, and that a "safety net" is needed to avoid missing the treatment of VT (increasing sensitivity but decreasing specificity). Thus a time-out feature may be used if there is a lack of confidence in the SVT discriminators; however, in the long run such a feature defeats the purpose of discrimination.

6.4 Sensitivity and specificity of an algorithm

When evaluating ICD tachycardia therapy, there are three crucial clinical questions to answer:
1. Does the algorithm detect all dangerous ventricular tachyarrhythmias?
2. If therapy is delivered, did the rhythm actually require treatment?
3. When therapy is withheld from a rapid rhythm, how safe was it to withhold therapy?

Sensitivity and specificity are statistical methods commonly used to compare different algorithms (Fig. 6.02). The *sensitivity* of a detection algorithm indicates the probability that VT/VF is detected when present. The *specificity* of a detection algorithm indicates the probability that VT/VF was not detected given that VT/VF was not present. New algorithms should therefore have a sensitivity and specificity as great as possible. Discriminators of SVT must be used carefully. It is not always a good idea to program all the discriminators because the ICD becomes more likely to inhibit needed therapy.

ICDs incorporate several detection processes, including:
1. initial detection that starts the first automatic therapy;
2. confirmation of the detected tachyarrhythmia during and/or upon completion of capacitor charging to determine the continuing presence of a sustained tachyarrhythmia;
3. synchronization with the ventricular EGM to ensure delivery of a shock during ventricular depolarization;
4. redetection of the same or possibly a different tachyarrhythmia after therapy;
5. detection of tachycardia termination according to a preset sequence of beats (Fig. 6.31).

ICDs with tiered therapy offer antitachycardia pacing (ATP), cardioversion for VT, and defibrillation for VF. Different tachycardias are best treated according to their mechanism and rate (Fig. 7.08). Tiered therapy attempts to treat sustained monomorphic VT at rates up to 250 bpm with less aggressive therapy such as ATP or, less frequently, low-energy cardioversion, reserving a maximum shock for VF. The introduction of potentially long delays before the delivery of a highvoltage shock represents a disadvantage of tiered therapy. However, new devices can charge the capacitor at the start of ATP thereby reducing the time to a potential shock.

7.1 Rhythm confirmation

Noncommitted function

Confirmation of continuing tachycardia may occur during or immediately after capacitor charging to verify that a detected tachycardia has not terminated spontaneously. When a noncommitted function is programmed, a device aborts therapy if it detects sinus rhythm after the initial diagnostic detection (either when charging or just before it delivers the shock) and, obviously, before delivery of the shock (Fig. 7.02).

When an ICD withholds therapy because of spontaneous tachycardia termination, a charged capacitor delays dissipation of its charge until the device

determines that tachycardia has not quickly restarted. This response facilitates rapid delivery of a shock in case of a quick return of tachycardia. In the case of an aborted shock, the device gradually "bleeds off" its charge painlessly and the capacitor becomes empty. The patient is unaware of this process and there is no damage to the ICD. The ICD records the number and EGMs of aborted shocks, which are important for diagnostic purposes.

Committed function

In an ICD programmed for a "committed shock" the confirmation process does not take place and the device delivers the shock at the completion of capacitor charging even if the tachycardia has terminated spontaneously (Fig. 7.01). Most devices allow the first shock to be noncommitted but all subsequent shocks are committed (Fig. 7.03). This behavior is based on the concept that a shock may be withheld should low-amplitude ventricular EGMs be unsensed during the "second look" period and the tachycardia then remains untreated. A committed shock may also occur in the case of a tachycardia that has spontaneously terminated during the confirmation "second look" phase, but has quickly recurred and been redetected. For example, if the ICD detects VT/VF and the shock is aborted, redetection will induce a committed shock. This response was designed to ensure VT/VF therapy in the case of intermittent undersensing.

7.2 Redetection

After therapy delivery (shock or ATP), the ICD determines whether the tachycardia has terminated (Fig. 7.04). Criteria for redetection of an unsuccessfully terminated tachycardia are often less rigorous than those for initial detection. Redetection is "trigger happy" for obvious reasons. Episode termination resets all sequences to basic values, and tachyarrhythmia detection resumes (Fig. 7.05).

Following a shock, redetection typically begins after an extended refractory period (of the order of 500–1000 ms). This period serves to prevent the shock energy itself from being detected as a ventricular event.

7.3 Antitachycardia pacing

7.3.1 Mechanism of antitachycardia pacing

Reentry underlies the primary mechanism of VTs. Antitachycardia pacing can terminate most sustained monomorphic tachycardias. During reentry in an anatomically defined circuit, there exists an excitable gap (Fig. 7.06). A reentrant VT can be terminated electrically if pacing stimuli induce ventricular depolarization in the excitable gap. In other words, pacing must capture the region of the circuit not yet activated by the oncoming circulating wavefront. A precisely timed ventricular extrastimulus during the excitable gap interferes with the circus movement and terminates the tachycardia by collision of the two wavefronts. However, if the extrastimulus comes too late, the oncoming circus movement may be blocked by refractoriness at the depolarized site but the wavefront induced by the pacing stimulus may perpetuate the tachycardia by traveling along the loop without encountering refractory tissue. In this situation, the tachycardia will persist but its timing will be temporarily "reset". A single critically timed extrastimulus may terminate "slow" VT, but in practice a burst or train of multiple stimuli is often required to interact with the VT circuit for termination. When the pacing site is far from the reentrant circuit, a train of stimuli works by "peeling back" the refractory periods to permit entry of activation into the excitable gap to terminate VT. Antitachycardia pacing is equally effective in nonischemic and ischemic cardiomyopathy (Fig. 7.07). In the setting of VT noninducibility in the electrophysiology laboratory, ATP can often be subsequently successful in clinical episodes.

7.3.2 Therapeutic use of antitachycardia pacing

Antitachycardia pacing delivers multiple pacing pulses in the VOO mode (much less frequently in the VVI mode according to the manufacturer and programmed type of ATP) with a high output (voltage and pulse duration) to ensure capture and propagation of pacing stimuli.

The pacing output for ATP and antibradycardia pacing are separately programmable. As the VT cycle length decreases, the probability of VT termination by pacing stimuli decreases. Shorter cycle lengths have a "protective" effect on the VT circuit because the excitable gap shortens with cycle length

thereby reducing the window of vulnerability. Shorter VT cycle lengths also reduce the probability that pacing stimuli delivered remotely can overcome the relatively long conduction time from the pacing site to the VT circuit before the stimulation site becomes refractory. As part of tiered therapy ATP may take longer to convert VT, but it leads to fewer shocks, less patient discomfort and less energy expenditure.

Slow VTs

Tiered therapy using initial ATP can reduce painful shocks and is highly effective in restoring sinus rhythm in about 90% of stable VT episodes up to around 200 b.p.m. (cycle length > 300–320 ms) (Figs 7.11 and 7.12). Moreover, acceleration occurs in 1–5% of cases (acceleration usually means > 10–25% change in VT cycle length, or the development of polymorphic VT or VF). Tiered therapy may take longer to convert the arrhythmia, but it leads to fewer shocks, less patient discomfort and less energy expenditure (Fig. 7.08). The cutoff rate for slow VT detection should ideally be above the patient's maximal rate to avoid therapy for sinus tachycardia.

Fast VTs

Antitachycardia pacing is now recommended for fast VTs with a cycle length up to 240–250 ms. Indeed, FVT episodes make up 75% of all ventricular arrhythmias previously programmed to shock (< 320 ms). Yet, about 60–70% of fast VTs (between a cycle length of 300 to 240 ms) are pace terminable (usual protocol is a single eight-pulse burst train at 88% of the VT cycle length, which may be followed by another burst with a cycle length shorter by 10 ms) without a substantial increase in acceleration compared with ATP for slower VTs. Episodes with a cycle length < 240 ms are considered as VF. Note that 250 b.p.m. corresponds to a cycle length of 240 ms whereas a rate of 240 b.p.m. gives a cycle length of 250 ms. ICDs other than Medtronic can be programmed for fast VTs as described above, with a detection rate of 230–250 b.p.m. with delivery of a single burst followed by a shock if unsuccessful.

Programming Medtronic ICDs for fast VT

Medtronic applies a "last eight intervals look-back" when fast VT via VF is programmed. This means that if 18/24 intervals are < 320 ms (fast VT detection interval, or FDI) then a separately running counter determines whether the last 8 of 18 intervals are < 320 ms but > 240 ms (minimum bound for fast VT detection) so that the rhythm can be classified as fast VT. This is important because many episodes of fast VT have a few short-cycle-length intervals at the onset before settling out into a stable rhythm. So, the "last eight intervals" look-back window enhances the rhythm classification for rapid, stable VT. If a single interval within the last eight is < 240 ms, a shock is delivered. Some find programming fast VT confusing because fast VT is programmed via VF. In this design VF is programmed at a cycle length of 320 ms but fast VT is programmed at a cycle length of 240 ms.

Antitachycardia pacing therapy for fast VT reduces the frequency of shocks without increasing time to VT termination or risk of acceleration. Even in patients who received an ICD for only VF, a VT detection zone should be programmed empirically because many patients will subsequently develop VT (as a prelude to VF), terminable with ATP (Figs 7.16 and 7.17). Aggressive ATP for VT with a cycle length of 240 ms or longer is now recommended in all patients with an ICD for primary and secondary prevention. In this way about three-quarters of the shocks using traditional ATP programming can be avoided. This positions an ICD primarily as an ATP device with backup defibrillation.

ATP programming

Antitachycardia pacing programming involves setting up a pattern of VT detection and stimulation. The number of burst attempts, the number of pulses within each burst, the coupling interval as a percentage of the VT cycle length, and the minimum pacing interval are all programmable (Figs 7.09 and 7.10). Programming the ICD to wait for 18 beats before treating an episode may reduce the number of episodes treated when compared with 12-beat detection. Burst and ramp pacing sequences have similar efficacy for slower VTs. For VTs with a cycle length of less than 300 ms, burst is more effective and less likely to result in acceleration (Fig. 7.11). Burst cycle lengths are adaptive and should be 85–90% of the VT cycle length for faster VTs and 70–80% of the VT cycle length for slower VTs (Figs 7.12–7.15). Routine electrophysiologic manipulation of ATP programming is not necessary because of the safety and effectiveness of empirical therapy. Furthermore, spontaneous VT is usually slower and more easily terminable than VT induced during programmed electrical stimulation.

Programming ATP in patients with an ICD for primary prevention

It is not clear whether patients fitted with an ICD for primary prevention should have a slow VT zone.

It is reasonable to program two zones in these patients: FVT and VF with a lower limit of about 182 b.p.m., sometimes 176 b.p.m. This may reduce inappropriate therapy for SVT. Then, programming a VT monitoring zone should indicate whether slow VT is really a clinical problem that requires treatment.

Types of ATP

Antitachycardia pacing can be programmed with a cycle length usually about 80–90% of that of the VT. Adaptive function automatically adjusts the coupling interval of the first stimulus to the VT $(R–S_1)$ as a programmed percentage of the cycle length of the detected VT, often as an averaged value. The cycle length of the burst is often the same as the coupling interval, but in some ICDs the coupling interval and the burst cycle length may be separately programmable (Figs 7.09 and 7.10). Pacing bursts can be fixed (constant cycle length within the burst) or autodecremental (ramp pacing) when the pacing burst accelerates (each cycle length within the burst decreases by a programmed intraburst step value so that the pacing rate increases progressively within a burst). Scanning refers to the change in the cycle length from one burst to the next one. A decremental scan step of 10 ms means that the cycle length of each successive burst will decrease by 10 ms (interburst decrement). Each burst (or ramp sequence) will thus be delivered at a faster rate. When this form of scanning is operative, the adaptive function works only with the first burst. In other words, if the cycle length of the first fixed burst is x and the scan step is 10 ms, the second burst will have a cycle length of $x – 10$ ms, and the third will have a cycle length of $x – 20$ ms. In summary, ramp pacing decreases the cycle length within a burst whereas scanning changes the cycle length from burst to burst. Some ATP protocols combine both fixed and ramp pacing (Figs 7.13–7.15). One system can add a single stimulus with each successive burst (burst decrement).

Number of bursts and maximum rate

For fast VT, as already discussed, one or occasionally two bursts may suffice. The number of burst attempts for slow VT depends on the hemodynamic stability of the tachycardia and the perceived risk. ICDs permit programming of the shortest burst cycle length or the maximum pacing rate. This ceiling applies to all ATP therapies. If the calculated pacing interval is shorter than the programmed minimum interval, the device will deliver pacing stimuli at the programmed minimum interval.

Backup

Antitachycardia pacing must always be backed by the next level of therapy – high-energy shocks with or without a low-energy shock – immediately after unsuccessful ATP. This safety feature is especially important if ATP causes an increase in the tachycardia rate. Should ATP fail, cardioversion (low-energy shocks) is given first to try to terminate VT. If a review of the stored VT episodes shows that ATP does not reliably terminate or accelerates VT, such therapy should be disabled and low-energy cardioversion should be considered as the initial VT therapy. Cardioversion also carries a similar risk of proarrhythmia.

7.3.3 Recent developments in ATP therapy

For the latest Medtronic ICDs (Entrust), one can select ATP delivery either before or during charging. This design provides flexibility for the treatment of fast VT (FVT).

It is important from the outset to realize that FVT programming preempts ATP during charging *as well as before charging* for VTs detected as FVT. This occurs because ATP during charging requires VF detection. In other words, a rhythm has to be declared as VF in order for ATP during charging to be delivered. Antitachycardia pacing during charging was probably intended to replace programming for FVT via VF – not to be used in conjunction with it. Therefore, FVT via VF should not be programmed ON if ATP during charging is also ON, with one exception discussed below. *The same rule applies to ATP before charging.*

1. *ATP delivery during capacitor charging.* ATP during charging (Figs 7.18 and 7.19) is available for only the first VF shock. As indicated above, this function precludes programming for FVT via VF. The device delivers a single sequence of ATP as it charges for VF therapy. ICD capacitors begin charging simultaneously with the delivery of ATP in preparation for release of the first shock should ATP fail to terminate the FVT or acceleration occurs. There is no delay in delivery of high-voltage therapy (should it be needed) because capacitors charge immediately upon initial tachycardia detection. ATP therapy in this setting requires that the last eight VV intervals be longer or equal to the programmed value. Review of the last eight R–R intervals for ATP during charging occurs immediately upon VF detection and coincidentally with the start of charging. The intent is to treat fast regular monomorphic VT (at the time of programming, the programmer would show: Deliver ATP if last 8 R–R greater or equal to . . .). As an example, the programmer might show 240 ms corresponding to a rate of 250 b.p.m.

(FVT for cycle length [CL] 300–240 ms is often programmed). The capacitor charges to the programmed energy as ATP is being delivered. To determine termination, the ICD looks at ventricular events only after charging has ended. If four of the last five ventricular intervals are "normal" (i.e. greater than the confirmation interval) the device cancels shock therapy (confirmation interval = programmed VT interval + 60 ms). If two consecutive VF intervals are seen during this window, high-voltage therapy is delivered. Thus, a shock can be delivered after arrhythmia conversion to sinus or a relatively slow basic rhythm. The potential risk of this inappropriate ICD discharge may outweigh the potential benefit of reduced time to tachycardia termination.

In some in instances, ATP during charging is being used in conjunction with FVT via VF programming, with FVT via VF programmed to 240 ms and "treat if last eight RR greater than" is programmed to 200 ms. Effectively, ATP during charging would be delivered if the last eight VV intervals were between 200 and 240 ms. This means that at least one attempt at ATP will be made for all ventricular rhythms in the VF zone. This allows standard "pain-free" or FVT via VF programming, which many have become accustomed to, while simultaneously allowing the device possibly to terminate faster VTs with cycle lengths between 200 and 240 ms painlessly without compromising time to high-voltage therapy for these hemodynamically unstable rhythms.

2. *ATP before charging.* ATP before charging can be programmed as the starting value but it makes little sense to do so. ATP before charging is a consequence of ChargeSaver operation. If ChargeSaver is enabled, the device will automatically switch from ATP during charging to ATP before charging operation. The change occurs when ATP has successfully terminated the detected arrhythmia on a programmable number of consecutive attempts. With ATP before charging a Medtronic ICD delivers one ATP sequence as soon as VT is detected. If VT is redetected, the device begins charging and delivers a second ATP sequence during charging. Review of VV intervals by the device to determine arrhythmia termination occurs after charging has ended, as in the ATP-during-charging algorithm.

7.4 Cardioversion

Cardioversion establishes the next programmable therapeutic level in a VT zone (Fig. 7.08). Each shock is synchronized to an R-wave. The shocks are almost always programmed to follow unsuccessful ATP therapies. In an ICD, cardioversion for VT typically delivers 5–10 J. Cardioversion energies less than 5 J should be avoided as they may precipitate atrial fibrillation. Backup defibrillation is mandatory because low-energy cardioversion can accelerate VT. Low-energy cardioversion is comparable to ATP in terms of efficacy and risk of VT acceleration. Antitachycardia pacing is generally used first, with low-energy cardioversion as backup.

7.5 High-energy shocks

Because VF defibrillation at any given shock energy depends on a probability function, the initial defibrillation energy should include an appropriate safety margin. A 10-J safety margin above the defibrillation threshold may be programmed for the first high-energy shock. Subsequent shocks are usually programmed at maximal output. A first shock lower than the maximum device output promotes faster capacitor charging to the programmed energy and thus faster shock delivery. However, many workers program the first shock for VF to the maximum output regardless of the DFT. Energy pathways, waveforms, tilt, pulse width and polarity are generally programmable.

7.6 Monitor zone

Finally, no therapy may be programmed in a VT zone to allow the ICD to record a previous occult arrhythmia, particularly in the slowest zone of VT detection.

7.7 Bradycardia pacing by the ICD

All ICDs incorporate antibradycardia pacing functions similar to those of a conventional pacemaker, but some features are different. Because VF sensing imposes a high ventricular sensitivity and a relatively short duration of the ventricular blanking periods, oversensing by an ICD is more difficult to avoid than with a standard pacemaker. Therefore ICDs utilize only bipolar leads. ICD devices allow multiple programmable modes, including DDDR, DDD, DDIR, DDI, AAIR, AAI, VVIR and VVI, according to the presence of an atrial lead.

Antibradycardia pacing in ICDs without cardiac resynchronization therapy (CRT)

In general, parameters are programmed basically in the same way as in conventional pacemakers, with

emphasis on minimizing RV pacing. Following a shock, the pacing threshold may be temporarily elevated. Consequently after a shock, the output (voltage and pulse duration) settings should be programmed to their maximal value (Fig. 7.20). The lower rate should be slower than the base rate and the post-shock pacing mode should be selected. After the shock a pause before the onset of pacing is programmed to allow the myocardium to recover because immediate antibradycardia pacing may be proarrhythmic. The duration of post-shock pacing (with different parameters from base pacing) is also programmable.

7.7.1 Minimizing right ventricular pacing

Much evidence has emerged recently about the harmful effects of chronic RV pacing (mostly apical) on LV function. Minimizing right ventricular pacing may reduce chronic changes in cellular structure and left ventricular geometry that contribute to impaired hemodynamic performance, mitral regurgitation and increased left atrial diameters, with the aim of reducing the risk of atrial fibrillation, congestive heart failure and death. On this basis, strategies to minimize RV pacing have become important where continual RV pacing may not be necessary (Fig. 7.21). At the time of follow-up, the percentage of right ventricular pacing can be determined from the diagnostic data. If the percentage is considered too high, reprogramming the ICD is required to reduce unnecessary RV pacing.

1. *Do not pace if it is not necessary.* Avoidance of RV pacing is especially important in ICD patients with a poor LV ejection fraction in the absence of sinus or AV nodal dysfunction. The VVI or DDI pacing mode (with a long AV delay) at a rate of 40 p.p.m. may be appropriate for many patients.
2. *Long fixed AV delay.* Using the DDDR (or DDIR) mode with a fixed long AV delay (250–300 ms) in patients with normal AV conduction is of limited value in preventing RV pacing. During AV block, pacing must occur with the programmed long AV delay. A long atrial refractory period may cause atrial undersensing and limits the programmable upper rate. A long AV delay favors endless loop tachycardia or repetitive non-reentrant VA synchrony with functional loss of atrial capture and pacemaker syndrome.
3. *Dynamic AV delay (AV search hysteresis, autointrinsic conduction search, search AV+).* These algorithms in the DDDR mode promote spontaneous AV conduction by allowing the functional AV delay to be longer than the programmed AV delay as long as AV conduction remains intact.

During AV block, the AV delay is physiologically more appropriate than with devices working with a fixed long AV delay (e.g. 200 vs 300 ms). In this algorithm the device periodically extends the AV (AP–V and AS–V) delay (gradually or suddenly) to a programmable value to search for AV conduction. If a conducted ventricular event is sensed during this extended AV delay, the pacemaker inhibits the ventricular output and continues to function (in the functional AAI or AAIR mode) with such an extended AV delay until no ventricular event is sensed. If there is a single cycle with no intrinsic ventricular event within the extended AV delay, the AV extension is canceled and the pacemaker reverts to the programmed (unextended) AV delay on the next cycle. The pacemaker then waits until the next search function (after a programmable time) is activated to look for the return of spontaneous AV conduction. This feature is particularly valuable in patients who would otherwise be suitable for permanent AAI or AAIR pacing.

A recent study tested the hypothesis that dual-chamber rate-responsive (DDDR) with AV search hysteresis (AVSH) 60-130 programming is not inferior to single-chamber (VVI)-40 programming in an ICD. All-cause mortality was not significantly different between the DDDR AVSH arm and the VVI arm.

4. *New pacing modes in which the algorithm maintains AAI or AAIR pacing (automatic mode switching DDDR → AAIR → DDDR).* The switch to AAIR from DDDR is achieved by periodic AV conduction checks by the device monitoring for a conducted ventricular sensed event. First- and second-degree AV block are tolerated in the AAIR mode up to a predetermined programmable limit. The permitted cycles of second-degree AV block are short but an occasional patient may become symptomatic. Supraventricular tachyarrhythmias activate automatic mode switching to the DDIR mode (AAIR → DDIR or DDDR → DDIR).

Pacemakers and ICDs with automatic mode switching DDDR → AAIR → DDDR according to AV conduction are effective in minimizing RV pacing, especially in patients with ICDs who often do not require rate support.

Medtronic's Managed Ventricular Pacing (MVP) has no AV interval (ending in VS) so that no ventricular pacing will occur after a long PR (AS–VS or AP–VS) interval. Sustained marked first-degree AV block may be hemodynamically important and symptomatic like retrograde VA conduction.

7.7.2 Post-shock pacing

Immediately after delivery of a shock, the ability of an ICD to sense intrinsic signals is diminished and the pacing threshold may rise temporarily with resultant loss of capture. Therefore, all ICDs offer special post-shock programmable features, in effect after a shock or ATP (Fig. 7.20). A pause (1–7 s) between therapy and onset of post-shock pacing can be programmed. A few seconds are allowed to elapse before starting post-shock pacing because immediate post-shock bradycardia pacing may be proarrhythmic. In pacemaker-dependent patients this period should be short.

Programming a temporary increase of the output settings with a higher pulse amplitude and width compensates for the high post-shock capture threshold. After the post-shock pacing period the ICD reverts automatically to the basic programmed bradycardia settings.

7.8 Atrial therapies

In patients with conventional indications for ICD implantation, atrial fibrillation (AF) may occur in more than 50% during the lifespan of the device and may lead to severe adverse events. About 25% of ICD recipients have a history of AF at the time of implantation. Organized atrial tachycardias (AT) are less common. Therefore, it was logical that the electrical management of AT/AF became an integral part of ICD and CRT-D devices. As the technology in these devices improves, it is likely that many more patients will be treated with these complex implantable systems in future years. Historically, an implantable stand-alone atrial defibrillator clearly demonstrated that the electrical treatment of AF was technically feasible using up to 6 J. However, the device was never commercially released for several reasons:

1. Tolerability: shock-induced discomfort. Multiple shocks were not uncommon because of very early recurrence after the first shock.
2. Lack of ventricular defibrillation for possible shock-induced ventricular arrhythmias.
3. Lack of painless therapies in the absence of atrial pacing.

Subsequently, dual-chamber atrial defibrillators were developed to allow independent detection and treatment of atrial and ventricular tachyarrhythmias (Figs 7.22 and 7.23). These dual-chamber defibrillators provided atrial antitachycardia functions, including prevention algorithms, arrhythmia detection capability and atrial therapy options. Device therapy for atrial tachyarrhythmias provides a sequential approach of tiered therapy starting with painless interventions such as atrial ATP (ramp or burst), then high-frequency (50-Hz) burst pacing, up to high-energy shocks. These functions come in the form of a device either with the conventional configuration used in ICDs implanted for ventricular tachyarrhythmias or with an atrial-specific configuration requiring a coronary sinus lead. The latter allows very low energies (< 4 J) for AF cardioversion. The atrial lead of such devices contains a defibrillation coil. Current devices favor a simple and common electrode system (without using a coronary sinus lead) for both atrial and ventricular defibrillation because the degree of pain with low-energy shock and that with high-energy shocks is not significantly different.

Atrial shock efficacy for AF is about 85% with the lead configuration described above when adequately programmed. The timing of the shock is programmable allowing a symptomatic patient to perform out-of-hospital cardioversion at the time of the patient's choosing. Prompt termination of atrial fibrillation may reduce the electrical and anatomic remodeling associated with persistent AF and may decrease the likelihood of recurrence. The efficacy of ATP for regular AT ranges from 30% to 66%. Nearly half of tachyarrhythmias start as regular AT and then accelerate and become less organized (AF) in few minutes. Thus, early delivery of atrial ATP for regular AT may increase the success rate, prevent AF, and decrease the need for a shock.

There is less urgency to treat AF as it is not immediately life threatening. It can occur much more frequently than VF and it can often terminate spontaneously. Consequently, atrial defibrillators were designed to deliver a shock manually by the patient or automatically after a few hours to ensure treatment of a sustained arrhythmia. Furthermore, AF often recurs shortly after a successful shock.

The use of atrial defibrillation with implantable devices is limited to a small number of patients. It is not widely accepted mainly because of patient discomfort. However, atrial defibrillation may be useful in highly symptomatic patients or those where AF precipitates heart failure.

The term pacemaker "refractory period" was originally used to describe the part of the pacemaker cycle when sensing was prevented. In other words, early pacemakers ignored signals falling in the refractory period, during which they could initiate neither a lower rate interval nor an AV delay. In fact, in early pacemakers the refractory period basically functioned as a blanking period. By definition, sensing in any form cannot take place during a blanking period. The original concept of the pacemaker refractory period remains valid for contemporary pacemakers and ICDs; because a signal within this special interval cannot begin a lower rate interval or AV delay.

The refractory period of a device now defines a timing cycle consisting of two phases:
1. an initial blanking period, occasionally called the absolute refractory period;
2. a second part, sometimes called the relative refractory period, during which sensing can occur to drive functions other than control of the lower rate and AV delay (Fig. 8.01).

During the blanking interval, which is either fixed or programmable, real-time or stored EGMs (but not their corresponding markers in older ICDs) can be faithfully recorded because they are processed outside the active sensing circuit. Some contemporary ICDs use special markers to indicate a signal detected within a blanking period. Blanking periods were designed to prevent a device from sensing its own discharge, myocardial activation, the polarization voltage at the lead–myocardial interface and crosstalk from the other electrical chamber. Blanking therefore starts coincidentally with stimulus delivery or a sensed event. Sensed data in the (relative) or unblanked refractory period are often used to regulate a number of timing cycles, diagnostic counting for automatic mode switching and other functions, except the initiation of a lower rate interval or AV

delay. A blanking period need not be followed by a refractory period, but a traditional refractory period always contains an initial blanking interval. Blanking periods after pacing are equal or longer than after sensing.

The terminology of refractory and blanking periods of ICDs is confusing. By contrast, the related ICD timing cycles of the ventricular channel are easier to understand because they all function as blanking periods. It is axiomatic that the ventricular channel of an ICD can only have blanking periods (provided one ignores the noise-sampling periods). The ventricular channel cannot have a refractory period (where sensing can occur but is processed differently) because it would defeat the concept that ICD sensing of ventricular activity must be uniform and unimpeded through as much of the cardiac cycle as possible. Thus, ICD ventricular blanking periods after a sensed ventricular event must be as short as possible to enhance sensing of fast ventricular rhythms. The duration of the ventricular blanking period was usually fixed in the past but it may be programmable in contemporary devices (Figs 8.02–8.07).

During antibradycardia pacing the atrial channel of dual-chamber ICDs functions basically like that of conventional pacemakers. The postventricular atrial refractory period (PVARP) begins with a programmable postventricular atrial blanking (PVAB) period used primarily to control far-field R-wave sensing by the atrial channel. However, some devices can detect atrial signals during most of this PVAB but the data are used only for arrhythmia detection and not for any of the antibradycardia functions such as counting for automatic mode switching. The duration of cross-chamber blanking (such as in the ventricular channel after an atrial event) must be known even if the duration is zero.

9 Complications of ICD therapy

The implantation technique for ICDs is basically similar to that for pacemakers but the complication rate is higher because of the complexity of lead function. Complications associated with ICD therapy may be related to venous access, the pocket or the hardware (lead and generator). They can occur early (perioperatively), or much later (Table 9.1).

9.1 Complications due to venous access

The risks of a complication related to subclavian vein puncture technique depend on operator skill and the difficulty of the subclavian puncture due to the patient's anatomy (Fig. 9.01). However, the use of the cephalic cut-down technique almost eliminates these complications. The use of the axillary vein is safer than subclavian puncture.

Pneumothorax is uncommon (1% in experienced hands) but it may occasionally occur in patients with emphysema or anatomic abnormalities. Pneumothorax may be asymptomatic and noted on routine follow-up chest X-ray, or it may be associated with pleuritic pain, respiratory distress or hypotension. A pneumothorax that involves less than 10% of the pleural space is mostly benign and resolves without intervention. A pneumothorax involving more than 10% or a tension pneumothorax requires the immediate placement of a chest tube.

Hemoptysis may occur if the lung is punctured and may be associated with a pneumothorax. Hemoptysis is usually self-limiting.

Hemothorax is a rare complication of subclavian puncture. It can be caused by laceration of the subclavian artery or by inadvertently introducing a large dilator or sheath into the artery. It is not caused by trauma to the lungs. In the absence of pneumothorax bleeding is usually controlled by lung pressure. However, if the ipsilateral lung is also collapsed, blood may escape freely into the pleural space (hemopneumothorax) and may result in substantial hemorrhage-associated hypotension and hemodynamic compromise necessitating draining.

Air embolism is a rare complication of subclavian vein puncture and mostly occurs when the lead is advanced through the introducer sheath because of the development of physiologic negative pressure. This complication can be avoided by using the deep Trendelenburg position during advancement of the introducer sheath or leads, by pinching the sheath when the trocar is withdrawn or by using sheaths with a hemostatic valve. The diagnosis of air embolism is obvious on fluoroscopy. Patients are mostly tolerant of this complication. However, respiratory distress, hypotension and arterial oxygen desaturation may occur with a large embolus. Therapy consists of 100% oxygen with inotropic support. Usually no therapy is required as the air is eventually absorbed into the lungs.

Perforation of the RV usually occurs without serious sequelae but cardiac tamponade may occur usually at the time of implantation. The latter requires emergency pericardiocentesis. Lead perforation usually becomes manifest only a few days after implantation but it may also occur several weeks after the initial procedure. It presents with a high pacing threshold, undersensing, and diaphragmatic stimulation. The diagnosis is made with telemetry of ventricular EGMs, chest X-rays, echocardiography and a computed tomography (CT) scan. Recording of an adequate ventricular EGM from the proximal RV electrode but an atypical one from the distal electrode should raise the suspicion of lead perforation. Gentle withdrawal of the lead (with surgical backup) and repositioning the tip to a different location is often successful when the procedure is done 24 hours or later after implantation.

Venous thrombosis or occlusion of the subclavian and brachiocephalic veins is common but frequently asymptomatic. Acute symptomatic thrombosis is relatively uncommon and may cause unilateral arm swelling usually several weeks after implantation. Superior vena cava syndrome (from occlusion) is more serious but rare, and causes facial edema and cyanosis as well as collateral veins on the thorax. Symptomatic thrombosis manifested by arm swelling can be treated conservatively with arm elevation and heparin followed by oral anticoagulation, or more aggressively with thrombolytic drugs. Superior vena cava syndrome requires vascular consultation for possible surgical correction.

Pulmonary embolism occurs rarely but the incidence may be underestimated, as it is usually unrecognized.

Table 9.1. Complications of ICD implantation

Venous access	Bleeding
	Pain
	Hemoptysis
	Pneumothorax
	Subcutaneous emphysema
	Hemothorax
	Thoracic duct injury
	Subclavian vein thrombosis
	Subclavian artery puncture
	Subclavian arteriovenous fistula
	Pulmonary embolism
	Air embolism
	Brachial plexus injury
Pocket	Hematoma
	Seroma
	Skin erosion
	Infection
Leads	Malposition
	Dislodgment
	Lead perforation
	Exit block without displacement
	Intracardiac thrombosis
	Infection
	Hemopericardium
	Cardiac tamponade
	Post-pericardiotomy syndrome
	Extracardiac stimulation
	Diaphragmatic stimulation
Leads: electrical problems	Insulator break
	Conductor break
	Lead disconnection
	Loose setscrew
	Connection problems
	Inadequate defibrillation threshold
	Undersensing

The presence of a symptomatic pulmonary embolism (potentially life threatening) in a patient with a device should raise the suspicion of a source from an ICD lead.

Brachial plexus injury may occur from the needlestick in the brachial plexus located close to the subclavian/axillary vein. This complication should be suspected postoperatively if the patient complains of pain or paresthesias of the upper extremity. There is usually complete recovery but neural injury may result in permanent muscle atrophy and impairment of shoulder motion.

9.2 Lead-related complications

Lead malposition

This may occur during transvenous lead placement. In patients with an atrial septal defect or a large patent foramen ovale, the ventricular lead may be advanced inadvertently into the left ventricle. This complication occurs because fluoroscopy is often limited to the anteroposterior (AP) projection during the procedure and LV placement may resemble RV placement. An LV lead position should be suspected when the tip of the lead is posterior on fluoroscopy and ventricular pacing gives rise to a right bundle branch block pattern.

Diaphragmatic stimulation

The potential for diaphragmatic stimulation should be tested at implantation by using the highest output from the generator. If diaphragmatic stimulation is negative on initial testing with a high output, subsequent diaphragmatic stimulation is rare. It may occur with slight or overt displacement of the RV lead or right atrial lead or RV perforation. Intractable diaphragmatic stimulation requires lead revision.

Lead dislodgment

This usually occurs in the first days after implantation and may occur up to 3 months after initial implantation. Right ventricular lead dislodgment occurs in 1–3% of cases. Lead displacement may be due to improper initial lead positioning, poor lead fixation or excessive arm/shoulder motions soon after surgery. Dislodgment of the lead may cause loss of capture and undersensing. The diagnosis is confirmed by device interrogation showing changes in the sensing and pacing thresholds compared with implantation data, and a chest X-ray in the case of macro-displacement. Immediate lead repositioning is mandatory.

Lead malfunction

Damage may occur during implantation. An insulation break may occur as a result of inadvertent placement of a suture around the lead without a protective sleeve, an overtight suture on the sleeve, or an accidental cut during surgery.

With increasing age of transvenous lead systems, a growing number of lead fractures and insulation defects have to be expected.

9.3 Pocket-related complications

Chronic severe pain may occur at the implantation-site in 1–2% of cases. A pocket *seroma* is due to fluid accumulation and is usually benign when not accompanied by signs of inflammation (Figs 9.01–9.03).

It is observed more commonly after ICD generator change when the new pulse generator is smaller than the pre-vious one. Aspiration should be discouraged because of the risk of introducing infection by contamination.

Pocket hematoma is relatively common. A hematoma is usually managed conservatively unless it expands in size and becomes tense and painful, whereupon evacuation becomes necessary with reoperation to identify and control the site of bleeding. The risk of postoperative bleeding is higher with heparin than warfarin.

Erosion is characterized by deterioration of tissue over an implanted pulse generator or movement of a lead toward or through the skin. Risk factors include an undersized pocket with tension on the overlying tissue, or implantation of the pulse generator too superficially or laterally in thin adults or children. When erosion is recognized at an early stage, signaled by redness and thinning of the skin, elective reoperation can be considered to relocate the pulse generator to a submuscular site. If any portion of the pulse generator or lead completely erodes through the skin, the site should be considered infected.

Infection occurs in about 0.5–1% of primary implantations but is more common after device replacement (2%). The mortality is very high if the leads and the ICD are not removed. The manifestations range from local reactions (redness, tenderness, swelling, abscess around the device) to uncommon life-threatening systemic sepsis with positive blood cultures. Early infections are usually caused by *Staphylococcus aureus*. Late infections, commonly caused by *Staphylococcus epidermidis*, are more indolent and may present months or years after implantation sometimes with only pain at the ICD site. The presence of infection mandates complete lead and device removal followed by antibiotics. Partial removal is associated with a high recurrence rate.

9.4 Generator-related complications

Normal functioning of an ICD system depends on proper connection between the leads and the generator. Care should be exercised to avoid misconnection of the leads in the port. A loose setscrew usually causes oversensing due to the generation of spurious signals, intermittent failure to pace or increased pacing threshold and lead impedance. When a defibrillation connector pin is loose, energy shunting may result in inadequate energy output and failure to defibrillate. To prevent this complication several steps should be performed routinely:

1. advance the lead pin past the metal contact points, all the way to the end of the receptacle;
2. tug on the lead to ensure that the set screws are tightened properly;
3. test the pacing threshold;
4. measure pacing and shocking impedances.

9.5 Inappropriate delivery of therapy

Inappropriate shocks most often occur due to supraventricular tachycardia (and sinus tachycardia), self-terminating VT (in committed systems), and sensing artifacts, for example myopotentials. T-wave oversensing is an uncommon cause of inappropriate shocks. Potential induction of fatal ventricular fibrillation by inappropriate shocks is rare. The commonest cause of inappropriate therapy is atrial fibrillation. In patients with symptomatic slow ventricular tachyarrhythmias, state-of-the-art ICD discrimination algorithms should be used to distinguish supraventricular arrhythmias from VT. Amiodarone plus beta-blocker therapy can prevent 75% of inappropriate shocks, and this combination is far superior to sotalol alone. With a low baseline DFT, amiodarone seems to increase the DFT only slightly.

9.6 Failure to deliver therapy or delay of therapy

Absent or delayed therapy may be caused by incorrect programming (including human error), ICD system performance, or a combination of the two. The most common causes are ICD inactivation, VT slower than the programmed detection interval, SVT–VT discriminators misclassifying VT or VF as SVT, undersensing, and problems with intradevice software (Fig. 9.05).

ICD inactivation

It is easily forgotten that when detection is programmed OFF for surgery using electrocautery, the ICD must be reprogrammed at the end of the procedure.

Ventricular tachycardia slower than the programmed detection rate

Spontaneous VT is often slower than induced VT. The VT detection interval should be programmed at least 40–50 ms longer than the slowest predicted VT for consecutive-interval counting, and 30–40 ms longer for x-of-y and the averaging St. Jude Medical algorithm. Patients with advanced heart failure who cannot tolerate prolonged slow VT require a long VT detection interval.

SVT–VT discriminators

SVT–VT discriminators may prevent or delay therapy if they misclassify VT or VF as SVT. The programmable SVT limit provides the highest rate for which the discriminators are active.
1. *Single-chamber discriminators.* Morphology discriminators may misclassify monomorphic VT.
2. *Dual-chamber discriminators.* If the atrial lead drops into the ventricle, the atrial channel senses a ventricular EGM. The ICD will therefore sense VT as a tachycardia with a 1:1 AV relationship and virtually simultaneous atrial and ventricular activation. Discriminators designed to withhold therapy from SVT with 1:1 AV conduction may then withhold VT therapy.

Duration-based "safety-net" features to override discriminators

These programmable features deliver therapy if an arrhythmia satisfies the ventricular rate criterion for a sufficiently long duration even if discriminators indicate SVT The decision to use a discriminator may be difficult as it depends on the probability that discriminators will prevent VT detection, the risk of failure to detect VT, and the likelihood of sustained SVT in the VT rate zone.

Undersensing

Clinically significant undersensing of VF is rare in modern ICD systems if the baseline R-wave amplitude is ≥ 5–7 mV. Ventricular fibrillation may be undersensed due to inappropriate programming, low-amplitude EGMs, rapidly varying EGM amplitude, drug effects and ischemia. Drug or hyperkalemic effects may slow VF into the VT zone causing undersensing of VF. Prolonged ischemia from sustained slow VT (longer than the VT detection interval) may cause deterioration of the ventricular signal and VF undersensing. Lead, connector, or generator problems may also present as undersensing.

9.7 Unsuccessful shock therapy

If an ICD classifies a shock as unsuccessful, stored EGMs must be reviewed to determine both if the shock was delivered for true VT/VF and if the shock actually failed to terminate VT/VF.

Misclassified therapy

ICDs misclassify effective therapy as ineffective if VT/VF recurs before the ICD determines the VT/VF episode as terminated and reclassifies the post-therapy rhythm as sinus. Decreasing the duration for redetection of sinus rhythm (as can be programmed with the St. Jude Medical device) might correct this classification error. ICDs may also misclassify shocks as ineffective if the post-shock rhythm is SVT in the VT rate zone (catecholamine-induced sinus tachycardia or shock-induced atrial fibrillation).

Patient-related factors

Factors that reversibly raise the DFT include hyperkalemia, antiarrhythmic drugs and ischemia. Pleural or pericardial effusions also raise the DFT, as can new myocardial infarction or progressive cardiac enlargement. Programming shock-pathway and waveform parameters may help in a few cases. Migration of an active-can ICD low on the chest wall can increase the DFT by altering the shock vector.

ICD system-related reasons

ICD-related causes of unsuccessful therapy include insufficient programmed shock strength or ATP sequences, battery depletion (usually due to inadequate clinical follow-up), generator component failure (hardware or software), lead failure, device–lead connection failures and lead dislodgment. Prolonged episodes caused by delayed detection and/or prolonged charge times may increase the shock strength required to convert VT or VF.

9.8 Proarrhythmia

Proarrhythmia, although rarely fatal, increases the morbidity associated with ICD therapy. Proarrhythmia seems to be related to suboptimal programming and technical limitations of devices. Proarrhythmia can be minimized by tailoring the "electrical prescription" to fit the clinical arrhythmia and ICD idiosyncrasies (Fig. 9.13). ICD-induced proarrhythmia may occur as a result of appropriate or inappropriate therapy. Manifestations include new tachycardias and also bradycardia, as in the post-shock situation. Drugs to prevent VT can also be proarrhythmic. Inappropriate ICD therapy remains a major clinical challenge resulting in poorer quality of life; device proarrhythmia occurs in spite of sophisticated algorithms for discrimina-

tion of supraventricular and sinus tachycardia from VT and VF. Examples of proarrhythmia include the induction of atrial fibrillation by a ventricular shock, and VT acceleration or degeneration into VF by ATP or a low-energy shock. Deceleration of VT by ICD therapy is also a form of proarrhythmia because the slower VT may not be detected by the ICD. Device proarrhythmia may be fatal. For example dislodgment of the ventricular lead to the level of the tricuspid annulus may cause sensing of the atrial signal during sinus tachycardia. An ICD may interpret this situation as VF and deliver inappropriate shocks. Ventricular fibrillation may not be sensed by the displaced lead resulting in death. The delivery of a noncommitted shock during nonsustained VT also carries the potential of causing a serious sustained ventricular tachyarrhythmia.

9.9 Electrical storm

Electrical storm in ICD patients is commonly defined as the detection of three or more ventricular tachyarrhythmias in 24 hours (Fig. 9.15). All appropriately detected VTs treated by ATP, one or more shocks or eventually untreated in a VT monitoring zone but sustained (> 30 s according to device memory) form part of the definition. To constitute an electrical storm, the VTs must consist of separate episodes. Consequently VT after unsuccessful therapy is not considered as a second episode. In contrast, incessant VT, that is, VT starting shortly (after ≥ 1 sinus cycle and within 5 min) after a technically successful therapy, forms part of the definition because it represents the most serious manifestation of electrical storm. Repetitive VT in the first week after ICD implantation should not be considered part of electrical storm because it has different clinical and prognostic implications.

9.9.1 Clinical manifestations

Obvious causes (ischemia, heart failure, hypokalemia) are evident in less than 20% of cases. Psychological stress may be an important trigger. Sympathetic activity appears to play an important role in the genesis of electrical storm.

Electrical storm seems to appear in approximately 25% of ICD patients, typically late (6–36 months) after implantation. Most patients present with monomorphic VT. The prevalence of VF (possibly reflecting other triggers such as acute ischemia) seems to be rather low at 3–20%. In this respect, it must be appreciated that the definition of VF based on stored bipolar EGMs has not been standardized.

9.9.2 Prognosis

Electrical storm may be associated with increased mortality, either on a short-term basis or as a predictor of impaired long-term prognosis. The prognosis of electrical storm is not clear when the device quickly terminates VTs by ATP. Thus ATP may render electrical storm a rather harmless event or it may carry a substantial risk if the underlying cause (e.g. ischemia, worsening of heart failure) is not treated.

9.9.3 Therapy

Treatment involves reduction of the elevated sympathetic tone with oral or intravenous beta-blockers, frequently combined with benzodiazepines for sedation (and occasionally propofol) Intravenous amiodarone has also been successful. Radiofrequency ablation holds great promise for electrical storm refractory to amiodarone. Magnesium and potassium may be helpful particularly in patients with prolonged QT intervals or hypokalemia. The number of VT cycles necessary for detection can be increased to allow spontaneous termination. Finally, overdrive pacing by increasing the lower rate of the ICD may terminate electrical storm in some patients.

9.10 Psychological problems

Many ICD recipients are able to resume their normal activities in the months after ICD implantation and successfully integrate the ICD into their life. However, in some patients ICD therapy may have adverse physical, social and psychological consequences. (Fig. 9.16) In survivors of cardiac arrest, cognitive processing may slow down and the patient may experience difficulties with intellectual activities requiring concentration. This may result in a decrease in social interaction causing isolation from family, friends and colleagues. Some ICD patients may show an overall reduction in physical activity, which may be due to discomfort in the shoulder and arm during the first weeks after ICD implantation. Patients may avoid exercise from the fear of receiving a shock with an increase in heart rate. Sometimes, when patients are instructed to avoid vigorous exercise, they respond overcautiously, assuming that even moderate exercise is dangerous. Fear of ICD discharge may also inhibit patients from resuming sexual activity. Other stress factors in ICD recipients include panic reactions or agoraphobia, a negative effect on body image, imaginary shocks, confrontation with death and uncertainty about the future, the unpredictability of shocks and loss of independence by driving restrictions.

The insecurities and doubts regarding living with an ICD are problems not easily discussed with the physician. At the outpatient clinic there is usually limited time for conversation beyond the physical check-up and interrogation of arrhythmic episodes and device parameters. A brief educational intervention given by a cardiac nurse targeting anxious patients and their family may alleviate unnecessary anxiety. Many ICD recipients misinterpret some of the information provided in the initial period after implantation. Early enrollment of patients into a cardiac rehabilitation program may improve quality of life and have a salutary effect. Meetings of support groups supervised by the implanting center may augment a patient's knowledge, dispel misconceptions, and enhance psychosocial adjustment by facilitating social exchange and emotional support. Cognitive behavioral therapy should be considered as it is designed to reduce stress and enhance coping with the potentially stressful effect of ICD therapy. All in all, about half of ICD patients experience depression or anxiety, and a psychiatric consultation is often necessary. The number of shocks is only one reason for depression and anxiety. Unexpected shock delivery is a stressful event, especially when it is repeated after a short time. This "near-death experience" may trigger a severe anxiety state. In the subset of patients receiving shocks, quality of life is worse, especially in those receiving five or more shocks. Therefore, activation of ATP for fast VTs should be performed in every ICD patient to minimize painful shocks that contribute to the deterioration of quality of life.

The physician must be prepared for a request from a patient or their surrogate to discontinue ICD therapy so as to avoid a long process of dying. It is ethically and legally permissible for a patient to request the withdrawal of any treatment. This situation is analogous to discontinuing other life-sustaining interventions according to a patient's wish. The alternatives must be discussed in detail with the patient and a psychiatric consultation is essential to rule out distorted judgment from depression and related problems.

When confronted with psychosocial issues the practitioner should keep the four As in mind:
1. ASK: assess concerns
2. ADVISE: anticipate psychosocial impact
3. ASSIST: be practical, educate, support, use experience
4. ARRANGE: psychosocial contact

10 ICD follow-up

Patients should be seen at regular intervals to monitor the implantation site, lead and device function, arrhythmia detection and therapy delivery (Fig. 10.01). The interval between routine follow-up visits may range from 3 to 6 months depending on the patient's condition and the time since implantation. There is usually more than one correct way to evaluate and program the ICD for each patient. Using a systematic approach ensures that no step is forgotten and no test unwittingly omitted. Fine-tuning the ICD for optimal results requires a detailed knowledge of the clinical status, concomitant medical conditions, and the ICD indication. Follow-up can be done remotely using specific equipment to interrogate and "upload" data to a secure website via the patient's telephone line. Remote follow-up systems permit device interrogation and retrieval of diagnostic data, but do not allow threshold testing or reprogramming.

Most emergency department visits by ICD patients are mostly related to the device or arrhythmia, but other common problems include acute coronary syndrome and congestive heart failure.

10.1 Patient instructions at time of discharge

Prior to discharge, a final check is performed to verify proper functioning of the ICD system so as to:
- ensure that the device is activated;
- perform final device programming;
- document lead position by chest X-ray and measure pacing threshold and R-wave amplitude to rule out early lead dislodgment;
- provide patient and family education;
- plan outpatient follow-up: 7 days and 1 month after implantation.

At the time of discharge, ICD patients must receive clear instructions for a smooth transition from the hospital environment to a daily routine at home (Fig. 9.01). Most manufacturers or hospitals provide a special ICD patient booklet explaining how the device works and giving information for the patient and family about living with an ICD.

10.1.1 General instructions

The manufacturer of the ICD will send the patient a permanent card (laminated) within 4–6 weeks. The patient should always carry his or her ICD identification card or wear a medic-alert bracelet or necklace. The ID card is very important in case of emergencies. It contains an emergency phone number and useful information about the ICD manufacturer, the type or model of the ICD and leads, serial numbers and date of implantation.

Following implantation, the patient should not take a shower or get the wound wet for 1 week, although bathing is permissible a few days after surgery as long as the incision is not submerged. Touching or rubbing the incision should be avoided. Steri-strips or tapes across the incision are allowed to fall off or a nurse can remove them at the first office visit 7–10 days after surgery.

The patient is instructed to monitor the ICD pocket and incision daily for several weeks while healing. The ICD will bulge slightly under the skin, but this bulge should decrease over the ensuing few weeks. The doctor's office should be notified if any of the following signs are observed, especially if they increase after the first days:
1. Any redness, heat, swelling or any kind of yellow, green or brown drainage from the site.
2. A soreness around the pulse generator or a bruise that does not go away.
3. A temperature of or above 100°F (38°C) or chills. The patient should check his or her temperature at home twice daily at the same time for 2 weeks and write it down on a piece of paper.

The patient may gradually resume his or her daily activities as tolerated and resume sexual activity once the incision has healed. Activities that involve rough contact with the ICD site should be avoided. Heavy lifting (over 5 kg or 10 pounds) should be avoided in the first 6 weeks. In the first month the range of shoulder motion should be restricted to up to 90° (putting elbow as high as the shoulder). Movement of the arm within the full extent of this range is encouraged to maintain shoulder mobility.

10.1.2 Special precautions

Driving is not allowed for 6 months. If no syncope has occurred in the 6 months after implantation, many experts favor resumption of driving. Strong magnetic fields should be avoided as they may "blind" the ICD preventing it from delivering life-saving therapy during exposure. When traveling by air the security agent should be informed about the presence of an ICD. Transient exposure to magnetic fields, including airport metal detectors, should cause no problem, especially if the patient walks briskly through the detector field. Magnetic fields may cause some ICDs to emit beeping tones until leaving the source. If the beep does not stop, the physician should be contacted.

When using a cellular phone it should be held up to the ear on the side opposite to the ICD. Cell phones should not be carried in a shirt pocket over the ICD.

10.1.3 Instructions on shocks

If, after receiving a single shock, the patient feels fine, there is no need for him or her to go to an emergency room (Fig. 9.18). The cardiologist should be notified and an office visit scheduled in a timely fashion. Alternatively the nature of the first shock can often be assessed by remote monitoring without the need for a follow-up visit. It is important for the patient to keep a record of the event, including date, time, symptoms and activities at the time. However, when two or more shocks are delivered within a short time, a family member or bystander should call an ambulance. The patient must not drive a car to go to the hospital.

When the patient receives a shock and becomes syncopal for longer than a minute, cardiopulmonary resuscitation (CPR) should be initiated immediately. A person in physical contact with the patient at the time of a shock may feel a low-amplitude electrical charge, but this is not dangerous in any way to a family member or bystander.

10.1.4 Outpatient follow-up and ICD device checks

Ask the patient if he or she is planning to move out of the area. There are two types of clinical follow-up for patients:
1. chronic surveillance every 3–6 months to assess and document routine device operation and clinical progress;
2. acute unexpected evaluations prompted by patient concerns, symptoms, shocks, unsuccessful therapy or presumed failure to deliver expected therapy.

When the ICD battery starts to show signs of depletion, evaluations need to be more frequent. Sound or audible alarms may be programmed to alert the patient when the battery voltage becomes critically low. The patient should be instructed to notify their physician if an alert sounds.

10.1.5 Remote monitoring

Today, remote follow-up systems allow clinicians to monitor their ICD patients away from the device clinic or hospital. These systems transmit device diagnostic data, stored EGMs and the presenting rhythm. In this way, they provide the same information as is obtained at an office visit. Remote interrogations complement and, in some cases, may even replace in-clinic ICD follow-up visits. Some workers use remote monitoring instead of visits on alternate follow-up sessions. Remote monitoring may also discover undocumented and asymptomatic arrhythmias, the detection of intermittent lead problems, and data helpful in optimizing device parameters and medical therapy. Remote monitoring should be considered as a form of intensified follow-up especially in cases where an advisory mandates careful follow-up. Patients should be told of the availability of remote monitoring. Failure to inform patients may eventually cause medicolegal problems in the case of late discovery of an ICD problem. Furthermore, patient consent is advised as the data pass through a third party. Reprogramming an ICD remotely is not available.

10.2 History and physical examination

The history involves questions about palpitations, dizziness, presyncope, syncope, ICD shocks and whether certain body positions triggered ICD therapy. Multiple shocks during intense physical effort suggest a shock for sinus tachycardia. A shock associated with repetitive movements may indicate a lead malfunction. Patients who report a single shock without sequelae can be evaluated by the physician during a routine office visit. Patients who have multiple shocks within a short period should be told to go to the hospital for evaluation.

At the first visit, the practitioner examines the ICD and lead insertion sites for hematoma, seroma, increased warmth, or erythema as indicators of possible early infection.

In patients with chronically implanted devices, arm swelling on the same side as the insertion site or the presence of excessive superficial venous collaterals may indicate large vein thrombosis and the possible need for anticoagulation or thrombolytic therapy. Overall assessment also focuses on the presence of congestive heart failure and myocardial ischemia, which might precipitate ventricular tachyarrhythmias.

A drug history (20–70% of ICD patients require concomitant antiarrhythmic drug therapy), especially any changes, should be sought because some drugs, especially antiarrhythmics, may alter pacing, sensing and defibrillation thresholds (Figs 9.09–9.11) or cause proarrhythmia (Figs 9.12 and 9.13). Antiarrhythmic drug therapy may cause sinus bradycardia and chronotropic incompetence, which may lead to pacing and pacemaker syndrome in patients with a single-chamber ICD. Amiodarone plus a beta-blocker is effective for preventing shocks and is more effective than sotalol but has an increased risk of drug-related adverse effects. Repeat defibrillation testing in the electrophysiology laboratory may be required to determine alterations in the DFT after starting a new antiarrhythmic drug. Drug-induced VT rate-slowing below the rate detection cutoff requires reprogramming of the ICD (Fig. 9.08). A slower VT rate generally makes ATP more effective.

10.3 Device interrogation

The session starts with device interrogation using a programming wand or wireless telemetry. Routine interrogation is mandatory even in the absence of shocks because interventions with ATP or aborted shocks may be asymptomatic. In this respect, it is important to avoid frequent aborted shocks because they decrease battery longevity. Interrogation provides the programmed ICD parameters. Measured and diagnostic data are then examined. The data package includes such features as real-time pacing lead impedance, shocking lead impedance, stored ventricular EGMs, device charge times (after a shock or automatic reforming of the capacitor: this represents the time required from arrhythmia diagnosis fully to charge an ICD and deliver its therapy) and battery-life indicators (voltage). The diagnostic data should always be printed out before programming. The therapy summary outlines the arrhythmic episodes since the last visit, how the ICD interpreted them and the corresponding type of therapy if any. These counters can be cleared after each visit to avoid confusion in the future. The degree of ventricular pacing has become important to prevent LV dysfunction. It is estimated from the event histograms that record the cardiac activity. The data may lead to reprogramming to minimize RV pacing.

10.4 Hardware identification

Rapid identification of an ICD model is useful when it is necessary to deactivate or reprogram the device. Patients should carry identification cards or a record from the implanting hospital with information regarding the manufacturer, ICD model, lead system and therapy options. An overpenetrated radiograph of the generator will show a radiopaque marker for identification of an unknown ICD.

10.5 Lead evaluation

The leads are the weakest part of the ICD system, and mechanical stresses are responsible for fracture and insulation problems. The major lead complications, in decreasing frequency, include: insulation defects (most common); lead fractures; loss of ventricular capture; abnormal lead impedance; and sensing failure (Figs 11.03 and 11.04).

Pacing and sensing

The ventricular sensing lead is evaluated for pacing impedance, R-wave amplitude and pacing threshold together with real-time recordings of the ventricular EGMs. The measured pacing impedance is compared with the chronic baseline value. Decreases of 30% or more, or pacing impedances below 200–250 Ω, may be indicative of insulation failure. Sudden and significant increases in pacing impedance may indicate conductor fracture. The atrial lead of a dual-chamber ICD is evaluated in the same way. Any major changes soon after implantation justify a chest X-ray for lead dislodgment. Many ICDs provide semiautomatic methods for determining the pacing threshold. The degree of pacemaker dependence should be estimated as in patients with standard pacemakers. The programmer measures the atrial and ventricular EGMs (as seen by the ICD) automatically. Alternatively, the signals can be determined directly from the telemetered EGM by measuring from the upper peak to the lower peak.

Defibrillation or shocking leads

Shocking-pathway impedance normally measures 20–80 Ω in transvenous systems. A high impedance suggests a conductor defect, and a low impedance suggests an insulation failure/short circuit. The impedance of the high-voltage electrodes is easily determined by using painless, weak test pulses delivered automatically by the device at periodic intervals and upon interrogation. High-voltage impedance measured by weak pulses correlates well with that measured by high-energy shocks. Newer ICD models report independent proximal and distal defibrillation coil impedances that closely approximate those of high-voltage shocks. Some ICDs require the delivery of a 12-V shock (felt by most patients) for shocking lead measurement rather than the painless system described above.

10.6 Ventricular electrograms

The ventricular EGM from the sensing lead during sinus rhythm should measure at least 5–7 mV to ensure reliable VF sensing. The amplitude of the ventricular EGM may be reduced, with the risk of undersensing VF, by antiarrhythmic drugs, myocardial infarction, shocks, fibrosis at the lead tip, new conduction defects and lead dislodgment. A low-amplitude ventricular EGM requires reprogramming of sensitivity and retesting of sensing with VF induction. Repositioning or replacement with a new separate bipolar sensing lead (no coils) may be required.

Many of the storage functions are programmable and include the number and duration of arrhythmic episodes, atrial or ventricular EGMs or both, and mode-switch episodes. ICDs store electrical measurements from delivered therapy such as capacitor charge time, delivered energy and high-voltage impedance recorded for each shock. These provide valuable information regarding battery and capacitor status and the integrity of the defibrillation lead system. Upon device interrogation, the programmer indicates whether new EGMs have been stored. Stored EGMs of tachyarrhythmia episodes provide the most important data for interpreting the causes and consequences of ICD shocks and other forms of therapy.

10.7 Types of electrograms

Near field electrograms

Recording of an EGM requires two electrodes. A near-field EGM (local electrogram) is recorded either between the tip and the ring electrodes of a bipolar lead or between the tip and the distal coil for an integrated lead. The near-field EGM records the local narrow bipolar EGM that reflects myocardial activation in the vicinity of the electrodes (Fig. 5.03). The ICD uses the near-field ventricular EGM for rate sensing and arrhythmia detection ("rate-sensing" channel).

Shock electrograms

A shock EGM records the electrical activity between two high-voltage defibrillation electrodes and is therefore a far-field EGM. For example, a shock EGM may record activity between the RV coil and the ICD can. Alternatively, it can record the potential difference between the ICD can and the proximal (SVC) defibrillation coil or the voltage between the two coils of a dual-coil defibrillation lead.

Far-field (hybrid) EGMs can also be recorded between one of the defibrillation coils and one of the sensing electrodes.

Tachycardias that are unidentifiable solely on the basis of cycle length are more easily discriminated by using EGM data from the widely spaced shock electrodes rather than recordings from the sensing electrodes. Far-field EGMs from the RV coil and the device generate a wider deflection that may closely resemble the surface ECG. Furthermore, far-field recordings may facilitate identification of atrial activity during a recorded event. These features are useful in single-lead ICDs without an atrial lead.

Real-time electrograms

These are recorded simultaneously with the surface ECGs, and annotated markers provide valuable information. The marker channel depicts how the device actually interprets cardiac activity. Annotations used by the marker channel vary according to the manufacturer, but there usually exists a legend key or description on the programmer screen or in the accompanying product manual.

Stored electrograms

Electrograms can be stored or recordings frozen in time and stored in the device memory for subsequent retrieval and analysis. The ICD records these EGMs after a specific triggered event, typically arrhythmia detection, diagnosis and outcome of therapy. A programmable pre-trigger interval immediately precedes the trigger; the longer the pre-trigger interval, the greater the likelihood of recording the initiating event of the tachyarrhythmia. The pre-trigger interval is programmable. ICDs possess a limited storage capacity, and a strategy of overwriting the oldest information means that only the most recent data may be retrievable (first in, first out). Obviously with a finite memory capacity, single-channel EGM recording can store more episodes than dual-channel recordings, which consume more memory. Representative strips of important stored EGMs should be printed and inserted into the patient's chart. It is important to erase diagnostic counters periodically to permit the availability of only the latest and most relevant information.

10.8 How to read stored electrograms

10.8.1 Analysis of single-chamber electrograms

Analysis of morphology, regularity and abruptness of tachycardia onset helps SVT–VT discrimination (Fig. 10.06).

Morphology

Morphologic features of the ventricular EGM enhance diagnosis because VT produces a change in the activation sequence and EGM configuration in about 90–95% of cases. The device classifies a rhythm as SVT if the R-wave morphology is identical to the baseline R-wave configuration stored in the device. A recording with the R-wave similar but not identical to the baseline R-wave morphology should be classified as VT, but SVT with rate-related aberrancy remains possible.

Regularity

Most VTs are regular. In a tachycardia with an irregular rhythm, atrial fibrillation (AF) should be suspected. But irregularity alone cannot reliably discriminate AF from VT because RR intervals during AF may become more regular with fast ventricular rates (rates > 170 b.p.m.). During ongoing AF, ventricular EGMs may occasionally show a subtle variability in morphology so that ventricular activity originating from multiple locations cannot be excluded.

Sudden onset

During exercise, the rate typically does not increase suddenly. The rate usually displays a progressive acceleration up to a level dictated by the workload. Sudden onset is indicative of VT, as opposed to sinus tachycardia, which does not start suddenly.

10.8.2 Analysis of dual-chamber electrograms

In dual-chamber ICDs, atrial and ventricular EGMs enhance the device's diagnostic capability (Figs 10.07

and 10.08). It should be borne in mind that VT can coexist with atrial flutter and atrial fibrillation. Ventricular tachyarrhythmia must be suspected with a completely regular fast rhythm unlike the baseline situation.

Most tachycardias with 1:1 AV association (V = A) are SVTs (Figs 1.09 and 1.10). Differentiation of SVT from VT with a 1:1 VA relationship is possible by using morphology criteria of the ventricular EGM, mode of onset and response to ATP.

Mode of onset

Atrial tachycardia (AT) typically starts with an early atrial beat. Therefore it usually starts with a short PP interval followed by a short RR interval. The atrial cycle length predicts the subsequent change in ventricular cycle length. However, VT usually starts with a ventricular premature beat and a short RR interval.

The common form (slow-fast) of AV nodal reentrant tachycardia (AVNRT) usually starts with a premature atrial complex. Typically, AVNRT shows nearly simultaneous activation of the atria and ventricles with unchanged ventricular EGMs (unless there is rate-related bundle branch aberrancy).

Diagnosis of supraventricular tachycardias by ventricular antitachycardia pacing

The response to ATP provides important diagnostic information about the mechanism of SVTs. A variety of responses may occur (Table 10.1; Fig. 1.15).

1. *No termination of tachycardia after ventricular ATP with atrial entrainment and an A–V response*
   Ventricular pacing during AVNRT or orthodromic reciprocating tachycardia (ORT) at a cycle length shorter than the tachycardia cycle, advances all the atrial EGMs to the pacing interval or rate (atrial entrainment) without terminating the tachycardia. Ventriculoatrial conduction occurs through the retrograde limb of the circuit. Therefore, after the last paced ventricular complex from the ATP sequence, the anterograde limb of the circuit remains nonrefractory, and the last retrograde atrial complex can conduct to the ventricle. This creates an A–V response.
   An *A–V response* after ATP with atrial entrainment is diagnostic of an AVNRT or an ORT and rules out an atrial tachycardia (Fig. 1.16).

2. *No termination of tachycardia after ventricular ATP with atrial entrainment and an A–A–V response*
   When ventricular pacing during atrial tachycardia produces 1:1 ventriculoatrial conduction, retrograde conduction occurs through the AV node. In this case, the last retrograde atrial

Table 10.1. Diagnosis of supraventricular tachycardia by response to ventricular antitachycardia pacing

	NO ACCELERATION of atrial rate	ACCELERATION of atrial rate
NO TERMINATION of tachycardia by ATP	Highly suggestive of AT *if* atrial rate remains constant	AT *if* A–A–V response
TERMINATION of tachycardia	Not AT	Not decisive

A = atrial electrogram; AT = atrial tachycardia; ATP = antitachycardia pacing; V = ventricular electrogram.

complex linked to ATP cannot conduct to the ventricle because the AV node is still refractory to anterograde conduction. This produces an A–A–V response (Fig. 1.17).

An *A–A–V response* is diagnostic of atrial tachycardia and excludes AVNRT and ORT.

3. *No termination of tachycardia after ventricular ATP and no atrial entrainment*

When a tachycardia does not terminate during ventricular ATP at a cycle length shorter than the tachycardia cycle and the atrial rate remains constant (no entrainment of the atria), atrial tachycardia becomes the most probable diagnosis (Fig. 1.18).

Dissociation between atrial activity and ventricular pacing *excludes ORT*.

4. *Termination of tachycardia after ventricular ATP and atrial entrainment*

No conclusions can be drawn when the tachycardia terminates after ATP at a cycle length shorter than the tachycardia cycle length and the atria are entrained.

5. *Termination of tachycardia after ventricular ATP without atrial entrainment*

Termination by ATP without depolarization of the atria excludes atrial tachycardia as a mechanism (Fig. 1.19).

10.9 Diagnostic data

ICD diagnostic data offer invaluable information regarding the functional status of the device and leads. The device itself determines atrial and ventricular sensing data and lead impedances at regular intervals. Significantly abnormal measurements of predetermined ranges or deviations from

previous measurements are usually highlighted on the programmer upon interrogation of the device.

10.10 Battery status

The telemetered information from the device includes a battery voltage indicator. The time required to charge the capacitors (charge time) to the maximum deliverable energy also acts as a index of battery status. The most common cause of asymptomatic premature battery depletion related to capacitor charging is repeated aborted shocks due to repetitive nonsustained VT or oversensing due to lead-connector problems.

A very long charge time alone (after reforming) requires ICD replacement even if the battery has not reached the ERI point.

10.11 Remote follow-up

Remote interrogation of ICDs provides frequent, convenient, safe and comprehensive device monitoring and reduces the frequency of outpatient visits. Although most patients with ICDs are followed routinely at intervals ranging from 3 to 6 months, many patients require additional nonscheduled visits to investigate a variety of problems; these problems can now be evaluated remotely thereby eliminating delayed detection of events associated with routine follow-up visits. Remote follow-up promises to reduce the time burden for patients and physicians. There are several systems that allow remote patient monitoring but all are manufacturer specific (Figs 10.15–10.17). These remote systems promise more efficient patient management at a time of rapidly increasing numbers of patients. Transmissions are via the internet. Implanted devices are interrogated with easy-to-use equipment in patients' homes (or elsewhere). Data collection is done with either a wand placed on the device or wirelessly to the patient's receiver-monitor. The equipment communicates stored and real-time data through standard telephone lines to secure computer servers that can be accessed by clinicians. Transmission to the pacemaker center can be activated by the patient (upon an audible alarm or symptoms) or done automatically (wirelessly in proximity to the receiver) according to predetermined circumstances (without an audible alarm) and prespecified limited data transmission. Technology using remote control software allows interrogation of the device memory, permits ICD monitoring by physicians or technical support from the manufacturer. Indeed, all the data obtained by device interrogation during a patient clinic visit may be just as easily retrieved remotely. These include battery longevity, the presence and appropriateness of device discharge, significance of an audible device alert, the development of new and often unsuspected arrhythmias, and the need for an earlier office visit for device reprogramming or drug therapy. Remote follow-up provides a convenient way for more frequent evaluation as a device approaches the ERI point.

Remote patient monitoring can thus virtually fulfill the requirements of an in-office follow-up but its main advantage is patient safety. Benefits include the ability to obtain an earlier diagnosis (and management) of arrhythmic events, increased safety, and reduced follow-up costs (by saving on transportation costs, particularly when the distance between home and the medical facility is more than 75 miles). Remote follow-up will probably reduce follow-up visits by more than 50%. Patients have expressed a high degree of satisfaction with the convenience and ease of use of remote ICD monitoring. They feel reassured that everything possible is being done to keep in touch with them. Finally, in heart failure patients with cardiac resynchronization devices and an ICD, remote monitoring is not a simple device check. Rather, it entails evaluation of the hemodynamic and pulmonary fluid status in the form of a disease management system.

10.12 Automatic monitoring and audible alarms

ICD technology allows automatic daily measurements of many parameters such as battery status, charge time, pacing and high-voltage impedance

(Table 10.2). Despite this sophistication, system-related complications occur in a significant proportion of patients. Measurements of pacing and high-voltage lead impedance are routinely performed at outpatient visits, but intermittent faults in lead integrity may be difficult to detect or confirm. Early detection is essential to avoid complications. Some ICDs contain a programmable audible alarm system to alert the patient that measured parameters are not within the normal range and prompt the patient to contact the physician. Some alerts are always on, whereas others can be programmed off. The alerts can be programmed to sound at the time of day selected by the clinician. A "silent" alarm feature can be selected with Medtronic ICDs. In such a case, the alarm signal is transmitted wirelessly to the patient's home monitor (whenever the patient is in close proximity) and then the alert is sent via a telephone line to the base server and then to the ICD center. The ICD center then calls the patient. Most alerts are lead-related. Thus, alerts are more common after device replacement using existing leads. As some patients do not hear the alarm, testing the alarm sound before discharge may be necessary. Conversely, some patients may perceive "phantom" alerts, pretending to have heard an alarm sound without a documented event in the device memory.

Implementation of automated monitoring with audible alarms may contribute to early detection of lead- and device-related complications such as lead fracture, insulation defect, dislodgment and sudden battery depletion. Although patient-alert features are a useful additional tool facilitating early detection of serious ICD complications, they do not substitute for regular ICD follow-up, because of their low sensitivity.

10.13 Emergency situations and magnet application

Most emergency department visits by ICD patients are related to the device or to arrhythmia. Acute coronary syndrome and congestive heart failure account for only 30% of visits. Application of the magnet over an ICD deactivates the tachycardia function. The antibradycardia function remains intact. The magnet response is useful in emergency situations, such as multiple inappropriate shocks where tachycardia therapy has to be turned off, or when using electrocautery in the operating room where a programmer may not be available. In such cases the magnet can be taped over the ICD. The Boston Scientific (Guidant) ICD provides several programmable functions. The device can be programmed to respond or not respond to magnet

Table 10.2. ICD alert sounds

Alert	Description
Low battery voltage	Battery voltage has reached early replacement indicator (ERI) voltage level
Excessive charge time	Charge time equals or exceeds charge time threshold
VF Detection/Therapy off	VF detection or VF therapy has been turned off
Atrial, RV, LV pacing impedance	Lead impedance is less or greater than minimum/maximum threshold
Shock lead impedance	Lead impedance is less or greater than minimum/maximum threshold
Number of shocks delivered in an episode	Number of shocks delivered in an episode is greater than or equal to the programmed number of shocks
All therapies in a zone exhausted for an episode	A specific arrhythmic episode was redetected after all programmed therapies for that type of episode were delivered
Electrical reset	The device has been reset and may require reprogramming
Pacing mode DOO or VOO	DOO or VOO mode is turned on
Active can off without SVC	Active can feature is turned off without a SVC lead in place
Beep during magnet application	Indicates presence of a strong magnet
Beep during capacitor charge	Feature may be useful during EP testing
Beep on sensed and paced ventricular events	Provides an R-wave synchronous tone

application. The ICD provides several functions when the "Enable Magnet Use" feature is programmed (Figs 10.20 and 10.21).

10.14 Turning off the ICD

Turning off an ICD may be necessary in the following circumstances:

1. During surgery using electrocautery. In this respect, it is easier to tape a doughnut magnet over the ICD for the duration of surgery.
2. In the presence of many inappropriate shocks.
3. Abiding by a patient's choice – usually when the patient is in a terminal condition.

11 Troubleshooting

Troubleshooting ICD problems encompasses all aspects of bradycardia pacemaker malfunction as well as evaluation of the appropriateness of therapies for ventricular arrhythmias.

11.1 Clinical history

Major symptoms such as palpitations, dizziness, near syncope or syncope or other prodromal symptoms suggest that shock therapy was for tachycardia but not necessarily VT/VF (Fig. 10.02). Shocks in a conscious or minimally symptomatic patient may arise from a hemodynamically tolerated VT, an SVT satisfying the detection criteria, a nonsustained VT with committed ICD function, or from oversensing of unwanted intracardiac or extracardiac signals. Shocks during heavy exertion suggest a response to sinus tachycardia.

11.2 Diagnosing the cause of shocks

The first step focuses on determining whether therapy was actually delivered. Some patients report ICD shocks when the ICD counters show no delivered therapy. This situation ("phantom shocks") may be caused by pacing-induced pectoral, diaphragmatic or intercostal muscle stimulation or spontaneous muscle contractions. Adapting the pacemaker output may solve the problem, and otherwise reassurance is all that is needed.

If an ICD discharge has occurred, it should be determined whether the shock was delivered in response to a true tachycardia or undesirable oversensing (Fig. 10.03). Stored EGMs with corresponding annotated markers will then easily reveal what triggered the shock. Inappropriate shocks occur in at least 20% of ICD patients, primarily for atrial fibrillation or other types of SVT. Inappropriate shocks also occur with lead failure, electromagnetic interference, and oversensing of T-waves or diaphragmatic potentials.

Management of a single shock

The approach consists of reassurance and evaluation in the next few days. If the shock is preceded by syncope, chest pain or severe dyspnea, the patient should be sent to the emergency department of a hospital. The antibradycardia function (with preservation of sensing) of an ICD is unaffected by application of a magnet.

Management of more than one shock

This requires hospitalization (Fig. 11.05). In the case of multiple inappropriate shocks, placing a magnet over the device can immediately disarm the antitachycardia function of an ICD.

11.3 Oversensing

11.3.1 Oversensing of intracardiac signals

Oversensing is more common than undersensing, which is very unusual. Oversensing may cause inappropriate treatment (shocks), which are disturbing to patients and carry the risk of inducing proarrhythmias that might be potentially fatal (Fig. 10.04). Oversensing of intracardiac signals is identified by characteristic alternation of intervals between sensed ventricular events and EGM morphology (PR vs RP, TQ vs QT, and short RR vs. long RR intervals separated by an isoelectric baseline).

P-wave oversensing

P-wave oversensing is rare but may occur if the distal coil of an integrated bipolar lead lies close to the tricuspid valve. If the PR interval exceeds the ventricular blanking period, the ventricular channel will sense both the P-wave and the QRS complex, a situation that may trigger a shock. This may occur in children or in adults if the RV lead becomes dislodged from the RV apex. Consistent oversensing of spontaneous P-waves often requires repositioning of the lead.

One amelioration strategy forces atrial pacing using DDDR pacing or dynamic overdrive modes. This procedure will shorten the ventricular cycle length and thereby prevent the ventricular sensitivity from reaching its maximum value (the minimum threshold expressed in millivolt).

R-wave double counting

Double counting of the R-wave occurs when split, fragmented or prolonged sensed ventricular EGMs emerge beyond the ventricular blanking period. Double counting of ventricular extrasystoles is not uncommon. Double counting of the basic QRS complex may be exacerbated by frequency-dependent sodium-channel blocking drugs, particularly at high rates. Interval plots gathered by device interrogation depict double R-wave counting in terms of a "railroad track" pattern with alternating short and long intervals.

R-wave double counting may result in shocks for SVT slower than the programmed VT detection rate. Because alternate RR intervals in any conducted rhythm also increment the VF counter, the ICD treats all detected VT or SVT episodes with shocks, regardless of true tachycardia cycle length. R-wave double counting may be treated by lead repositioning or by lengthening the ventricular blanking period (if programmable) or reducing the ventricular sensitivity provided that sensing of VF/VT remains adequate.

T-wave oversensing

T-wave oversensing typically displays alternating sensed intervals, but the magnitude of alternation may be small. Postpacing T-wave oversensing is relatively benign and results in bradycardia pacing below the programmed lower rate.

T-wave sensing can be corrected by decreasing the sensitivity of the ventricular channel provided that VF/VT sensing remains satisfactory. A decrease in sensitivity requires retesting the ICD with VF induction to confirm continuing proper sensing. Occasionally the sensing lead needs to be repositioned or replaced to achieve larger R-wave amplitudes. The latter reduces T-wave sensing based on the automatic sensing algorithms of ICDs. "Slow" automatic gain control in Guidant ICDs (Fig. 5.07) seems particularly effective in reducing the likelihood of T-wave oversensing of large R-waves. St. Jude Medical ICDs provide a programmable "threshold start" and "decay delay" (Figs 5.05 and 5.09) to contain the oversensed T-wave, but this function must be used cautiously because it may impair VT/VF sensing.

Far-field R-wave oversensing

Far-field R-wave oversensing on the atrial channel impairs dual-chamber SVT–VT discrimination but it does not cause inappropriate detection of VT when the ventricular rate remains in the sinus zone. Far-field R-wave oversensing often shows a pattern of alternating short and long atrial cycle length. The marker depicting the oversensed R-wave remains close to the ventricular EGM. Control of far-field R-wave sensing can be achieved in several ways:
1. prolongation of the postventricular blanking period or its equivalent;
2. decrease of baseline atrial sensitivity without jeopardizing sensing of atrial fibrillation;
3. algorithmic rejection by identifying a specific pattern of atrial and ventricular events (Medtronic PR Logic);
4. automatic decrease of atrial sensitivity after ventricular events (Fig. 5.10).

11.3.2 Oversensing of extracardiac signals

Sensed extracardiac signals can precipitate inappropriate ICD therapies (Fig. 10.05). These signals replace the isoelectric baseline with high-frequency noise.

Myopotential oversensing

Diaphragmatic myopotentials. Myopotential oversensing usually occurs after long diastolic intervals or after paced events when the amplifier sensitivity or gain becomes maximal (Fig. 11.02). Diaphragmatic myopotentials are most prominent on the sensing EGM. Myopotential oversensing should be suspected when symptoms develop during movement. The presence of myopotential interference can be confirmed during follow-up by monitoring the ventricular EGM during deep breathing, Valsalva maneuver, arm movement or by forcefully pushing the hands together.

Persistent oversensing of low-amplitude high-frequency myopotential signals may cause inappropriate VT detection and inhibition of bradycardia pacing in pacemaker-dependent patients. Oversensing of myopotentials can be treated by decreasing the ventricular sensitivity, but proper sensing of VF should be retested. Repositioning of the lead or replacement of an integrated lead with a true bipolar lead may be necessary. Myopotential oversensing due to a lead insulation failure requires lead replacement.

Pectoral myopotentials. Pectoral myopotentials are more prominent on the far-field EGM that includes the ICD can, but these EGMs are not used for rate counting with the exception of a VT–SVT discrimination system linked to a morphology algorithm.

Other sources of myopotentials

Reversal of the coils in a dual-coil integrated lead should be suspected if there is noise (myopotentials) in both the sensing and shocking EGMs (Fig 13.73, Case 62). This problem may cause sensing of thoracic pectoral myopotentials and atrial activity with resultant ICD inhibition and/or inappropriate therapy (shocks).

A loose setscrew to the distal defibrillation coil of an integrated ICD lead may cause the detection of noise and pectoral myopotentials recordable in both the near-field and far-field ventricular EGMs.

Lead/connector problems

The "make and break" or false signals of a defective lead or connection often become manifest intermittently. Lead interference due to contact of the sensing lead with an abandoned lead creates another source of intermittent oversensing. Some ICDs record the number of extremely short nonphysiologic ventricular intervals (120–140 ms) labeled as RR interval by the ICD. Such data suggest an occult lead problem barring double R-wave counting of ventricular extrasystoles. In other ICDs, heart rate intervals can be evaluated for possible nonphysiologic intervals.

The most common site of a fracture (or insulation break) is between the first rib and clavicle or around the site of the anchoring sleeve. A suspected lead failure requires evaluation of all EGMs, pacing threshold, pacing impedance and painless HV electrode impedance; other sources of evidence include chest X-ray, stored episode EGMs and data logs.

Ventricular lead problems usually present either as oversensing, resulting in inappropriate shocks, or as abnormal diagnostic measurements (impedance) at follow-up. A lead problem may also present less commonly as VF undersensing or unsuccessful therapy, often fatal.

Repeated shocks associated with motion of the ipsilateral arm or certain body positions should raise the suspicion of lead fracture or lead instability (Fig. 11.03). Deep respiration, coughing or a Valsalva maneuver while monitoring the VEGM at follow-up may differentiate myopotentials from false signals, but both may coexist.

Manipulation of the device pocket may elicit electrical noise artifacts consistent with lead conductor fracture or a loose connection of the setscrew in the ICD header. In this respect it is important also to record the shock EGM. Noise only on the shock (far-field) EGM but sparing the sensing (near-field) EGM, indicates a defect in the shocking lead. High-voltage impedance measured by painless weak pulses correlates well with values measured by high-energy shocks. Shocking impedance normally measures 25–80 Ω. A high HV shocking impedance indicates a fracture, a low value an insulation defect

in the shocking circuit (Fig. 11.04). A low pacing impedance indicates an insulation defect, whereas a high pacing impedance indicates a complete or partial interruption of the sensing/pacing lead, a loose setscrew or a defective adapter.

11.4 Electromagnetic interference

Electromagnetic interference occurs when electrical signals of noncardiac or nonphysiologic origin affect ICDs. The larger the space between the electrodes, the larger the amplitude of the interfering signals. Therefore, the signal amplitude will be larger on the high-voltage EGM recorded from widely spaced electrodes than on the sensing EGM from closely spaced electrodes (Fig. 11.06). Electromagnetic interference (EMI) may provoke spurious tachyarrhythmia detection with consequent inappropriate shocks (inhibition of shocks is also possible). In dual-chamber ICDs using atrial channel information to discriminate between VT and SVT, simultaneous oversensing of EMI in both channels could result in varied and unpredictable arrhythmia detection.

As mentioned above, spacing between the electrodes determines the effect of EMI. With the proliferation of electronics and microprocessors in all kinds of devices the impact of EMI on ICD function has become clinically important.

Electromagnetic compatibility (EMC) problems always encompass three essential elements:
1. a victim (here the implanted ICD) malfunctioning because of unwanted signals;
2. a culprit or source emitting electromagnetic energy;
3. a coupling path linking source and victim.
To improve the compatibility between ICDs and their environment, these three elements have to be controlled.

The amplitude of most disturbing EMI fields attenuates rapidly with distance (measured in wavelengths). The larger the distance between source and victim, the lower the field strength directed at the victim (in most situations, doubling the distance halves the field strength) (Fig. 11.07).

Electromagnetic susceptibility of ICDs

ICDs are strikingly more vulnerable to EMI than pacemakers. ICD sensing amplifiers are more susceptible to EMI by design to detect very small signals during VF in conjunction with automatic threshold adaptation and very high sensitivities. The band-pass filters in ICDs contain broader bandwidths to detect the higher frequencies during VF, again increasing susceptibility to EMI. ICDs cannot use long refractory periods after sensed events. Some ICDs do not have any noise reversion capability. Others contain a very short noise-sampling window giving only an imperfect protection from EMI.

All contemporary ICDs are hermetically shielded in a titanium housing, a conducting metal case forming a Faraday cage to avoid the direct influence of electromagnetic radiation on ICD electronics. Filtering can eliminate a lot of the high-frequency signals, for example the use of small ceramic feed-through capacitors in the header renders ICDs nearly immune to most cellular phones. Bipolar leads with a small distance between ring and tip electrodes also reduce sensing of spurious low-frequency signals; special interference rejection circuits further eliminate these signals. Digital signal processing combined with multielement feed-through filters shows promise for complete device immunity!

11.4.1 Sources of electromagnetic interference

Potential sources of EMI include numerous circumstances at work in an industrial environment, situations in daily life and in conjunction with many medical diagnostic or therapeutic procedures (Fig. 11.08).

Medical sources

Magnetic resonance imaging (MRI) produces a static magnetic field, followed by application of rapidly varying magnetic and electromagnetic (radiofrequency pulses emitted during scanning) fields. Exposure to the static magnetic field results in activation of the reed-switch with asynchronous pacing in pacemakers and suspension of arrhythmia detection in most ICDs. Magnetic attraction may displace the device. The RF fields can induce EMI in the device circuitry with inhibition of pacing, spurious tachyarrhythmia detection, electrical reset and rapid pacing. Heating around the lead tip may increase the capture thresholds (Fig. 11.09). Therefore, MRI is contraindicated in ICD patients.

RF (shortwave) or microwave diathermy is contraindicated in patients with an ICD and should absolutely be avoided in the vicinity of an ICD.

If *cardioversion or defibrillation* is required in ICD patients, internal cardioversion via the device with a commanded shock is preferable. If external cardioversion/defibrillation is necessary, the degree of pacemaker dependency and stability of the intrinsic cardiac rhythm should be evaluated. A programmer and a transcutaneous external pacemaker should be available. Prior to shock a high-voltage output should be programmed to counteract a transient elevation in the pacing threshold. External cardioversion/defibrillation should be performed with the lowest possible energy using a biphasic waveform that requires less energy. Whenever possible, an anteroposterior configuration of the self-adhesive patches or paddles should be employed. The shocking electrodes should be at least 5–10 cm away from the device. After cardioversion, complete analysis of the device should be performed to ensure that the system has sustained no damage. An increase in capture threshold requires repeat determination of the pacing and sensing thresholds 24 hours later.

Procedures involving *electrosurgery* are particularly hazardous in ICD patients. Sensing of the cautery output signal (pulsed RF) may either trigger ICD therapy for a presumed ventricular arrhythmia or inhibit the pacing output. Moreover, the ICD may potentially be reprogrammed or even damaged. To prevent such problems, the tachyarrhythmia detection/therapy should be disabled and rate-response features deactivated during surgery (via the programmer). Alternatively for some ICDs, the tachycardia therapies (but not antibradycardia pacing) can be inactivated by simple magnet application over the ICD during surgery followed by removal after the procedure. Note that in some devices prolonged magnet application turns off therapies until a reactivation maneuver is performed by repeated magnet application or with a programmer. *Electrocautery* may induce a power-on-reset situation, and a rise in the pacing threshold. When tachyarrhythmia detections/therapies are turned off, continuous monitoring of the ECG is necessary and an external defibrillator should always be immediately available. Pacemaker-dependent patients require programming, if possible, to an asynchronous or triggered mode to prevent inhibition. After termination of the surgical procedure, the device has to be interrogated in detail and all parameters for pacing, sensing, tachyarrhythmia detection and tachyarrhythmia therapies checked and confirmed.

Radiotherapy may cause permanent damage of electronic circuit components from ionizing radiation. Direct irradiation should be avoided and the device should be shielded with lead during the radiation treatment or even removed and reimplanted away from the field if necessary. Shock coil failure due to structural lead damage after high-dose radiation treatment is possible. EMI generated by the machinery might close the reed switch, causing unexpected reversion to an OFF mode and requiring restoration to the therapy mode.

Radiofrequency ablation. As the RF current (500–1000 kHz) for arrhythmia ablation frequently switches on/off, it acts like a pulse-modulated source and the interaction with an implanted ICD becomes unpredictable (even runaway has been reported for older systems). The hazards and precautions are generally the same as for electrosurgery and electrocautery although problems are infrequent.

Lithotripsy is not a real EMI threat in itself because it does not use electromagnetic waves (however, positioning and controlling the machinery and activating the shock are done electrically, which produces EMI). Lithotripsy uses acoustic shockwaves to disintegrate renal or gallbladder stones. These strong mechanical shocks can break down some electronic components so that lithotripsy has to be avoided in the vicinity of the ICD. However, the general contraindication for lithotripsy is perhaps overly conservative.

Endoscopy with a wireless video-capsule (e.g. PillCam, Given Imaging Ltd, Yoqneam, Israel) uses a capsule that contains an image-capturing system, a power source and a telemetry system transmitting data at 434 MHz. Most ICDs do not show any influence from EMI involved in the video capsule but some may demonstrate oversensing and delivery of inappropriate therapy. Therefore, the Pill-Cam should be used only in a hospital, after suspension of ICD therapy and in conjunction with monitoring.

Sources of EMI in daily life

Home appliances such as electric razors, mixers, induction ovens, vacuum cleaners and washing machines are essentially benign if used in accordance with the international standards (ISO-IEC).

Electric tools in close contact with the body may affect an ICD if a current (frequency 50 Hz or 60 Hz) passes through the body in the vicinity of the device. The leakage current is very small ($< 50\,\mu A$) for electric tools complying with the international standards. Nevertheless, some tools need to be properly grounded and EMI is possible with interruption of the ground connection (earth), although the danger of electrocution appears higher than the EMI risk. Because of the typical 60 Hz noise pattern, EMI due to leakage current is easily recognized in stored EGMs (Fig. 11.11).

Cellular phones. Interactions are rare in contemporary ICDs. State-of-the-art devices are protected by so-called feed-through filters between the header and the hermetically sealed can. These low-pass filters prevent unwanted signals from entering the ICD housing. Nevertheless, digital devices (PCS, Personal Communication Service; and GSM, Global System for Mobile communication) still provide potential EMI especially at maximum output power (0.6 W in the USA and 2 W in Europe at the beginning of a call, just before the first audible ring). Therefore the US Food and Drug Administration (FDA) recommendations remain valid: the distance between an activated phone and an ICD should not be less than 6 inches (15 cm) and the patients should avoid carrying their activated cellular phone in a breast or shirt pocket overlying the implanted device. According to some reports, cellular phones do not interfere with the remote monitoring functions of recent ICDs and pacemakers.

Other *wireless communication devices* such as laptop computers in a wireless network, DECT (Digital Enhanced Cordless Telecommunications) phones and remote controls are usually no threat to ICDs in view of their low radiated power.

Antitheft devices (EAS, electronic article surveillance) and *security systems* (AMDG, airport metal detector gates) are widespread. Most pacemakers interact with high-energy pulsed low-frequency EAS systems such as acoustomagnetic systems. Asynchronous pacing, atrial as well as ventricular oversensing, pacemaker inhibition and pacemaker triggering have been reported. Yet, there are no reports in the real world of serious patient harm. Although EAS systems could trigger spurious ICD shocks in the older "Ventak AV" type, neither false arrhythmia detections nor shocks have been reported for recent state-of-the-art ICDs. Obviously, the pacing function may be disturbed depending upon the degree of exposure (time and distance).

Some patients walk briskly through a store entrance, whereas others amble slowly. The worst-case scenario deals with an occasional patient unwittingly leaning against one of the theft deterrent pylons or gates. Patients should be reminded not to linger near any equipment or areas that may involve electromagnetic emissions. In situations where the presence of EAS or AMDG equipment is not apparent to a lay observer, warning notices should be posted for device patients.

Slot machines represent another source of EMI. ICD patients receiving shocks while playing with slot machines have been observed. Although that report is not confirmed by others or by simulation, it is prudent to warn ICD patients of this potential interaction.

Stun guns (e.g. Taser) are electrical self-defense and immobilization weapons used by law enforcement agencies. These weapons shoot darts (i.e. electrodes) into the victim. The darts remain connected to the gun via insulated wires that conduct trains of 15 to 20 pulses per second. The pulses have a duration of 40–100 μs and a peak voltage of up to

50,000 V. An ICD patient immobilized in this way (because of uncontrolled violent behavior) almost always shows no immediate adverse effects.

Sources of EMI in the industrial environment.

Among the myriad potential sources of EMI, some industrial equipment raises concern (Fig. 11.10).
- high-voltage power lines
- industrial transformers and motors
- electric melting furnaces (induction)
- electric welding equipment (arc or spot welders)
- large RF transmitters (broadcasting, radar)
- degaussing coils

Some of these sources emit energy in the radiofrequency spectrum; others generate strong magnetic fields that could close the reed switch in ICDs.

ICD patients returning to work in an environment suspected of harboring high-level EMI represent a challenge. In general, true bipolar sensing leads are mandatory. On-site evaluation by a technical consultant from the device manufacturer is highly desirable (however, this service is seldom available due to liability concerns).

11.4.2 Possible responses to EMI

Exposure to EMI may have various consequences for a patient fitted with an ICD.
- *Pacing inhibition* is potentially catastrophic in patients dependent on their ICD for bradycardia pacing (e.g. after AV junction ablation to prevent spurious shocks for SVT). Because asynchronous pacing may not occur, due to lack of reliable noise reversion modes, prolonged inhibition remains a potential problem. Depending on the duration of the inhibition and the emergence of escape rhythms, lightheadedness, syncope or even death may result.
- *Triggering of rapid or premature pacing* from EMI oversensing by the atrial channel induces ventricular pacing at the upper tracking rate limit and/or causes unnecessary mode switching. EMI can also disturb the proper function of a nonatrial sensor for rate-adaptive pacing and increase the pacing rate up to the sensor-triggered upper rate limit.

- EMI may provoke *spurious tachyarrhythmia detection* with consequent inappropriate shocks (inhibition of shocks is also possible).
- *Power-on reset* elicited by EMI resets the DDD(R) mode to the VVI or VOO mode causing hypotension in patients susceptible to pacemaker syndrome. In the reset mode, devices function only with basic factory-preset instructions stored in the nonvolatile read-only memory (ROM). Electric reset in ICDs generally results in a "shock-box" configuration with maximum energy shocks for rates above a fixed maximum (145–170 b.p.m.) and backup pacing in the VVI mode at a fixed base rate (60 p.p.m.). The power-on reset mode does not revert back when the EMI ceases but it does not represent device malfunction. The solution requires a specific programmer command to restore the proper indices. In some devices, the pacing mode and rate during power-on reset resemble the ERI point. Telemetry of battery voltage and impedance can differentiate electric reset from battery depletion. An electric reset due to EMI should display a normal battery voltage.
- Strong magnetic fields may induce *closure of the reed switch* (e.g. large stereo speakers, decorative neodymium magnets, industrial transformers, etc.). A closed reed switch causes temporary suspension of tachyarrhythmia detection and therapy. Normal function returns upon removal of the magnetic field. Older ICD models from CPI (Guidant–Boston Scientific) were deactivated by continuous application of a strong magnet of more than 10 gauss for more than 30 s. Reactivation required a programmer command or the application of a magnet for more than 30 s. In newer devices, magnet application is used to trigger specific behavior (EGM storage, event markers, replay of alert tones).
- *Damage to the generator* is rare. In the majority of cases, the effects of EMI are temporary and disappear when the device moves out of range from the EMI source. Very strong EMI (external defibrillation, electrosurgery, etc.) can cause permanent damage such as output failure, pacemaker runaway, etc. Physical damage to some electronic components also occurs under the influence of ionizing radiation and strong acoustic waves.

12 Cardiac resynchronization

12.1 Indications

Cardiac resynchronization therapy (CRT) with biventricular pacing (RV and LV) is now established therapy for patients with dilated cardiomyopathy (severe systolic LV dysfunction on the basis of ischemic or nonischemic etiology) and congestive heart failure (with New York Heart Association [NYHA] class III or IV symptoms) associated with major left-sided intraventricular conduction delay such as left bundle branch block (see appendix). Many CRT patients (almost all in the United States) also receive an ICD (ICD-CRT) device. The European guidelines (2007) recommend that the use of CRT without an ICD should be based on:

1. the patient's expectation of survival of less than 1 year;
2. health-care logistical constraints and cost considerations.

The intraventricular conduction disorder causes an inefficient or uncoordinated pattern of LV activation resulting in mechanical LV dyssynchrony with segments contracting at different times. LV dyssynchrony typically arises from electrical delay translated into mechanical delay between the septal and lateral walls.

Enrollment in most of the major trials included: congestive heart failure (CHF) in NYHA III or IV functional class despite optimal pharmacologic therapy; LV ejection fraction (LVEF) < 35%, LV end-diastolic diameter > 55 mm, and QRS duration > 120 or 150 ms. Currently, patients are selected mainly on electrocardiographic criteria. However, the severity of mechanical systolic dyssynchrony is a much better predictor of a CRT response after CRT. Echocardiography has provided direct evidence of wall motion resynchronization in patients receiving CRT. Although many workers have searched for the best echocardiographic index to identify LV dyssynchrony so as to predict responders to CRT before the device implantation, this issue is still debatable. For this reason the US and European guidelines for CRT do not require echocardiographic proof of mechanical LV dyssynchrony.

The US guidelines for biventricular pacing include medically refractory symptomatic NYHA class III or IV patients with idiopathic dilated or ischemic cardiomyopathy, QRS ≥ 130 ms, LV end-diastolic diameter > 55 mm and LVEF < 35%. The European guidelines are similar except for a QRS ≥ 120 ms and evidence of LV dilatation. As far as the US guidelines are concerned, it is reasonable to consider patients with a QRS complex of 120 ms because many of the trials have shown benefit in this group of patients.

12.2 CRT in patients with a narrow QRS complex

Small noncontrolled studies have demonstrated that heart failure patients with a narrow QRS (< 0.12 s) may benefit from CRT. Despite the growing body of evidence suggesting that echocardiographic criteria may be a better method to evaluate mechanical LV dyssynchrony so as to predict benefit from CRT, such therapy remains controversial in the absence of randomized trials in the setting of a narrow QRS complex.

12.3 Impact of CRT

The improved sequence of electrical activation with CRT, which has no positive inotropic effect as such, improves cardiac efficiency by restoring the near-normal LV contraction pattern. This translates into beneficial acute and long-term hemodynamic effects by virtue of more coordinated and efficient LV contraction and function. Long-term hemodynamic improvement by reverse LV remodeling causes an increase in LVEF (usually up to 6% in randomized trials) and a decrease in LV systolic and diastolic volumes. These changes occur progressively and may take 3 to 6 months or longer (> 1 year) to become established. Cardiac resynchronization therapy also reduces functional mitral regurgitation both acutely and on a long-term basis by superimposed LV reverse remodeling. Cardiac output increases whereas ventricular filling pressure decreases without increasing myocardial oxygen consumption. Cardiac resynchronization therapy improves NYHA functional class (0.5–0.8 in randomized trials), exercise tolerance (20% mean increase in distance walked in 6 min in randomized trials), quality of life and morbidity. Long-term reverse remodeling of the failing LV results in reductions in CHF hospitalizations and mortality independent of defibrillator therapy when combined with optimal pharmacotherapy. There is also a reduction of sympathetic/parasympathetic imbalance, attenuating the chronic sympathetic activation of heart failure and of neurohumoral activation due to increased systolic blood pressure and improved LV filling time. The benefits of CRT are similar in magnitude to those of angiotensin-converting enzyme (ACE) inhibitors and beta-blockers, and are superimposed on the benefits of medical therapy.

12.4 Percentage of biventricular pacing

It is necessary to ensure that biventricular pacing takes place 100% of the time. The percentage of biventricular pacing and ventricular sensing must be carefully checked in the stored memorized data retrieved from the device. Remote home monitoring is particularly helpful for this assessment. Devices must be programmed carefully to prevent "electrical" desynchronization. Troubleshooting loss of resynchronization may be difficult and requires a thorough knowledge of biventricular pacemaker function, timing cycles and complex algorithms.

12.5 Failure of CRT benefit

The transvenous implantation success rate is about 90–95%, but about 30% of patients do not respond to CRT. A number of factors may be responsible for this failure. The two major causes are placement of the LV lead at a suboptimal location and the limitation of ECG-based patient selection criteria. In about one-third of heart failure patients with left bundle branch block or intraventricular conduction delay, ECG patterns are not associated with significant LV mechanical dyssynchrony. This observation correlates with the incidence of the nonresponder rate in clinical trials of CRT. Because retiming to recoordinate LV contraction is the primary goal of CRT, it is therefore unlikely that CRT will benefit patients with wide QRS complexes in the absence of mechanical dyssynchrony. Echocardiography with tissue Doppler imaging (TDI) can detect the direction and velocity of the contracting or relaxing myocardium (Fig. 12.02). Tissue Doppler imaging is a reproducible technique

to detect regional myocardial function and timing of events by measuring the time to peak systolic velocity during the ejection phase in several myocardial segments. It is emerging as a useful tool to improve the selection of patients for CRT.

12.6 What is a CRT responder?

There is no standardized definition of when a patient should be considered a nonresponder. Neither is there a consensus on whether indices of LV reverse remodeling or clinical status should be used as endpoints for assessing response to CRT. This is compounded by the observations that CRT recipients may have clinical improvement without echocardiographic improvement and vice versa. Improvement in NYHA functional class or increased distance walked in 6 min or improved heart failure-related quality of life is considered by some workers as an adequate response, but these parameters may be influenced by spontaneous changes and/or a placebo effect. Others would consider an adequate response in terms of changes in oxygen uptake at anaerobic threshold during exercise or reduction of LV systolic and diastolic volumes along with improvement in NYHA functional class. The LVEF and LV end-systolic volume (LVESV) are commonly used parameters of LV reverse remodeling in assessing improvement in systolic function. A change in LVESV (reduction of LVESV > 15%) after 3–6 months is the single best predictor of a good prognosis, lower long-term mortality and reduced incidence of heart failure events, and theoretically is less subject to the placebo effect. Some patients who have no or minimal acute changes in any assessment modality may show gradual or delayed improvement after a few months. As a rule patients without reverse remodeling are more symptomatic.

12.7 Complications of CRT implantation

Left ventricular lead dislodgment

The dislodgment rate for LV leads is higher (2–5%) than that for atrial or RV leads, and dislodgment tends to occur soon after implantation.

Infection

The incidence of infection with a primary implantation should be 0.5–1% but a long procedure increases the risk.

Coronary sinus dissection and perforation

Coronary sinus (CS) dissection may be caused by too vigorous advancement of the guiding catheter or by injection of the contrast medium through an angiographic catheter with its tip pressed against the vessel wall. The incidence of coronary sinus dissection is 2–5%. However, CS dissection usually heals well and CS perforation is rare. Some workers believe that lead manipulation and placement should be abandoned if the dissection is distal in the coronary sinus. Implantation of the LV lead can then be performed several weeks later. A lead can usually be passed through a proximal coronary sinus dissection by finding the true lumen of the coronary sinus for satisfactory passage of the LV lead. With a dissection, an echocardiogram should be performed to rule out a pericardial effusion.

Phrenic nerve stimulation and diaphragmatic pacing

Phrenic nerve stimulation is a common problem and can be difficult to demonstrate during implantation in the sedated and supine patient. It may become evident only when the patient becomes active and changes body positions (Fig. 12.04). This complication is related to the anatomic vicinity of the left phrenic nerve to the LV pacing site, especially when the LV lead is implanted into a posterior or posterolateral coronary vein. It may also be related to LV lead dislodgment. Occasionally after implantation, phrenic nerve stimulation can be controlled by lowering the LV voltage (maintaining capture) provided the capture threshold for phrenic nerve stimulation is much higher than that of LV capture. Special programmable options and leads allow programming of lead function in terms of true bipolar LV pacing as well as using the RV ring as an anode and the LV tip or ring as the cathode. These manipulations alter the LV–RV pacing vector noninvasively (electronic repositioning). This function enables more flexibility to overcome problems with high LV pacing thresholds and phrenic nerve stimulation.

12.8 Programming of CRT devices

Many of the CRT failures in randomized trials (about 20–30%) can be attributed to improper patient selection, suboptimal LV lead placement, inadequate medical therapy and device programming. As CHF patients represent a heterogeneous group, the best performance of CRT can be achieved by optimal programming of the device for each individual. Figure 12.20 outlines the basic approach to programming CRT devices. The details are discussed later in the text.

12.9 ECG patterns recorded during LV pacing from the coronary venous system

A right bundle branch block (RBBB) pattern in correctly positioned lead V_1 occurs when the stimulation site is in the posterior or posterolateral coronary vein (the traditional sites for resynchronization). Leads V_2 and V_3 may or may not be positive. With apical sites, leads V_4–V_6 are typically negative. With basal locations leads V_4–V_6 are usually positive as with the concordant positive R-waves during overt preexcitation in left-sided accessory pathway conduction in the Wolff–Parkinson–White syndrome. Pacing from the depth of the middle cardiac vein or the great (anterior) vein, which are unsatisfactory sites for LV pacing, produces a LBBB pattern of depolarization.

Thus, when lead V_1 shows a negative QRS complex during LV pacing, consideration should be given to incorrect ECG lead placement (lead V_1), location in the middle or great (anterior) cardiac vein, or an undefined mechanism involving severe intramyocardial conduction abnormality. The frontal plane axis during LV pacing at the best site often points to the right inferior quadrant (right axis deviation) and less commonly to the right superior quadrant. In an occasional patient with uncomplicated LV pacing with a typical RBBB pattern in lead V_1, the axis may point to the left inferior or left superior quadrant. The reasons for these unusual axis locations are unclear.

12.10 ECG patterns and follow-up of CRT

Loss of capture in one ventricle will cause a change in the morphology of ventricular paced beats in the 12-lead ECG similar to that of either single-chamber RV pacing or single-chamber LV pacing. A shift in the frontal plane axis may be useful to corroborate loss of capture in one of the ventricles (Fig. 12.06). If both the native QRS complex and the biventricular paced complex are relatively narrow, then a widening of the paced QRS complex will identify loss of capture in one chamber with effectual capture in the other.

Paced QRS duration and status of mechanical ventricular resynchronization

The paced QRS during biventricular pacing is often narrower than that of monochamber RV or LV pacing. Thus, measurement of QRS duration during follow-up is helpful in the analysis of appropriate biventricular capture and fusion with the spontaneous QRS. If the biventricular ECG is virtually similar to that recorded with RV or LV pacing alone and no cause is found, it should not be concluded, without a detailed evaluation of the pacing system, that one of the leads does not contribute to biventricular depolarization. Chronic studies have shown that the degree of narrowing of the paced QRS duration is a poor predictor of the mechanical cardiac resynchronization response. In this respect some patients with monochamber LV pacing exhibit an equal or superior degree of mechanical resynchronization compared with biventricular pacing despite a very wide paced QRS complex.

Biventricular pacing with the RV lead located at the apex

The frontal plane QRS axis usually moves superiorly from the left (RV apical pacing) to the right superior quadrant (biventricular pacing) in an anticlockwise fashion if the ventricular mass is predominantly depolarized by the LV pacing lead. The frontal plane axis may occasionally reside in the left superior rather than the right superior quadrant during uncomplicated biventricular pacing (Fig. 12.08).

The QRS is often positive in lead V_1 during biventricular pacing when the RV is paced from the apex. A negative QRS complex in lead V_1 may occur under the following circumstances:

- incorrect placement of lead V_1 (too high on the chest);
- lack of LV capture;
- LV lead displacement or marked latency (exit block or delay from the LV stimulation site);
- ventricular fusion with the conducted QRS complex;
- coronary venous pacing via the middle cardiac vein (also the anterior cardiac vein);
- unintended placement of two leads in the RV.

A negative QRS complex in lead V_1 during uncomplicated biventricular pacing probably reflects different activation of a heterogeneous biventricular substrate (ischemia, scar, His–Purkinje participation in view of the varying patterns of LV activation in spontaneous LBBB, etc.) and does not necessarily indicate a poor (electrical or mechanical) contribution from LV stimulation.

Biventricular pacing with the RV lead in the outflow tract

During biventricular pacing with the RV lead in the outflow tract, the paced QRS in lead V_1 is often negative and the frontal plane paced QRS axis is often directed to the right inferior quadrant (right axis deviation) (Fig. 12.09).

Ventricular fusion beats with native conduction

In patients with sinus rhythm and a relatively short PR interval, ventricular fusion with competing native conduction during biventricular pacing may cause misinterpretation of the ECG – a common pitfall in device follow-up (Fig. 12.11). Marked QRS shortening mandates exclusion of ventricular fusion with the spontaneous QRS complex especially in the setting of a relatively short PR interval. The presence of ventricular fusion should be ruled out by observing the paced QRS morphology during progressive shortening of the AS–VP (atrial sensing–ventricular pacing) interval in the VDD mode or the AP–VP (atrial pacing–ventricular pacing) interval in the DDD mode.

Long-term ECG changes

Many studies have shown that the paced QRS duration does not vary over time as long as the LV pacing lead does not move from its initial site. Yet, surface ECGs should be performed periodically because the LV lead may become displaced into a collateral branch of the coronary sinus. Dislodgment of the LV lead may result in loss of LV capture with the ECG showing an RV pacing QRS pattern with an increased QRS duration and superior axis deviation.

12.11 Anodal stimulation in biventricular pacemakers

Although anodal capture may occur with high-output traditional bipolar RV pacing, this phenomenon is almost always not discernible electrocardiographically. Biventricular pacing systems may utilize a unipolar lead for LV pacing via a coronary vein. The tip electrode of the LV lead is the cathode and the proximal electrode of the bipolar RV lead often provides the anode for LV pacing. This arrangement creates a common anode for RV and LV pacing. A high current density (from two sources) at the common anode during biventricular pacing may cause anodal capture manifested as a paced QRS complex with a somewhat different configuration from that derived from pure biventricular pacing (Fig. 12.13). Anodal capture during biventricular pacing disappears by reducing the LV output of the pacemaker or when the device (even at high output) is programmed to a true unipolar system with the common anode on the pacemaker can, a function that is available only in devices without an ICD.

Anodal capture was recognized in first-generation transvenous biventricular pacemakers (without separately programmable RV and LV outputs) when three distinct pacing morphologies were observed exclusive of fusion with the spontaneous QRS complex:

- biventricular with anodal capture (at a high output);
- biventricular (at a lower output);
- RV (with loss of LV capture) or rarely LV (with loss of RV capture) (Fig. 12.14).

This form of anodal stimulation may also occur during biventricular pacing with contemporary devices only if there is a common anode on the RV lead.

A different form of anodal capture involving the ring electrode of the bipolar RV lead can also occur with contemporary biventricular pacemakers with *separately programmable ventricular outputs*. During monochamber LV pacing at a relatively high output, RV anodal capture produces a paced QRS complex identical to that registered with biventricular pacing. Occasionally this type of anodal capture prevents electrocardiographic documentation of pure LV pacing if the LV pacing threshold is higher than that of RV anodal stimulation. Such anodal stimulation may complicate threshold testing and should not be misinterpreted as pacemaker malfunction. Furthermore, if the LV threshold is not too high, appropriate programming of the pacemaker output should eliminate anodal stimulation in most cases. The use of true bipolar LV leads eliminates all forms of anodal stimulation.

12.12 ECG of biventricular pacemakers with varying VV intervals

Contemporary biventricular devices permit programming of the interventricular interval usually in steps from + 80 ms (LV first) to − 80 ms (RV first) to optimize LV hemodynamics. In the absence of anodal stimulation, increasing the VV interval gradually to 80 ms (LV first) will progressively increase the duration of the paced QRS complex, and alter its morphology with a larger R-wave in lead V_1 indicating more dominant LV depolarization. The varying QRS configuration in lead V_1 with different VV intervals cannot be correlated with the hemodynamic response.

Right ventricular anodal stimulation during biventricular pacing (Fig. 12.12) interferes with a programmed interventricular (VV) delay (often programmed with the LV preceding the RV) aimed at optimizing cardiac resynchronization, because RV anodal capture causes simultaneous RV and LV activation (the VV interval becomes zero). In the presence of anodal stimulation, the ECG morphology and its duration will not change if the device is programmed with VV intervals of 80, 60 and 40 ms (LV before RV). The delayed RV cathodal output (80, 60, 40 ms) then falls in the myocardial refractory period initiated by the preceding anodal stimulation. At VV intervals ≤ 20 ms, the paced QRS may change because the short LV–RV interval prevents propagation of activation from the site of RV anodal capture in time to render the cathodal site refractory. Thus, the cathode also captures the RV and contributes to RV depolarization, which then takes place from two sites, RV anode and RV cathode.

12.13 Upper rate response of biventricular pacemakers

The upper rate response of biventricular pacemakers exhibits two forms according to the location of the P-wave in the pacemaker cycle:

1. A pre-empted Wenckebach upper rate response with AS–VS (AS = atrial sensed event, VS = ventricular sensed event) sequences and the P-waves tracked beyond the postventricular atrial refractory period (PVARP).
2. AR–VS (AR = atrial event sensed in the pacemaker atrial refractory period) sequences containing the P-waves detected (but not tracked) within the PVARP.

Pre-empted Wenckebach upper rate response

In patients with a biventricular pacemaker, the Wenckebach upper rate response (or more precisely the manifestation of upper rate interval > total atrial refractory period) may not be immediately recognizable because no paced beats are evident. Patients undergoing CRT tend to have near-normal sinus node function and AV conduction.

In the setting of a relatively short PVARP, the Wenckebach upper rate response of a biventricular pacemaker creates a repetitive pre-empted process in the form of an attempted Wenckebach upper rate response with each cycle (Fig. 12.18). There is a partial or incomplete extension of the programmed AV (AS–VP) interval in each pacemaker cycle but the device cannot release VP because the conducted spontaneous QRS complex continually occurs before completion of the upper rate interval when VP is expected. The spontaneous QRS complex is therefore sensed by the pacemaker, and ventricular pacing is pre-empted. This form of upper rate response tends to occur in patients with relatively normal AV conduction, a short programmed AV delay, a relatively slow programmed (atrial-driven) upper rate, and a sinus rate faster than the programmed (atrial-driven) upper rate. It is therefore more likely to emerge on exercise or during times of distress when adrenergic tone is high. Because patients with CHF are susceptible to sinus tachycardia (especially during decompensation despite beta-blocker therapy), it is particularly important to program a relatively fast upper rate during biventricular pacing to avoid an upper rate response manifested by the emergence of the patient's spontaneous conducted QRS complex.

Upper rate limitation with P-wave in the PVARP: atrial refractory block

When the P–P interval < total atrial refractory period (TARP) during biventricular pacing (in the setting of relatively normal sinus node function and AV conduction), a 2:1 block response does not usually occur because every spontaneous P-wave falls in the PVARP (depicted in the marker channel as a atrial event sensed in the pacemaker refractory period) where they cannot be tracked (or initiate the programmed AS–VP interval). The conducted QRS complex (VS) linked to the preceding P-wave (in the PVARP) initiates a PVARP that will contain the succeeding P-wave. This sequence ensures the perpetuation of functional atrial undersensing. Thus, no P-wave can be tracked (Fig. 12.19). In this situation, the prevailing AV delay (or the spontaneous PR interval or AR–VS) is longer than the programmed AS–VP. There are no pauses, and no pacemaker stimuli are evident as in the pre-empted Wenckebach upper rate response.

12.14 Programming the upper rate

An inappropriately low-programmed upper rate is an important cause of ventricular desynchronization in heart failure (HF) patients, who often have normal sinus and AV nodal function. Loss of atrial tracking above the programmed upper rate causes loss of biventricular pacing (pre-excitation) and permits the emergence of the spontaneous QRS complex related to spontaneous AV conduction. Thus, a relatively low upper rate can deny HF patients the benefit of resynchronization at high sinus rates, which are not uncommon in this patient population during exercise or situations associated with increased circulating catecholamines (especially during decompensation despite beta-blocker therapy). In other words, one must avoid "breakthrough" ventricular sensing within a patient's exercise zone. An initial upper rate of 140 p.p.m. or faster is often appropriate. The risk of tracking rapid

atrial rates by a biventricular device (as occurs with antibradycardia pacemakers) is not an important issue in the presence of normal sinus and AV conduction. Relatively low upper rates must also be avoided even in patients with symptomatic angina because loss of resynchronization can itself precipitate cardiac ischemia by increasing maximum oxygen uptake (MVO$_2$).

The maximum spontaneous rate may be attenuated by larger doses of beta-blockers (often better tolerated with device therapy) or other drugs that depress sinus node function. In difficult or refractory cases, especially in patients with marked first-degree AV block, ablation of the AV junction should be considered to ensure continual ventricular depolarization by the implanted device.

Exit from upper rate response and delayed restoration of P-wave tracking

When the upper rate response pushes the P-wave into the PVARP with resultant loss of ventricular resynchronization, a biventricular pacemaker may not resume 1:1 atrial tracking when the sinus rate drops immediately below the programmed upper rate (Figs 12.15 and 12.16). The P-wave can remain locked in the PVARP (as an AR event) even when the P–P interval is longer than the upper rate interval dictated by the programmed TARP (AS–VP + PVARP). The explanation for this response lies in the fact that the prevailing TARP is longer than the programmed TARP, which is the sum of the programmed (AS–VP + PVARP). The AR–VS interval (spontaneous AV conduction or PR interval) is longer than the programmed AS–VP interval. Based on the different durations of the AV delay (AR–VS > AS–VP), the prevailing TARP during AR–VS operation [(AR–VS) interval + PVARP] must therefore be longer than the programmed TARP [(AS–VP) interval + PVARP]. As the atrial rate drops below the programmed upper rate, the pacemaker will continue to operate with "desynchronized" AR–VS cycles below the upper rate (dictated by the programmed TARP) until the P–P or sinus interval becomes longer than the sum of (AR–VS) interval + PVARP, thereby allowing escape of the trapped sinus P-wave out of the PVARP. Thus, restoration of resynchronization (AS–VP) will occur at a rate substantially slower than the programmed upper rate (dictated by the programmed TARP). These considerations are important in HF patients who may occasionally develop substantial increases in sinus rates despite beta-blocker therapy.

The postponed restoration of atrial tracking upon emergence from the upper rate is worse in patients with first-degree AV block.

Loss of resynchronization below the programmed upper rate: locking of P-waves inside the PVARP

Desynchronized AR–VS, AR–VS . . . sequences containing trapped or locked P-waves within the PVARP can also occur outside situations where a fast atrial rate (above the programmed upper rate) gradually drops below the programmed upper rate. There are many causes of electrical desynchronization capable of starting at rates slower than the programmed upper rate (Table 12.1). For example, during sinus rhythm and synchronized biventricular pacing (below the upper rate), a ventricular premature complex (or T-wave oversensing, which produces the same effect) by initiating a regular PVARP, shifts pacemaker timing so that the succeeding undisturbed sinus P-wave now falls in the PVARP. This P-wave inside the PVARP conducts to the ventricle producing a spontaneous QRS complex, which is sensed by the device. The sinus P-waves will remain trapped in the PVARP as long as the P–P interval is less than [(AR–VS) + PVARP]. In other words, biventricular pacing remains inhibited until either the occurrence of a nonrefractory sensed atrial depolarization or delivery of an atrial pacing pulse outside the TARP. Loss of atrial synchrony may extend over a period of time (e.g. seconds to hours) depending on the pacemaker's programmed rate settings and the sinus rate. Such forms of electrical desynchronization (AR–VS sequences) may be symptomatic and can be precipitated by a variety of mechanisms. Based on these considerations, the aim should be to program a short PVARP. The PVARP extension after a ventricular premature complex should be turned off as well as the pacemaker-mediated tachycardia termination algorithm based on PVARP prolongation for one cycle.

Similarly, an undersensed atrial event that conducts to the ventricle resulting in an R-wave can be interpreted as a "pacemaker-defined" premature ventricular complex (PVC). The sensed "PVC" generates a PVARP, which then contains the next atrial event (AR). This arrangement brings about a second

---

Table 12.1. Loss of cardiac resynchronization during DDD or DDDR pacing in the presence of preserved biventricular pacing

Intrinsic	1. Atrial undersensing from low-amplitude atrial potentials 2. T-wave oversensing and other types of ventricular oversensing such as diaphragmatic potentials 3. Long PR interval 4. Circumstances that push the P-wave into the PVARP such as a junctional or idioventricular rhythm 5. New arrhythmia such as atrial fibrillation with a fast ventricular rate 6. Short runs of unsustained, often relatively slow, ventricular tachycardia. Such arrhythmias are common and often asymptomatic 7. First-generation devices with a common sensing channel: ventricular double counting and sensing of far-field atrial activity

Extrinsic	1. Inappropriate programming of the AV delay or any function that prolongs the AV delay such as rate smoothing, AV search hysteresis, etc.
	2. Low maximum tracking rate
	3. Slowing of the atrial rate upon exit from upper rate behavior
	4. Functional atrial undersensing below the programmed upper rate:
	  A. Precipitated by an atrial premature beat or ventricular premature beat
	  B. Long PVARP including automatic PVARP extension after a premature ventricular complex and single beat PVARP extension related to algorithms for automatic termination of endless loop tachycardia
	5. Inappropriately slow programmed lower rate permitting junctional escape (cycle length < lower rate interval) in patients with periodic sinus arrest
	6. Intraatrial conduction delay where sensing of AS is delayed in the right atrial appendage. A short AS–VP interval may not be able to achieve biventricular pacing

AS = atrial sensed event; AV = atrioventricular; PVARP = postventricular atrial refractory period; VP = ventricular paced event.

conducted R-wave. The AR–VS pattern will continue if the patient's atrial rate is fast enough.

Automatic unlocking of P-waves from the PVARP

Special algorithms can be programmed to restore 1:1 atrial tracking at rates slower than the programmed upper rate. The algorithms automatically identify an AR–VS pattern of cardiac activity and activate PVARP shortening. These algorithms do not function when the atrial rate is faster than the programmed upper rate or during automatic mode switching. This function promotes 1:1 atrial tracking whenever the "effective or prevailing TARP" [(AR–VS) + PVARP] prevents atrial tracking at rates below the programmed upper rate. A device can detect AR–VS, AR–VS . . . sequences suggestive of ventricular desynchronization whereupon temporary PVARP abbreviation permits the device to sense a sinus P-wave beyond the PVARP and restore atrial tracking and ventricular resynchronization. In other words, the algorithm shortens the TARP. A P-wave falling in the postventricular atrial blanking period (for pacing) cannot activate the special algorithm.

These algorithms are particularly useful in patients with sinus tachycardia and first-degree AV block, in whom prolonged locking of P-waves inside the PVARP is an important problem.

12.15 Atrial fibrillation

Some devices have programmable algorithms that increase the percentage of biventricular pacing during atrial fibrillation so as to promote some degree of rate regularization (without an overall increase in the ventricular rate) by dynamic matching with the patient's own ventricular responses (up to the programmed maximum tracking rate). Activation of this algorithm does not result in control of the ventricular rate, and should not be a substitute for ablation of the AV junction in patients with drug-refractory rapid ventricular rates. In the absence of AV junction ablation if the ventricular rate is controlled pharmacologically, it is important not to overestimate the percentage of biventricular pacing because a device logs fusion and pseudo-fusion beats as ventricular paced beats.

12.16 Ventricular-triggered mode

The ventricular-triggered mode in some resynchronization devices automatically attempts to provide resynchronization in the presence of ventricular

sensing. A ventricular-sensed event initiates an immediate emission of a ventricular or usually a biventricular output (according to the programmed settings) in conformity with the programmed upper rate interval. For example, Medtronic devices offer this function in the VVIR mode, but in dual-chamber devices triggering occurs upon sensing only within the programmed AV delay. The ventricular output will be ineffectual in the chamber where sensing was initiated because the myocardium is physiologically refractory. The stimulus to the other ventricle thus attempts to capture and provide a measure of resynchronization. Ventricular triggering may be helpful in some patients but its true benefit is difficult to assess as the ventricles may be activated in an order that may not be hemodynamically favorable.

12.17 Programming the optimal AV delay

The atrioventricular (AV) interval during AV sequential pacing influences LV systolic performance by modulating preload. The majority of the acute and long-term benefit from CRT is independent of the programmed AV interval. The influence of the AV delay appears to be less important than the proper choice of LV pacing site. Nevertheless, programming of the left-sided AV delay is important in CRT patients. AV timing can, if appropriate, maximize the benefit of CRT, but if programmed poorly it has the potential to curtail the beneficial effects. Optimization will not convert a non-responder to a responder, but may convert an under-responder to improved status.

The optimal AV delay in CRT patients exhibits great variability from patient to patient. This suggests that an empirically programmed AV delay interval is suboptimal in many patients. Thus, empiric programming of the AV delay is generally not recommended.

The aim should always be for atrial sensing, which is, as a rule, hemodynamically more favorable than atrial pacing. Thus, the lower rate is often programmed to a relatively slow value. In the occasional patient with an accelerated idioventricular or junctional rhythm inhibiting ventricular pacing and CRT, the lower rate should be increased to suppress the interfering rhythm.

Optimized AV synchrony is achieved by the AV delay setting that provides the best left atrial contribution to LV filling, the maximum stroke volume, shortening of the isovolemic contraction time, and the longest diastolic filling time in the absence of diastolic mitral regurgitation (in patients with a long PR interval). In clinical practice there are many techniques for optimizing the AV delay in CRT patients as well as great variability in their use. The techniques include invasive (LV or aortic dP/dt max) and noninvasive techniques (largely echocardiography). AV interval optimization in DDD(R) pacemakers has traditionally been achieved using noninvasive Doppler echocardiography, which still remains widely used in CRT patients for acute and long-term hemodynamic assessment (Figs 12.21 and 12.22). However, Doppler echocardiographic methods for AV optimization in CRT patients vary substantially in performance. They include analysis of mitral, LV outflow tract and aortic blood-flow velocity profiles using conventional pulsed and continuous-wave Doppler techniques and determination of dP/dt as derived from the continuous-wave Doppler profile of mitral regurgitation. Apart from echocardiography, other techniques include radionuclide angiography, impedance cardiography, plethysmography and data from a peak endocardial acceleration sensor incorporated into a pacing lead. Echocardiographic techniques for AV (and VV) optimization require experienced personnel, and are time-consuming. Furthermore, CRT optimization by echocardiography is sensitive to intra- and inter-observer variability. The best method of measuring or assessing the effects of AV interval programming in terms of accuracy, cost, rapidity, ease and perhaps full automaticity remains to be defined, but a recently developed semiautomatic method holds great promise (discussed later).

Consideration should be given to promoting fusion of LV pacing with right bundle branch activation (short AV delay) on a trial basis if the absence of fusion yields a suboptimal CRT response.

12.18 Intraatrial and interatrial conduction delay

Some patients have intraatrial conduction delay so that the atrial channel senses the atrial EGM from the atrial appendage late and during the isoelectric portion of the PR interval. The AS–VS interval (as seen by the device) during spontaneous AV conduction becomes quite short and can measure only 50–60 ms. Such patients may not tolerate an AS–VP interval of 40 ms or less to produce biventricular pacing, which in all likelihood might be associated with some degree of fusion with the spontaneous conducted QRS complex. This situation calls for one of two options:

1. Using the ventricular-triggered mode upon sensing the QRS complex after the sensed P-wave. A trial of the triggered mode might produce the desired clinical improvement.

2. Ablation of the AV junction with subsequent optimization of the AV delay.

12.19 Programming the interventricular (VV) interval

The usefulness of programming the VV interval is controversial in view of two recent trials showing no benefit. Nevertheless it may prove beneficial in patients with a suboptimal CRT response or HF. Programming the VV interval is guided by the same techniques as AV delay optimization. Determination of the extent of residual LV dyssynchrony after VV programming requires more sophisticated echocardiographic techniques. The benefit of VV programming is additive to AV delay optimization. Contemporary biventricular ICD devices permit programming of the VV interval usually in steps from +80 ms (LV first) to −80 ms (RV first) to optimize LV hemodynamics. This design is based on mounting evidence that simultaneous activation of the two ventricles for CRT is illogical and that the best mechanical efficiency may be achieved by sequential rather than simultaneous pacing of the two ventricles. Interventricular interval programmability may partially compensate for a less than optimal LV lead position by tailoring ventricular timing and may also correct for individual heterogeneous ventricular activation patterns commonly found in patients with LV dysfunction and HF.

Interventricular interval programmability has shown a heterogeneous response with great variability of the optimal VV delay from patient to patient. The optimal VV delay cannot be identified clinically in the majority of patients. Consequently adjustment of the VV delay, like the AV delay, must be individualized. Although VV programmability produces a rather limited improvement in LV function or stroke volume, the response is important in patients with a less than desirable response to CRT. The optimal VV delay should decrease LV dyssynchrony and provide a more homogeneous LV activation with faster LV emptying and improved and longer diastolic filling. Interventricular interval programmability may increase LV ejection fraction and other indices of LV function, and may also reduce mitral regurgitation in some patients, but overall improvement is only moderate.

The range of optimal VV delay is relatively narrow and most commonly involves LV pre-excitation by 20 ms. LV pre-excitation is required in most patients.

Right ventricular pre-excitation should be used cautiously because advancing RV activation may cause a decline of LV function. Consequently

RV pre-excitation should be reserved for patients with LV dyssynchrony in the septal and inferior segments provided there is hemodynamic proof of benefit. Patients with ischemic cardiomyopathy (with slower conducting scars) may require more pre-excitation than those with idiopathic dilated cardiomyopathy. Interventricular interval programming is of particular benefit in patients with a previous myocardial infarction.

12.20 Semiautomatic optimization of AV and VV intervals

QuickOpt Timing Cycle Optimization (St. Jude Medical) runs an automatic sequence of intracardiac EGM measurements, and displays on the programmer the optimal AV and VV intervals in 90 s. The system uses an exclusive algorithm to calculate the optimal timing values (Figs 12.23 and 12.24). These values are then programmed manually into the CRT device. QuickOpt optimization was found to be consistently comparable with a traditional echocardiographic procedure for determining optimal AV and VV delays. Most patients do not undergo AV and VV optimization by traditional methods because echocardiographic optimization typically takes much longer and is expensive. QuickOpt optimization, which allows efficient and frequent optimization of AV and VV intervals, can even be used when the device is being programmed before leaving the surgical suite.

Another system (SmartAVDelay™), recently introduced by Boston Scientific (Guidant), also permits rapid programmer-based determination of the AV delay. The algorithm also uses a formula based on intracardiac electrograms that accurately predicts the AV delay associated with the maximum LV dP/dt. The device measures the sensed and paced AV delays (AS-VS and AP-VS). It also measures the interventricular conduction interval between the RV and LV electrograms in the case of a bipolar LV lead whereupon the system provides the optimal AV delay automatically. The duration of the surface QRS complex is used in the semi-automatic function if the LV lead is unipolar. A further programming adjustment is required if the LV lead is not in the correct site. This system does not evaluate the V-V delay which has to be programmed before determining the optimal AV delay. The sensed and paced AV delays are individually determined in contrast to the St Jude system that calculates the paced AV delay by adding 50 ms to the optimal sensed AV delay.

Most CRT patients do not undergo AV and V-V optimization by traditional methods because echocardiographic optimization typically takes a long time and is expensive. These new systems based on intracardiac electrograms allow efficient and frequent optimization of AV and V-V interval can even be used when the device is being programmed before leaving the surgical suite. Although preliminary data are encouraging further study of these automatic or semi-automatic AV optimization based on intracardiac electrograms is needed.

12.21 Congestive heart failure after CRT

Reduction of diuretics is important after CRT in patients with near-optimal LV filling pressures and an adequate diuresis to prevent prerenal azotemia, which may mask or delay the benefit of CRT. The dose of beta-blockers can be increased after CRT; moreover, these agents may be successful in patients with previous intolerance. Cardiac resynchronization therapy cannot substitute for medical management. The combination of device therapy and optimal medical therapy provides synergistic effects to enhance reverse LV remodeling, and long-term survival (Fig. 12.05).

1. A CRT nonresponder should initially be evaluated for the development of atrial fibrillation, or of cardiac ischemia with a view to revascularization. Rate control, including AV node ablation or electrical cardioversion to restore normal sinus rhythm, is essential in patients who develop atrial fibrillation.
2. Evaluate LV lead for loss of capture.
3. Optimization of AV and VV intervals may provide some improvement within a short period of time.
4. Echocardiographic evaluation of LV dyssynchrony: if significant intraventricular dyssynchrony is still present, then lead repositioning should be considered using epicardial placement if necessary.
5. Persistence of symptoms despite correction of LV dyssynchrony requires evaluation for severe mitral regurgitation. Mitral valve surgery offers symptomatic improvement to patients, even ones with poor LV function, and should be considered in selected patients with persistent significant mitral regurgitation.

12.21.1 Device monitoring of heart failure

Various measurements by an ICD can be very useful in the management of HF patients. It is believed that early diagnosis and treatment of impending HF may retard progression of LV dysfunction and reduce mortality. Hence the importance of periodic remote monitoring. In this respect, it is interesting that patients may experience rather subtle symptoms 7–21 days before the clinical development of HF. During this period, remote monitoring a number of parameters permits early diagnosis before clinical manifestations. One manufacturer provides the capability for remote transmission of blood pressure and weight.

Intrathoracic impedance

Fluids conduct electricity more easily than solids. Fluid accumulation in the lungs leads to decreased intrathoracic impedance and increased conductivity (Fig. 12.25). A Medtronic device can track thoracic fluid status by the emission of low-amplitude electrical pulses to measure transthoracic impedance between the coil of the RV lead and the can of a CRT device or ICD (OptiVol). This measurement is made multiple times each day. The OptiVol fluid status monitoring system collects impedance signals between 12.00 am and 6.00 am, as this time period was shown earlier to best reflect fluid accumulation. Measures of LV end-diastolic pressure correlate inversely with impedance values. This impedance level is averaged once per day to create a reference range, known as the OptiVol Fluid Index which is a surrogate of impedance. The OptiVol Fluid Index represents the accumulation of consecutive day-to-day differences between the daily and reference impedance. The physician can select a threshold for notification of decreased impedance for each patient based on stored values. The fluid index rises as the impedance level drops from increased fluid in the lungs. An audible alert is available when the OptiVol Fluid Index reaches a certain threshold. Abnormal values can occur 2 weeks before clinical deterioration. The cause of the abnormal findings must be investigated as it may be due to recent-onset atrial fibrillation. Remote monitoring with the OptiVol feature can result in early treatment during the preclinical stage of heart failure decompensation and a consequent significant reduction in hospital admissions for HF. The ICD provides a Heart Failure Management Report with 14-month trends of AT/AF burden, ventricular rate during AF, heart rate variability, patient activity and night/day heart rates.

Heart rate variability

Heart rate varies from heartbeat to heartbeat. Heart rate variability (HRV) is the beat-to-beat variation in heart rate (between successive heartbeats, i.e. R–R intervals), and provides an indirect indicator of autonomic status and neurohormonal activation,

an important pathophysiologic factor in a number of cardiovascular disease states and HF. Heart rate variation of a well-conditioned heart is generally large at rest. During exercise, HRV decreases as the heart rate and exercise intensity increase. A reduction in HRV is a marker for reduced vagal activity. A reduction in HRV implies enhanced sympathetic activity. HRV is lower in patients with high mortality and hospitalization risk. Heart rate variability software is incorporated into many of the newer CRT devices, which can record daily measures of HRV. With a dual-chamber device HRV is calculated from atrial-sensed activity, whereas in a single-chamber ICD HRV is calculated from the RR intervals. As the neurohormonal system responds to detected changes in LV function before the patient experiences symptoms, HRV data may be useful for predicting a worsening condition and possibly preventing a hospital admission. Device-measured HRV parameters and patient outcomes improve significantly after CRT. Lack of HRV improvement 4 weeks after CRT identifies patients at higher risk for major cardiovascular events. One must remember that new AF can also cause abnormal HRV. At this time, HRV is not much used in the real world.

Activity

An activity sensor (piezoelectric or accelerometer) detects body movement and reflects the patient's daily physical activity. The data can be registered even if the rate-adaptive pacing mode is not programmed. The accuracy of using activity data to predict heart failure is dependent on the patient, and partly on the type of activities. The level of activity may not decrease early enough before the onset of decompensation, especially in patients with severe heart failure who are mostly sedentary. In CRT patients, an increase in recorded activity represents a good symptomatic response and CRT efficiency associated with a parallel improvement in the quality-of-life and NYHA class. Activity data may be important when deciding whether a patient can go back to work.

Nocturnal heart rate

Nocturnal heart rate is important in patients with CHF. An increase in nocturnal heart rate may be a sign of impending decompensation. If the sinus rate is higher than expected (e.g. 90 b.p.m.), a CHF patient requires more beta-blocker therapy. Nocturnal rate monitoring may also pick up unsuspected episodes of atrial fibrillation.

12.21.2 Special testing for CRT patients

Special testing for CRT patients includes assessment of percentage ventricular sensing; optimization of AV and VV intervals; evaluation of intrathoracic impedance data about pulmonary fluid status; and exercise testing in selected patients to look for abnormalities such as atrial undersensing or threshold problems not apparent at rest.

12.22 Ventricular proarrhythmia after CRT

Ventricular proarrhythmia after CRT may present either as sustained monomorphic VT or polymorphic VT (torsades de pointes, TdP) precipitated mainly by epicardial (in the coronary venous system) LV and to a lesser degree biventricular pacing. Ventricular tachycardia induced by LV pacing alone can be eliminated by turning off LV pacing, and some cases of LV-induced VT may sometimes be suppressed during biventricular pacing. In some patients, the induction of monomorphic VT by LV or biventricular pacing represents an exacerbation of a previously controlled arrhythmia, but in others it appears de novo. In contrast TdPs (polymorphic VT) are caused by a different mechanism related to amplified transmural dispersion of repolarization associated with QT prolongation. This is due to enhanced transmural dispersion of repolarization (as in the long QT syndrome) induced by LV epicardial pacing.

13 APPENDIX A

American College of Cardiology/American Heart Association/European Society of Cardiology

2006 Guidelines for the Management of Patients with Ventricular Arrhythmias and the Prevention of Sudden Death

13.1 Definitions

13.1.1 Levels of evidence

- *Level of evidence A:* Data derived from multiple randomized clinical trials or meta-analyses.
- *Level of evidence B:* Data derived from a single randomized trial, or nonrandomized studies.
- *Level of evidence C:* Only consensus opinion of experts, case studies, or standard of care.

13.1.2 Classification of recommendations

- Class I: Conditions for which there is evidence and/or general agreement that a given procedure/treatment is beneficial, useful and effective.
- Class II: Conditions for which there is conflicting evidence and/or a divergence of opinion about the usefulness/efficacy of a procedure or treatment.
  - Class IIa: Weight of evidence/opinion is in favor of usefulness/efficacy.
  - Class IIb: Usefulness/efficacy is less well established by evidence/opinion.
- Class III: Conditions for which there is evidence and/or general agreement that a procedure/treatment is not useful or effective and in some cases may be harmful.

13.2 Ventricular arrhythmia and sudden cardiac death related to specific pathology

13.2.1 Left ventricular dysfunction due to prior myocardial infarction

Class I

1. Aggressive attempts should be made to treat heart failure (HF) that may be present in some patients with LV dysfunction due to prior myocardial infarction (MI) and ventricular tachyarrhythmias. (*Level of evidence: C*)
2. Aggressive attempts should be made to treat myocardial ischemia that may be present in some patients with ventricular tachyarrhythmias. (*Level of evidence: C*)
3. Coronary revascularization is indicated to reduce the risk of sudden cardiac death (SCD) in patients with VF when direct, clear evidence of acute myocardial ischemia is documented to immediately precede the onset of VF. (*Level of evidence: B*)
4. If coronary revascularization cannot be carried out and there is evidence of prior MI and significant LV dysfunction, the primary therapy of patients resuscitated from VF should be the implantable cardioverter defibrillator (ICD) in patients who are receiving chronic optimal medical therapy and those who have reasonable

expectation of survival with a good functional status for more than 1 year. (*Level of evidence: A*)

5. ICD therapy is recommended for primary prevention to reduce total mortality by a reduction in SCD in patients with LV dysfunction due to prior MI who are at least 40 days post-MI, have an LVEF less than or equal to 30–40%, are New York Heart Association (NYHA) functional class II or III, are receiving chronic optimal medical therapy, and who have reasonable expectation of survival with a good functional status for more than 1 year. (*Level of evidence: A*) [See Section 1.2 in the original full-text guideline document.]

6. The ICD is effective therapy to reduce mortality by a reduction in SCD in patients with LV dysfunction due to prior MI who present with hemodynamically unstable sustained VT, are receiving chronic optimal medical therapy, and who have reasonable expectation of survival with a good functional status for more than 1 year. (*Level of evidence: A*)

Class IIa

1. Implantation of an ICD is reasonable in patients with LV dysfunction due to prior MI who are at least 40 days post-MI, have an LVEF of less than or equal to 30–35%, are NYHA functional class I on chronic optimal medical therapy, and who have reasonable expectation of survival with a good functional status for more than 1 year. (*Level of evidence: B*) [See Section 1.2 in the original full-text guideline document.]

2. Amiodarone, often in combination with beta-blockers, can be useful for patients with LV dysfunction due to prior MI and symptoms due to VT unresponsive to beta-adrenergic-blocking agents. (*Level of evidence: B*)

3. Sotalol is reasonable therapy to reduce symptoms resulting from VT for patients with LV dysfunction due to prior MI unresponsive to beta-blocking agents. (*Level of evidence: C*)

4. Adjunctive therapies to the ICD, including catheter ablation or surgical resection, and pharmacological therapy with agents such as amiodarone or sotalol, are reasonable to improve symptoms due to frequent episodes of sustained VT or VF in patients with LV dysfunction due to prior MI. (*Level of evidence: C*)

5. Amiodarone is reasonable therapy to reduce symptoms due to recurrent hemodynamically stable VT for patients with LV dysfunction due to prior MI who cannot or refuse to have an ICD implanted. (*Level of evidence: C*)

6. Implantation is reasonable for treatment of recurrent ventricular tachycardia in patients post-MI with normal or near-normal ventricular

function who are receiving chronic optimal medical therapy and who have reasonable expectation of survival with a good functional status for more than 1 year. (*Level of evidence: C*)

Class IIb

1. Curative catheter ablation or amiodarone may be considered in lieu of ICD therapy to improve symptoms in patients with LV dysfunction due to prior MI and recurrent hemodynamically stable VT whose LVEF is greater than 40%. (*Level of evidence: B*)

2. Amiodarone may be reasonable therapy for patients with LV dysfunction due to prior MI with an ICD indication, as defined above, in patients who cannot or refuse to have an ICD implanted. (*Level of evidence: C*)

Class III

1. Prophylactic antiarrhythmic drug therapy is not indicated to reduce mortality in patients with asymptomatic nonsustained ventricular arrhythmias. (*Level of evidence: B*)

2. Class IC antiarrhythmic drugs in patients with a past history of MI should not be used. (*Level of evidence: A*)

13.2.2 Valvular heart disease

Class I

Patients with valvular heart disease and ventricular arrhythmias should be evaluated and treated following current recommendations for each disorder. (*Level of evidence: C*)

Class IIb

The effectiveness of mitral valve repair or replacement to reduce the risk of SCD in patients with mitral valve prolapse, severe mitral regurgitation, and serious ventricular arrhythmias is not well established. (*Level of evidence: C*)

13.2.3 Congenital heart disease

Class I

1. ICD implantation is indicated in patients with congenital heart disease who are survivors of cardiac arrest, after evaluation to define the cause of the event and exclude any reversible causes. ICD implantation is indicated in patients who are receiving chronic optimal medical therapy and who have reasonable expectation of survival with a good functional status for more than 1 year. (*Level of evidence: B*)

2. Patients with congenital heart disease and spontaneous sustained VT should undergo invasive hemodynamic and electrophysiologic (EP) evaluation. Recommended therapy includes catheter ablation or surgical resection to eliminate VT. If that is not successful, ICD implantation is recommended. (*Level of evidence: C*)

Class IIa

Invasive hemodynamic and EP evaluation is reasonable in patients with congenital heart disease and unexplained syncope and impaired ventricular function. In the absence of a defined and reversible cause, ICD implantation is reasonable in patients who are receiving chronic optimal medical therapy and who have reasonable expectation of survival with a good functional status for more than 1 year. (*Level of evidence: B*)

Class IIb

EP testing may be considered for patients with congenital heart disease and ventricular couplets or nonsustained ventricular tachycardia (NSVT) to determine the risk of a sustained ventricular arrhythmia. (*Level of evidence: C*)

Class III

Prophylactic antiarrhythmic therapy is not indicated for asymptomatic patients with congenital heart disease and isolated PVCs. (*Level of evidence: C*)

13.2.4 Metabolic and inflammatory conditions

Myocarditis, rheumatic disease and endocarditis

Class IIa

1. ICD implantation can be beneficial in patients with life-threatening ventricular arrhythmias who are not in the acute phase of myocarditis, who are receiving chronic optimal medical therapy, and who have reasonable expectation of survival with a good functional status for more than 1 year. (*Level of evidence: C*)

Class III

ICD implantation is not indicated during the acute phase of myocarditis. (*Level of evidence: C*)

Infiltrative cardiomyopathies

Class I

In addition to managing the underlying infiltrative cardiomyopathy, life-threatening arrhythmias should be treated in the same manner that such arrhythmias are treated in patients with other cardiomyopathies, including the use of ICD in patients who are receiving chronic optimal medical therapy and who have reasonable expectation of survival with a good functional status for more than 1 year. (*Level of evidence: C*)

Endocrine disorders and diabetes

Class I

1. Persistent life-threatening ventricular arrhythmias that develop in patients with endocrine disorders should be treated in the same manner that such arrhythmias are treated in patients with other diseases, including use of ICD and pacemaker implantation as required in those who are receiving chronic optimal medical therapy and who have reasonable expectation of survival with a good functional status for more than 1 year. (*Level of evidence: C*)
2. Patients with diabetes with ventricular arrhythmias should generally be treated in the same manner as patients without diabetes. (*Level of evidence: A*)

End-stage renal failure

Class I

Life-threatening ventricular arrhythmias, especially in patients awaiting renal transplantation, should be treated conventionally, including the use of ICD and pacemaker as required, in patients who are receiving chronic optimal medical therapy and who have reasonable expectation of survival with a good functional status for more than 1 year. (*Level of evidence: C*)

Obesity, dieting and anorexia

Class I

Life-threatening ventricular arrhythmias in patients with obesity, anorexia or when dieting should be treated in the same manner that such arrhythmias are treated in patients with other diseases, including ICD and pacemaker implantation as required. Patients receiving ICD implantation should be receiving chronic optimal medical therapy and have reasonable expectation of survival with a good functional status for more than 1 year. (*Level of evidence: C*)

Class IIa

Programmed weight reduction in obesity and carefully controlled refeeding in anorexia can effectively reduce the risk of ventricular arrhythmias and SCD. (*Level of evidence: C*)

Class III

Prolonged, unbalanced, very-low-calorie, semistar-vation diets are not recommended; they may be harmful and provoke life-threatening ventricular arrhythmias. (*Level of evidence: C*)

Pericardial diseases

Class I

Ventricular arrhythmias that develop in patients with pericardial disease should be treated in the same manner that such arrhythmias are treated in patients with other diseases, including ICD. Patients receiving ICD implantation should be receiving chronic optimal medical therapy and have reasonable expectation of survival with a good functional status for more than 1 year. (*Level of evidence: C*)

Pulmonary arterial hypertension

Class III

Prophylactic antiarrhythmic therapy generally is not indicated for primary prevention of SCD in patients with pulmonary arterial hypertension (PAH) or other pulmonary conditions. (*Level of evidence: C*)

Transient arrhythmias of reversible cause

Class I

See section 8.7 in the original full-text guideline document.

13.2.5 Ventricular arrhythmias associated with cardiomyopathies

Dilated cardiomyopathy (DCM) (nonischemic)

Class I

1. An ICD should be implanted in patients with nonischemic dilated cardiomyopathy (DCM) and significant LV dysfunction who have sustained VT or VF, are receiving chronic optimal medical therapy, and who have reasonable expectation of survival with a good functional status for more than 1 year. (*Level of evidence: A*)
2. ICD therapy is recommended for primary prevention to reduce total mortality by a reduction in SCD in patients with nonischemic DCM who have an LV ejection fraction (LVEF) less than or equal to 30–35%, are NYHA functional class II or III, who are receiving chronic optimal medical therapy, and who have reasonable expectation of survival with a good functional status for more

than 1 year. (*Level of evidence: B*) [See Section 1.2 in the original full-text guideline document.]

Class IIa

1. ICD implantation can be beneficial for patients with unexplained syncope, significant LV dysfunction, and nonischemic DCM who are receiving chronic optimal medical therapy and who have reasonable expectation of survival with a good functional status for more than 1 year. (*Level of evidence: C*)
2. ICD implantation can be effective for termination of sustained VT in patients with normal or near-normal ventricular function and nonischemic DCM who are receiving chronic optimal medical therapy and who have reasonable expectation of survival with a good functional status for more than 1 year. (*Level of evidence: C*)

Class IIb

1. Placement of an ICD might be considered in patients who have nonischemic DCM, LVEF of less than or equal to 30–35%, who are NYHA functional class I receiving chronic optimal medical therapy, and who have reasonable expectation of survival with a good functional status for more than 1 year. (*Level of evidence: C*) [See Section 1.2 in the original full-text guideline document.]

Hypertrophic cardiomyopathy (HCM)

Class I

ICD therapy should be used for treatment in patients with HCM who have sustained VT and/or VF and who are receiving chronic optimal medical therapy and who have reasonable expectation of survival with a good functional status for more than 1 year. (*Level of evidence: B*)

Class IIa

1. ICD implantation can be effective for primary prophylaxis against SCD in patients with HCM who have one or more major risk factor for SCD and who are receiving chronic optimal medical therapy and in patients who have reasonable expectation of survival with a good functional status for more than 1 year. (*Level of evidence: C*)

Arrhythmogenic right ventricular cardiomyopathy (ARVC)

Class I

ICD implantation is recommended for the prevention of SCD in patients with ARVC with documented sustained VT or VF who are receiving chronic optimal medical therapy and who have reasonable expectation of survival with a good functional status for more than 1 year. (*Level of evidence: B*)

Class IIa

1. ICD implantation can be effective for the prevention of SCD in patients with ARVC with extensive disease, including those with LV involvement, one or more affected family members with SCD, or undiagnosed syncope when VT or VF has not been excluded as the cause of syncope, who are receiving chronic optimal medical therapy, and who have reasonable expectation of survival with a good functional status for more than 1 year. (*Level of evidence: C*)

Neuromuscular disorders

Class I

Patients with neuromuscular disorders who have ventricular arrhythmias should generally be treated in the same manner as patients without neuromuscular disorders. (*Level of evidence: A*)

13.2.6 Heart failure

Class I

1. ICD therapy is recommended for secondary prevention of SCD in patients who survived VF or hemodynamically unstable VT, or VT with syncope and who have an LVEF less than or equal to 40%, who are receiving chronic optimal medical therapy, and who have a reasonable expectation of survival with a good functional status for more than 1 year. (*Level of evidence: A*)
2. ICD therapy is recommended for primary prevention to reduce total mortality by a reduction in SCD in patients with LV dysfunction due to prior MI who are at least 40 days post-MI, have an LVEF less than or equal to 30–40%, are NYHA functional class II or III receiving chronic optimal medical therapy, and who have reasonable expectation of survival with a good functional status for more than 1 year. (*Level of evidence: A*) [See Section 1.2 in the original full-text guideline document.]
3. ICD therapy is recommended for primary prevention to reduce total mortality by a reduction in SCD in patients with nonischemic heart disease who have an LVEF less than or equal to 30–35%, are NYHA functional class II or III, are receiving chronic optimal medical therapy, and who have reasonable expectation of survival

with a good functional status for more than 1 year. (*Level of evidence: B*) [See Section 1.2 in the original full-text guideline document.]

Class IIa

1. ICD therapy combined with biventricular pacing can be effective for primary prevention to reduce total mortality by a reduction in SCD in patients with NYHA functional class III or IV, who are receiving optimal medical therapy, in sinus rhythm with a QRS complex of at least 120 ms, and who have reasonable expectation of survival with a good functional status for more than 1 year. (*Level of evidence: B*)
2. ICD therapy is reasonable for primary prevention to reduce total mortality by a reduction in SCD in patients with LV dysfunction due to prior MI who are at least 40 days post-MI, have an LVEF of less than or equal to 30–35%, are NYHA functional class I, are receiving chronic optimal medical therapy, and have reasonable expectation of survival with a good functional status for more than 1 year. (*Level of evidence: B*) [See Section 1.2 in the original full-text guideline document.]
3. ICD therapy is reasonable in patients who have recurrent stable VT, a normal or near-normal LVEF, and optimally treated HF and who have a reasonable expectation of survival with a good functional status for more than 1 year. (*Level of evidence: C*)
4. Biventricular pacing in the absence of ICD therapy is reasonable for the prevention of SCD in patients with NYHA functional class III or IV HF, an LVEF less than or equal to 35%, and a QRS complex equal to or wider than 160 ms (or at least 120 ms in the presence of other evidence of ventricular dyssynchrony) who are receiving chronic optimal medical therapy and who have reasonable expectation of survival with a good functional status for more than 1 year. (*Level of evidence: B*)

Class IIb

1. Amiodarone, sotalol, and/or beta-blockers may be considered as pharmacological alternatives to ICD therapy to suppress symptomatic ventricular tachyarrhythmias (both sustained and nonsustained) in optimally treated patients with HF for whom ICD therapy is not feasible. (*Level of evidence: C*)
2. ICD therapy may be considered for primary prevention to reduce total mortality by a reduction in SCD in patients with nonischemic heart disease who have an LVEF of less than or equal to 30–35%, are NYHA functional class I receiving

chronic optimal medical therapy, and who have a reasonable expectation of survival with a good functional status for more than 1 year. (*Level of evidence: B*) [See Section 1.2 in the original full-text guideline document.]

13.2.7 Genetic arrhythmia syndromes

Long QT syndrome (LQTS)

Class I

1. Implantation of an ICD along with use of beta-blockers is recommended for LQTS patients with previous cardiac arrest and who have reasonable expectation of survival with a good functional status for more than 1 year. (*Level of evidence: A*)

Class IIa

Implantation of an ICD with continued use of beta-blockers can be effective to reduce SCD in LQTS patients experiencing syncope and/or VT while receiving beta-blockers and who have reasonable expectation of survival with a good functional status for more than 1 year. (*Level of evidence: B*)

Class IIb

Implantation of an ICD with the use of beta-blockers may be considered for prophylaxis of SCD for patients in categories possibly associated with higher risk of cardiac arrest such as LQT2 and LQT3 and who have reasonable expectation of survival with a good functional status for more than 1 year. (*Level of evidence: B*)

Brugada syndrome

Class I

An ICD is indicated for Brugada syndrome patients with previous cardiac arrest receiving chronic optimal medical therapy and who have reasonable expectation of survival with a good functional status for more than 1 year (*Level of evidence: C*)

Class IIa

1. An ICD is reasonable for Brugada syndrome patients with spontaneous ST-segment elevation in V_1, V_2 or V_3 who have had syncope, with or without mutations demonstrated in the *SCN5A* gene and who have reasonable expectation of survival with a good functional status for more than 1 year. (*Level of evidence: C*)

2. An ICD is reasonable for Brugada syndrome patients with documented VT that has not resulted in cardiac arrest and who have reasonable expectation of survival with a good functional status for more than 1 year. (*Level of evidence: C*)

Catecholaminergic polymorphic ventricular tachycardia (CPVT)

Class I

Implantation of an ICD with use of beta-blockers is indicated for patients with CPVT who are survivors of cardiac arrest and who have reasonable expectation of survival with a good functional status for more than 1 year. (*Level of evidence: C*)

Class IIa

Implantation of an ICD with the use of beta-blockers can be effective for patients affected by CPVT with syncope and/or documented sustained VT while receiving beta-blockers and who have reasonable expectation of survival with a good functional status for more than 1 year. (*Level of evidence: C*)

13.2.8 Arrhythmias in structurally normal hearts

Idiopathic ventricular tachycardia

Class IIa

ICD implantation can be effective therapy for the termination of sustained VT in patients with normal or near-normal ventricular function and no structural heart disease who are receiving chronic optimal medical therapy and who have reasonable expectation of survival for more than 1 year. (*Level of evidence: C*)

Alcohol

Class I

Persistent life-threatening ventricular arrhythmias despite abstinence from alcohol should be treated in the same manner that such arrhythmias are treated in patients with other diseases, including an ICD, as required, in patients receiving chronic optimal medical therapy and who have reasonable expectation of survival for more than 1 year. (*Level of evidence: C*)

14 APPENDIX B

American College of Cardiology/American Heart Association/Heart Rhythm Society

2008 Guidelines for ICD and CRT

14.1 Recommendations for ICD therapy

Class I

1. ICD therapy is indicated in patients who are survivors of cardiac arrest due to VF or hemodynamically unstable sustained VT after evaluation to define the cause of the event and to exclude any completely reversible causes. *(Level of Evidence: A)*
2. ICD therapy is indicated in patients with structural heart disease and spontaneous sustained VT, whether hemodynamically stable or unstable. *(Level of Evidence: B)*
3. ICD therapy is indicated in patients with syncope of undetermined origin with clinically relevant, hemodynamically significant sustained VT or VF induced at electrophysiological study. *(Level of Evidence: B)*
4. ICD therapy is indicated in patients with LVEF less than 35% due to prior MI who are at least 40 days post-MI and are in NYHA functional Class II or III. *(Level of Evidence: A)*
5. ICD therapy is indicated in patients with non-ischemic DCM who have an LVEF less than or equal to 35% and who are in NYHA functional Class II or III. *(Level of Evidence: B)*
6. ICD therapy is indicated in patients with LV dysfunction due to prior MI who are at least 40 days post-MI, have an LVEF less than 30%, and are in NYHA functional Class I. *(Level of Evidence: A)*
7. ICD therapy is indicated in patients with non-sustained VT due to prior MI, LVEF less than 40%, and inducible VF or sustained VT at electrophysiological study. *(Level of Evidence: B)*

Class IIa

1. ICD implantation is reasonable for patients with unexplained syncope, significant LV dys-function, and nonischemic DCM. *(Level of Evidence: C)*
2. ICD implantation is reasonable for patients with sustained VT and normal or near-normal ventricular function. *(Level of Evidence: C)*
3. ICD implantation is reasonable for patients with HCM who have 1 or more major risk factors for SCD. *(Level of Evidence: C)*
4. ICD implantation is reasonable for the prevention of SCD in patients with ARVD/C who have 1 or more risk factors for SCD. *(Level of Evidence: C)*
5. ICD implantation is reasonable to reduce SCD in patients with long-QT syndrome who are experiencing syncope and/or VT while receiving beta blockers. *(Level of Evidence: B)*
6. ICD implantation is reasonable for non hospitalized patients awaiting transplantation. *(Level of Evidence: C)*
7. ICD implantation is reasonable for patients with Brugada syndrome who have had syncope. *(Level of Evidence: C)*
8. ICD implantation is reasonable for patients with Brugada syndrome who have documented VT that has not resulted in cardiac arrest. *(Level of Evidence: C)*
9. ICD implantation is reasonable for patients with catecholaminergic polymorphic VT who have syncope and/or documented sustained VT while receiving beta blockers. *(Level of Evidence: C)*
10. ICD implantation is reasonable for patients with cardiac sarcoidosis, giant cell myocarditis, or Chagas disease. *(Level of Evidence: C)*

Class IIb

1. ICD therapy may be considered in patients with nonischemic heart disease who have an LVEF of less than or equal to 35% and who are in NYHA functional Class I. *(Level of Evidence: C)*

2. ICD therapy may be considered for patients with long-QT syndrome and risk factors for SCD. *(Level of Evidence: B)*

3. ICD therapy may be considered in patients with syncope and advanced structural heart disease in whom thorough invasive and noninvasive investigations have failed to define a cause. *(Level of Evidence: C)*

4. ICD therapy may be considered in patients with a familial cardiomyopathy associated with sudden death. *(Level of Evidence: C)*

5. ICD therapy may be considered in patients with LV noncompaction. *(Level of Evidence: C)*

Class III

1. ICD therapy is not indicated for patients who do not have a reasonable expectation of survival with an acceptable functional status for at least 1 year, even if they meet ICD implantation criteria specified in the Class I, IIa, and IIb recommendations above. *(Level of Evidence: C)*

2. ICD therapy is not indicated for patients with incessant VT or VF. *(Level of Evidence: C)*

3. ICD therapy is not indicated in patients with significant psychiatric illnesses that may be aggravated by device implantation or that may preclude systematic follow-up. *(Level of Evidence: C)*

4. ICD therapy is not indicated for NYHA Class IV patients with drug-refractory congestive heart failure who are not candidates for cardiac transplantation or CRT-D. *(Level of Evidence: C)*

5. ICD therapy is not indicated for syncope of undetermined cause in a patient without inducible ventricular tachyarrhythmias and without structural heart disease. *(Level of Evidence: C)*

6. ICD therapy is not indicated when VF or VT is amenable to surgical or catheter ablation (e.g., atrial arrhythmias associated with the Wolff-Parkinson-White syndrome, RV or LV outflow tract VT, idiopathic VT, or fascicular VT in the absence of structural heart disease). *(Level of Evidence: C)*

7. ICD therapy is not indicated for patients with ventricular tachyarrhythmias due to a completely reversible disorder in the absence of structural heart disease (e.g., electrolyte imbalance, drugs, or trauma). *(Level of Evidence: B)*

14.2 Recommendations for cardiac resynchronization therapy in patients with severe systolic heart failure

Class I

1. For patients who have LVEF less than or equal to 35%, a QRS duration greater than or equal to 0.12 seconds, and sinus rhythm, CRT with or without an ICD is indicated for the treatment of NYHA functional Class III or ambulatory Class IV heart failure symptoms with optimal recommended medical therapy. *(Level of Evidence: A)*

Class IIa

1. For patients who have LVEF less than or equal to 35%, a QRS duration greater than or equal to 0.12 seconds, and AF, CRT with or without an ICD is reasonable for the treatment of NYHA functional Class III or ambulatory Class IV heart failure symptoms on optimal recommended medical therapy. *(Level of Evidence: B)*

2. For patients with LVEF less than or equal to 35% with NYHA functional Class III or ambulatory Class IV symptoms who are receiving optimal recommended medical therapy and who have frequent dependence on ventricular pacing, CRT is reasonable. *(Level of Evidence: C)*

Class IIb

1. For patients with LVEF less than or equal to 35% with NYHA functional Class I or II symptoms who are receiving optimal recommended medical therapy and who are undergoing implantation of a permanent pacemaker and/or ICD with anticipated frequent ventricular pacing, CRT may be considered. *(Level of Evidence: C)*

Class III

1. CRT is not indicated for asymptomatic patients with reduced LVEF in the absence of other indications for pacing. *(Level of Evidence: B)*

2. CRT is not indicated for patients whose functional status and life expectancy are limited predominantly by chronic noncardiac conditions. *(Level of Evidence: C)*

Note: page numbers in **bold** refer to tables

415